D1257713

THE
UNIVERSITY OF WINNIPEG
PORTAGE & BALMORAL
WINNIPEG, MAN.   R3B 2E9
CANADA

DISCARDED

DISCARDED

CATECHOLAMINES AND BEHAVIOR · 2

Neuropsychopharmacology

QP
981
.C25C37
1975
v.2

CATECHOLAMINES AND BEHAVIOR · 2

Neuropsychopharmacology

Edited by

Arnold J. Friedhoff

Millhauser Laboratories of
  the Department of Psychiatry
New York University School of Medicine
New York, New York

PLENUM PRESS • NEW YORK AND LONDON

Library of Congress Cataloging in Publication Data

Main entry under title:

Catecholamines and behavior.

Includes bibliographies and indexes.
CONTENTS: v. 1. Basic neurobiology. — v. 2. Neuropsychopharmacology.
1. Catecholamines. 2. Psychopharmacology. I. Friedhoff, Arnold J. [DNLM: 1.
Behavior — Drug effects. 2. Catecholamines — Physiology. QV129 C357]
QP981.C25C37   599'.01'88   75-11697
ISBN 0-306-38412-4 (v. 2)

© 1975 Plenum Press, New York
A Division of Plenum Publishing Corporation
227 West 17th Street, New York, N.Y. 10011

United Kingdom edition published by Plenum Press, London
A Division of Plenum Publishing Company, Ltd.
Davis House (4th Floor), 8 Scrubs Lane, Harlesden, London, NW10 6SE, England

All rights reserved

No part of this book may be reproduced, stored in a retrieval system, or transmitted,
in any form or by any means, electronic, mechanical, photocopying, microfilming,
recording, or otherwise, without written permission from the Publisher

Printed in the United States of America

Preface

This volume is intended to provide students and investigators of brain–behavior relationships with an understanding of the current concepts of the role of catecholamines in the regulation of behavior. Catecholamines are now believed to be modulators or transmitters in systems regulating a number of important aspects of behavioral function. The present intense interest in catecholamines is reflected by the large number of scientific reports dealing with these compounds. Even those reports which are relevant to behavior are staggering in number. The contributors to this book have drawn on the salient literature, as well as on their own work, with a view toward clarifying relationships between the basic neurobiology of catecholaminergic neural systems and normal and abnormal behavioral function. Current work in this field is heavily dependent on the use of psychotropic drugs to produce model behavioral states, or as biological probes. As a result psychopharmacological studies are generously represented. In the last chapter of Volume 2 the editor has attempted to further relate and develop the material in the two volumes from the conceptual and theoretical standpoint.

New York   AJF

Contributors to Volume 2

Wagner H. Bridger, *Department of Psychiatry, Albert Einstein College of Medicine, Bronx, New York*

Thomas R. Bozewicz, *Department of Psychiatry, Albert Einstein College of Medicine, Bronx, New York*

Doris H. Clouet, *Testing and Research Laboratory, New York State Drug Abuse Control Commission, Brooklyn, New York*

John M. Davis, *Illinois State Psychiatric Institute, and Associate Professor of Psychiatry, University of Chicago, Pritzker School of Medicine, Chicago, Illinois*

Richard P. Ebstein, *Neurochemistry Laboratories, Department of Psychiatry, New York University Medical Center, New York, New York*

Lewis S. Freedman, *Neurochemistry Laboratories, Department of Psychiatry, New York University Medical·Center, New York, New York*

Arnold J. Friedhoff, *Millhauser Laboratories, New York University Medical Center, New York, New York*

Menek Goldstein, *Neurochemistry Laboratories, Department of Psychiatry, New York University Medical Center, New York, New York*

David A. Gorelick, *Department of Pharmacology, Albert Einstein College of Medicine, Bronx, New York*

Ronald Kuczenski, *Department of Psychiatry, School of Medicine, University of California, San Diego, La Jolla, California*

James W. Maas, *Department of Psychiatry, Yale University School of Medicine, New Haven, Connecticut*

Arnold J. Mandell, *Department of Psychiatry, School of Medicine, University of California, San Diego, La Jolla, California*

Dennis L. Murphy, *Laboratory of Clinical Science, National Institute of Mental Health, Bethesda, Maryland*

Dong H. Park, *Neurochemistry Laboratories, Department of Psychiatry, New York University Medical Center, New York, New York*

D. E. Redmond, Jr., *Laboratory of Clinical Science, National Institute of Mental Health, Bethesda, Maryland*

David S. Segal, *Department of Psychiatry, School of Medicine, University of California, San Diego, La Jolla, California*

Eric A. Stone, *Millhauser Laboratories of the Department of Psychiatry, New York University Medical Center, New York, New York*

Contents

Chapter 4

**Catecholamines and Depression: A Further Specification of the
Catecholamine Hypothesis of the Affective Disorders**

James W. Maas

Chapter 5

Catecholamines and Psychosis

John M. Davis

Chapter 6

Serum Dopamine-β-Hydroxylase in Various Pathological States

Menek Goldstein, Richard P. Ebstein, Lewis S. Freedman, and
Dong H. Park

Chapter 7

Possible Roles of Catecholamines in the Action of Narcotic Drugs

Doris H. Clouet

Chapter 8

Metabolic Adaptation to Antidepressant Drugs: Implications for Pathophysiology and Treatment in Psychiatry

Arnold J. Mandell, David S. Segal, and Ronald Kuczenski

Chapter 9

Integration and Conclusions

Arnold J. Friedhoff

Chapter 1

The Role of Catecholamines in Animal Learning and Memory*

David A. Gorelick, Thomas R. Bozewicz,
and Wagner H. Bridger

Departments of Pharmacology and Psychiatry
Albert Einstein College of Medicine
Bronx, New York

1. DEFINITIONS

1.1. Catecholamines ⌐

Since the locus of learning and memory is presumably within the CNS, we will consider only the two catecholamines (CA) which are important putative CNS neurotransmitters in mammals, dopamine (DA) and norepinephrine (NE). We exclude epinephrine, which is found chiefly in the peripheral nervous system (PNS), because little CNS pharmacological work has been done with it, although recent evidence suggests that it may function as a CNS neurotransmitter (Hökfelt *et al.*, 1974; Koslow and Schlumpf, 1974).

1.2. Learning and Memory

For the purposes of this chapter, we will use an empirical definition of learning: the process by which experience or practice leads to a relatively

* During the preparation of this chapter David A. Gorelick was supported by NIH training grant 5T5 GM 1674 from the National Institute of General Medical Sciences; Thomas R. Bozewicz was supported by NIMH grant MH 06418.

permanent change in behavior (Kimble, 1961). Thus, we exclude from consideration changes in behavior which are due to factors other than experience, e.g., maturation, senescence, or nutrition, or factors which are not relatively permanent, e.g., sensitization or fatigue. As so defined, the concept of learning includes that of memory, since the former could not occur without the latter. However, we will reserve the word "learning" for the acquisition of behavioral change and use the word "memory" to refer to the persistence of learning over time so that it can be expressed in later behavior. Memory can be subdivided into three separate processes: (i) consolidation, the entry of the information into storage, (ii) retention, the storage process itself, and (iii) retrieval, the bringing of the information out of storage.

2. PROBLEMS OF SPECIFICITY

2.1. Behavioral Specificity

In any behavioral experiment, the learning process is not observed directly. What is observed is a change in the behavior or performance of an animal in a particular task. Such a change can be caused not only by learning, but also by changes in other processes which contribute to the performance of the behavior, such as perception, motivation, or motor ability. A behavioral change can be attributed to learning only after establishing its independence from changes in other behavioral processes. This is particularly important when studying the relation between CA and learning, because CA play a role in many behavioral processes besides learning (see other chapters of these volumes).

Two types of control experiments are important in ruling out effects on behavioral processes other than learning. One type is to show that the treatment used to affect behavior does not affect the particular perceptual, motivational, and motor variables used in that experiment. This is usually done by showing that conditioned or spontaneous behavior involving these variables is unaffected. The other type of control experiment is to show that the behavioral effect of the treatment is consistent even when completely different variables are used. Examples of such variables include, for perception, the sensory modality of the conditioned stimulus (CS); for motivation, the type of reinforcement; for motor ability, the response requirements of the task. Ideally, one should parametrically alter these variables to ensure that they are equivalent in their ability to control the animal's behavior.

An experimental example may help clarify how a change in behavior can be attributed to learning by use of proper controls. Cooper *et al.* (1973)

trained rats in a discriminated shuttlebox escape/avoidance task. The task involved presenting the rat with a CS, in this case a light plus a tone, followed after 10 sec by an unconditioned stimulus (UCS), continuous 0.8 mA electric shock to the feet. If the rat made a conditioned response (CR), crossing to the other side of the shuttlebox within 10 sec of CS onset, the UCS was avoided. A CR made after UCS onset resulted in escape from the UCS. Rats given a 6-hydroxydopamine (6-OHDA) treatment which decreased brain CA levels during training made significantly fewer avoidance responses than did control rats given saline. Does this difference in performance reflect a difference in learning because of altered brain CA levels?

One alternate possibility is that the treatment altered the perceptual process. A rat whose vision was impaired would obviously do poorly in a task involving a visual CS. A general visual perceptual deficit could be ruled out by showing that unconditioned responses to a visual CS, e.g., orienting, photophobic, visual cliff, or startle responses, were not impaired by the treatment. Another necessary control would be to show that similar behavioral effects were obtained when using CS of different sensory modalities, e.g., auditory or tactile. Since CS of different modalities may differ in the extent to which they can control behavior, a parametric comparison should be done. The finding of a consistent effect with different stimulus modalities would suggest that the treatment's behavioral effect was not due to visual impairment.

Another possibility is that the treatment altered motivation. If an electric shock were less painful or produced less fear in a treated rat, the rat would be less motivated to exert effort to avoid or escape the shock. One way to rule out a specific deficit of fear motivation would be to test the effect of the treatment on different unconditioned responses (UCR) elicited by the UCS, e.g., freezing, jumping, squealing. Another way would be to use completely different aversive UCS such as an air blast or sudden loud noise, instead of electric shock. The use of other motivational states, such as hunger, thirst, or sex, provides a further necessary control to ensure that the treatment is not affecting this process. Each type of motivation used should be tested parametrically to ensure that equivalent motivational states are induced in the animal. The finding of a consistent effect with different levels and types of reinforcers would suggest that the treatment's behavioral effects were not due to a motivational alteration.

A third possibility is that the treatment affected motor ability. A rat could have learned the appropriate CR but still be unable to perform it because of a motor deficit. This possibility could be ruled out by showing that the treatment does not affect similar responses when made spontaneously or as UCR. Cooper *et al.* (1973) found that neither spontaneous motor activity in an activity cage nor crossings in the shuttlebox between trials (no CS present) were affected by the treatment. Another necessary control would be to show that the treatment has similar behavioral effects on tasks requiring different types of responses. Some important comparisons would be between tasks requiring active *vs.* passive responses and between tasks requiring a certain response rate or latency for a correct response (strict requirements) *vs.* tasks with broader requirements such as making a correct choice (e.g., discrimination task). The finding of a consistent effect on tasks with these different response requirements would suggest that the treatment's behavioral effects were not due to alteration of motor ability. Cooper *et al.* (1973) found that their treatment did not affect the acquisition of a one-trial passive avoidance task. This difference in behavioral effect between active (shuttlebox) and passive avoidance tasks suggests that the treatment does not affect learning, but does have some effect on the ability to make this type of active learned response. This effect appears to be limited to learned responses because, as mentioned above, unconditioned and spontaneous active motor responses were not affected by the treatment. Another explanation for the absence of a deficit on the passive avoidance task may be that this task is not of equivalent difficulty to the active task. If the passive task were much easier to learn than the active (as suggested by the fact that significant learning occurs in one trial), the lower level of CA activity remaining after the treatment might still be sufficient to maintain performance without a deficit.

The time at which a treatment is active in relation to the time the behavior is measured affects the behavioral specificity of the results (McGaugh, 1973). Only experiments where the treatment is active during training (acquisition) can provide information about learning, *per se*. A key criterion for the occurrence of a learning effect is whether the behavioral change persists after the effects of the experimental treatment have worn off, since learning, by definition, must involve a relatively permanent change in behavior. However, there are several difficulties in interpreting such results. A learning effect might occur but not be reflected in later behavior because of state dependency effects, i.e., an impairment of performance because of the difference in "brain states" during training and during later performance caused by the treatment (Overton, 1974). A behavioral change may persist after training and yet not be due to an effect of the treatment on learning. Instead, the treatment might have altered other behavioral variables during training (e.g., arousal, number of reinforcements received) in such a way as to change later behavior. Experiments where the treatment is active only immediately (seconds to hours) after training can provide information about consolidation and retention. However, possible state-dependency effects must be controlled (Wright, 1974). Information about retention alone can be provided by experiments where the treatment is active a sufficient time (days) after acquisition and before later performance to avoid any effects on consolidation or retrieval and nonlearning processes, respectively. Postacquisition studies, where the treatment is active during performance, are hard to interpret because many behavioral processes are involved. Observed behavioral changes could be due to effects on retention, retrieval, the expression of learning, or on nonlearning processes such as perception, motivation, or motor ability. State dependency is an additional possible confounding factor. Unfortunately, most CA-affecting treatments have been used only in this postacquisition paradigm.

2.2. Chemical Specificity

Few, if any, biological treatments have only one known effect on neurotransmitters, and there always exists the possibility of unknown side effects. Thus, it is impossible to know for certain that the behavioral effect of any treatment is due to its effects on CA. The best approach is to use several treatments which affect CA by different mechanisms, since it is unlikely that all of these would have the same side effects in common. In addition, one can test whether treatments which affect CA oppositely (e.g., agonists and antagonists) have opposite behavioral effects. Another approach is to correlate the intensity and time course of the treatment's effects on CA with its effects on behavior. A further problem is that a treatment which initially affects only CA may eventually alter other neurotransmitters by feedback or feed-forward effects. This can make demonstration of chemical specificity very difficult, especially *in vivo*.

2.3. Anatomical Specificity

We use this term to refer to the problem of specifying the site of action of a treatment. Treatments given peripherally will affect only the peripheral nervous system (PNS) unless they can cross the blood–brain barrier. Treatments which do cross the barrier will still reach and potentially affect the entire CNS, as will treatments given into the CSF (e.g., intraventricularly). Only treatments administered directly into CNS tissue (e.g., chemical implantation, electrical stimulation, or lesioning of specific neurons) offer some degree of anatomical specificity. Such treatments help achieve behavioral and chemical specificity by affecting only a limited number (hopefully only one) of behavioral or neurotransmitter systems. Such specificity helps avoid multiple effects on other behavioral processes which may confound effects on learning. For example, it has been hypothesized that a specific NE system in the medial forebrain bundle (MFB) is essential for motivated learning (Stein, 1969). Overall changes in CNS NE may not only produce changes in this MFB motivational system, but also in the NE systems mediating arousal and motor function. These changes in other NE systems could confound the effects of the hypothesized MFB motivational system.

3. EXPERIMENTAL APPROACHES

3.1. CA Activity as Independent Variable

Two different experimental approaches have been used in studying the relation between catecholamines and learning. The first approach considers CA activity in the CNS as the independent variable, manipulating it and measuring consequent changes in behavior. Many manipulations have been used which affect every step in the natural metabolic cycle of CA, ranging from biosynthesis, storage, and presynaptic release, through reuptake, catabolism, and postsynaptic receptor activation and blockade. In addition, techniques for specifically destroying catecholaminergic neurons have been used.

3.2. Behavior as Independent Variable

The second approach considers the organism's behavior as the independent variable, manipulating it and measuring consequent changes in CNS catecholaminergic activity. Many different learning paradigms have been used with either positive or negative reinforcement. Techniques for detecting changes in catecholaminergic activity range in sophistication from measuring whole brain levels of CA to measuring turnover in specific brain regions *in vivo* with radioactive labeling.

4. CA AS INDEPENDENT VARIABLE

4.1. Chemical Specificity

4.1.1. Treatments Which Decrease CA Activity

Four main techniques have been used to decrease CA activity within the CNS in learning and memory experiments: (i) synthesis inhibition, either at the tyrosine hydroxylase or dopamine-β-hydroxylase steps; (ii) disruption of presynaptic storage; (iii) blockade of postsynaptic CA receptors; and (iv) selective destruction of CA neurons, either electrolytically or chemically.

4.1.1.a. Synthesis Inhibition. CA synthesis at the tyrosine hydroxylase step is usually inhibited with α-methyl-p-tyrosine (AMPT) (Moore and Dominic, 1971). This treatment decreases both NE and DA (Weissman and Koe, 1965; Rech *et al.*, 1966), but does not affect serotonin (Weissman and Koe, 1965; Tagliamonte *et al.*, 1971). Synthesis at the dopamine-β-hydroxylase step is usually inhibited with disulfiram (Goldstein, 1966). This treatment decreases only NE, leaving serotonin unchanged (Maj *et al.*, 1970; Johnson *et al.*, 1972) and DA either unchanged or increased (Goldstein and Nakajima, 1967). Other dopamine-β-hydroxylase inhibitors may affect serotonin (Johnson *et al.*, 1972).

4.1.1.b. Disruption of Presynaptic Storage. Reserpine and most reserpinelike drugs (e.g., tetrabenazine) have little chemical specificity because they disrupt storage of serotonin and histamine as much as CA (Sulser and Bass, 1968). An exception to this is prenylamine, which at low doses can affect CA without affecting serotonin (Obianwu, 1965; Juorio and Vogt, 1965). Some specificity in the use of reserpine is introduced by attempting to reverse the effect with a treatment which will increase only CA. This is usually done by systemic administration of L-dopa, often in conjunction with a peripheral amino acid decarboxylase inhibitor so that more L-dopa reaches the CNS. However, when L-dopa is so administered it has widespread neurochemical effects (see section 4.1.2.c below) which make interpretation of results difficult. Therefore, we will not discuss further experiments using reserpine or L-dopa.

4.1.1.c. Postsynaptic CA-Receptor Blockers. Three types of postsynaptic CA-receptor blockers have been used: α-adrenergic blockers, including phentolamine and phenoxybenzamine; β-adrenergic blockers, including dichlorisoproterenol, pronethalol, and propranolol; and dopamine blockers, including pimozide. All of these blockers can block histamine and acetylcholine receptors in the PNS (Furchgott, 1972; Janssen *et al.*, 1968). The α- and β-adrenergic blockers have other effects in the PNS, including blocking serotonin receptors (Furchgott, 1972), inhibiting neuronal and extraneuronal NE uptake (Euler, 1972) and decreasing NE synthesis (Stjarne and Lishajko, 1966). Some of the β-adrenergic blockers (dichloroisoproterenol, pronethalol) have a partial β-agonist effect and many, including propranolol, have a membrane-stabilizing effect similar to that of local anesthetics (Fitzgerald, 1969). Within the CNS, phenoxybenzamine appears to be the most specific CA receptor blocker. Other α-adrenergic blockers and propranolol can block DA receptors (Andén *et al.*, 1966;

Kebabian *et al.*, 1972; Andén and Strombom, 1974) and pimozide and halo-peridol can block NE receptors (Blumberg and Sulser, 1974).

    4.1.1.d. Destruction of CA Neurons. The specificity of electrolytic lesions depends on limiting their extent to areas containing only CA neurons. This problem does not occur with 6-OHDA, which, when administered into the CSF (intraventricularly or intracisternally), is rather selectively taken up by CA neurons (Schubert *et al.*, 1973) and destroys CA nerve terminals (Thoenen and Tranzer, 1973). This treatment usually does not affect levels of other putative neurotransmitters (Breese and Traylor, 1970; Jacks *et al.*, 1972; Grewaal *et al.*, 1974); however, recent evidence suggests that it may sometimes affect serotonergic (Juge *et al.*, 1972; Hery *et al.*, 1973; Cooper *et al.*, 1973) or cholinergic (Ho and Loh, 1972) neurons. Furthermore, it does have a nonspecific neurotoxic effect when administered directly into brain tissues, even at microgram doses (Poirier *et al.*, 1972; Butcher and Hodge, 1973). One advantage of 6-OHDA is that it can be given in such a way as to decrease NE levels significantly more than DA levels, or *vice versa* (Breese and Traylor, 1971).

4.1.2. Treatments Which Increase CA Activity

    Five main techniques have been used to increase CA activity in the CNS in learning and memory experiments: (i) presynaptic release; (ii) blockade of presynaptic reuptake; (iii) administration of CA agonists or their precursors; (iv) electrical stimulation of CA neurons; and (v) inhibition of CA catabolism, either at the monoamine oxidase (MAO) or catechol-*O*-methyltransferase (COMT) steps.

    4.1.2.a. Presynaptic Release. The chief drug used to cause presynaptic release of CA is amphetamine. This drug can affect CA activity by several mechanisms, including MAO inhibition, blockade of presynaptic reuptake, and presynaptic release, but the latter is the most important in producing behavioral effects (Sulser and Sanders-Bush, 1971; Azzaro and Rutledge, 1973; Philippu *et al.*, 1974). The releasing effect not only increases spontaneous presynaptic release of CA, but also stimulation-induced release (Farnebo, 1971). Amphetamine, in doses greater than 5 mg/kg, can also release serotonin presynaptically (Fuxe and Ungerstedt, 1970; Azzaro and Rutledge, 1973) and inhibit serotonin synthesis (Schubert *et al.*, 1970; Knapp *et al.*, 1974) and catabolism (Schubert *et al.*, 1970).

    4.1.2.b. Blockade of Presynaptic Reuptake. The chief drugs used to block presynaptic reuptake are the tricyclic antidepressants. These drugs vary in specifcity: the secondary amines (e.g., desipramine, nortriptyline, protriptyline) have a greater effect on NE than on DA, while the tertiary amines (e.g., imipramine, amitriptyline) have a greater effect on DA and also significantly affect serotonin (Sulser and Sanders-Bush, 1971; Meek *et al.*, 1970; Lidbrink *et al.*, 1971). The tricyclics also have anticholinergic and antihistaminic activity, as well as some local anesthetic properties (Sigg, 1968). Because of their effects on both CA and serotonin, we will not discuss further experiments using tertiary amine tricyclics.

4.1.2.c. Administration of CA Agonists and Precursors. Three types of postsynaptic CA-receptor agonists have been used: α-adrenergic agonists, including clonidine; β-adrenergic agonists, including isoproterenol; and dopamine agonists, including apomorphine. These agonists have rarely been used in experiments on learning and memory. NE itself is largely an α-adrenergic agonist, at least in the PNS (Innes and Nickerson, 1970). The precursor most often used is L-dopa, which is usually administered peripherally. When L-dopa is so administered it can be taken up by serotonergic neurons (Barrett and Balch, 1971) and can cause decreased brain levels of serotonin (Bartholini *et al.*, 1968; Butcher and Engel, 1969; Everett and Borcherding, 1970; Karobath *et al.*, 1971; Langelier *et al.*, 1973; Algeri and Cerletti, 1974), and increased levels of 5-hydroxyindole acetic acid (Bartholini *et al.*, 1968; Everett and Borcherding, 1970), possibly by displacing serotonin from serotonergic neurons. Furthermore, L-dopa has been shown to inhibit serotonin synthesis in rat striatum and brain stem slices (Goldstein and Frenkel, 1971). L-Dopa also causes a wide variety of neurochemical changes in the CNS (Wurtman and Romero, 1972), including decreased brain levels of tryptophan and tyrosine (Karobath *et al.*, 1971), decreased brain turnover of histamine (Thoa *et al.*, 1972), decreased brain levels of S-adenosylmethionine (Wurtman *et al.*, 1970) and altered brain glucose metabolism (Tyce, 1971). In view of these widespread effects, the chemical specificity of L-dopa is unclear. Therefore, we will not discuss further experiments using L-dopa.

4.1.2.d. Inhibition of CA Catabolism. Because MAO is involved in the catabolism of serotonin as well as CA, MAO inhibitors affect both kinds of biogenic amines (Marley and Stephenson, 1972). This makes studies using MAO inhibitors difficult to interpret, and we will not discuss any such studies. The chief COMT inhibitor used is pyrogallol, which increases brain CA levels when given *in vivo* (Marley and Stephenson, 1972).

4.2. Anatomical Specificity

4.2.1. Treatments Which Decrease CA Activity

Except for 6-OHDA, most treatments which decrease CNS CA activity are usually administered peripherally. The synthesis inhibitors do cross the blood–brain barrier and act within the CNS to decrease CA levels. The fact that the extent and time course of their behavioral effects parallels that of the CA depletion in the CNS suggests that the latter is their important site of action (Rech *et al.*, 1966; Osborne and Kerkut, 1972). The postsynaptic CA-receptor blockers also cross the blood–brain barrier and appear in the CNS (Mayer, 1962; Masuoka and Hansson, 1967; Nickerson and Hollenberg, 1967; Janssen and Allewijn, 1968). There is some evidence that this is their important site of action after peripheral administration (Murmann *et al.*, 1966; Janssen *et al.*, 1968).

4.2.2. Treatments Which Increase CA Activity

Amphetamine, the tricyclic antidepressants, and pyrogallol are almost always administered peripherally. When so administered, these drugs do cross the blood–brain barrier and exert effects in the CNS (Grossman and Sclafani, 1971; Sigg, 1968; Marley and Stephenson, 1972). The CA themselves do not cross the blood–brain barrier when administered peripherally (Marley and Stephenson, 1972), and so we will only discuss experiments in which CA are given centrally.

4.3. Acquisition

4.3.1. Treatments Which Decrease CA Activity

Decreased CNS CA activity may sometimes impair acquisition of tasks with strict active response requirements, but does not impair, and may sometimes facilitate, acquisition of tasks with less strict requirements. Treatment with 6-OHDA (doses which decrease brain CA levels 75–80% or 90%) impairs acquisition of active positively or negatively reinforced conditioned responses in rats (Cooper *et al.*, 1973; Fibiger *et al.*, 1974; Howard *et al.*, 1974; Mason and Iversen, 1974; Zis *et al.*, 1974), often at doses which do not impair postacquisition performance. Changes in motor activity or consummatory behavior do not appear to account for these results. In the one case where it was studied, retention of the conditioned response after it had been acquired was not affected by 6-OHDA (Mason and Iversen, 1974). Treatment with prenylamine (dose which decreases brain CA levels 50–60%) impairs acquisition of an active escape/avoidance response in rats, but also decreases motor activity (Gregory, 1968). When the decrease in motor activity is corrected for by analysis of covariance, the apparent impairment of avoidance acquisition disappears (Gregory, 1968). Treatment with AMPT (dose which decreases brain CA level 40%) does not affect acquisition of an active shuttlebox escape/avoidance response in mice, nor is spontaneous motor activity affected (Ahlenius, 1973). However, AMPT (dose which decreases brain CA levels, but extent not measured) facilitates acquisition, as measured by a decrease in number of trials to a criterion of nine correct responses in ten trials, in a thirst-motivated discrimination task with broad response requirements in rats, even though response latency was increased (Saper and Sweeney, 1973). Treatment with 6-OHDA (doses identical to those which impair active avoidance acquisition) does not affect acquisition of a one-trial passive avoidance response in rats (Cooper et al., 1973).

The evidence is somewhat contradictory as to whether decreased NE activity or decreased DA activity is responsible for impairment of the ability to make an active learned response. Treatment with a dopamine-β-hydroxylase inhibitor has been found to either impair or have no effect on acquisition of an active shuttlebox escape/avoidance response. Osborne and Kerkut (1972) found that disulfiram (dose which decreased brain NE 50%) impaired acquisition in rats, while Ahlenius (1973) found that FLA-63 (dose which decreased brain NE 50%, DA unchanged) did not affect acquisition in mice. In neither experiment was there an effect on spontaneous motor activity, as measured by intertrial crossings of the shuttlebox. Support for the idea that decreased NE impairs active learned responding comes from an experiment by Anlezark et al. (1973). They made bilateral electrolytic lesions in the locus coeruleus of rats which decreased cerebral cortex NE levels by 70% (this nucleus consists of NE-containing cell bodies). Such lesions impaired acquisition of an active, hunger-motivated response, but did not affect weight gain or spontaneous motor activity. There is also evidence that decreased NE facilitates active responding. Treatment with 6-OHDA which decreases brain NE levels much more than DA levels (50% vs. 25%, respectively) facilitates acquisition of an active shuttlebox escape/avoidance response in rats, probably because of the greatly increased motor activity which also occurs (Cooper et al., 1973). Reduction of brain NE activity with the β-adrenergic receptor blockers dichloroisoproterenol (5–10 mg/kg, ip) or pronethanol (10 mg/kg, ip) also facilitates acquisition of an active avoidance response in rats, although the α-adrenergic blocker phentolamine (10 mg/kg, ip) has no effect (Merlo and Izquierdo, 1965). There is much evidence for the idea that decreased DA impairs active learned responding. A 6-OHDA treatment which decreases brain DA levels much more than NE levels (85% vs. 25%, respectively) impairs acquisition of an active shuttlebox escape/avoidance response in rats (Cooper et al., 1973). Acquisition of a food-reinforced active T-maze response in rats is impaired by 6-OHDA treatments which decrease brain DA levels more than NE levels, but is less impaired by 6-OHDA treatments which decrease both CA levels about equally (Howard *et al.*, 1974). Injection of 6-OHDA into the substantia nigra of rats, which decreases striatal DA 90% and hypothalamic NE 65%, impairs acquisition of positively or negatively reinforced active conditioned responses, while 6-OHDA injection into the ventral NE pathway, which also decreases hypothalamic NE 65% but does not affect DA, has no effect on acquisition (Fibiger *et al.*, 1974).

4.3.2. Treatments Which Increase CA Activity

Nearly all the acquisition studies we will discuss used amphetamine to increase CNS CA activity. Different effects of amphetamine are observed depending upon the response requirements of the task used. In most experiments using tasks with strict active response requirements, amphetamine improves performance during acquisition (Grossman and Sclafani, 1971). Several lines of evidence suggest that this effect is not due to increased learning, but rather to amphetamine's facilitation of the ability to make an active response. In most cases where it has been studied, unconditioned motor activity increases in parallel with the improved conditioned responding (e.g., Barrett *et al.*, 1974; Coyle *et al.*, 1973; Gupta and Holland, 1972; Sansone and Renze, 1971). When animals are tested without the drug, performance declines to nondrug control levels, suggesting that the drug effect is not permanent (Barrett and Steranka, 1974; Kulkarni and Job, 1967; Sansone and Renze, 1971). However, Barrett and Steranka (1974) found that when amphetamine was withdrawn gradually (i.e., decreasing doses on successive days) performance did not decline. This result suggests that the performance decline might be due to state-dependency effects, which can occur with amphetamine (Lal, 1969). In tasks with passive response requirements, where an increase in motor activity would impair performance, amphetamine produces impairment (Bohdanecky and Jarvik, 1967; Grossman and Sclafani, 1971; Novick and Pihl, 1969).

There is some evidence suggesting that increased motor activity is not the only reason for amphetamine's facilitation of performance during acquisition. Gupta and Holland (1972) did a multivariate analysis of the factors responsible for amphetamine's facilitation of active avoidance and found that increased motor activity accounted for only 21% of the variance in avoidance performance. The remainder of the variance was due to a factor they called "conditionability" which was increased by amphetamine. Furthermore, Rahmann (1970) has found that methamphetamine can cause long-lasting improvement in performance of a food-motivated visual discrimination task with broad active response requirements. Wolthuis (1971) has found that methamphetamine can improve performance of a light–dark discrimination task where responses during the light are rewarded with

water, and responses in the dark are punished with electric shock. Methamphetamine had no effect on total water consumption or reactivity to shock.

Several acquisition studies have used treatments other than amphetamine. Yen *et al.* (1971) found that desipramine (3 mg/kg ip) caused a
50% increase in acquisition performance on an active avoidance task in mice,
but suggested that this might be due to increased motor activity. Izquierdo
and coworkers found that acquisition of an active avoidance task in rats is
impaired by isoproterenol (β-adrenergic agonist) (Vasquez *et al.*, 1967;
Merlo and Izquierdo, 1967) and not affected by pyrogallol (12.5 mg/kg ip)
(Merlo and Izquierdo, 1965). Isoproterenol's effect was blocked by
phentolamine or pronethalol (Merlo and Izquierdo, 1967), while isoproterenol itself blocked amphetamine-produced facilitation (Vasquez *et al.*,
1967).

4.3.3. Interpretation

The most consistent finding in acquisition studies is that significant
decreases of CA activity lead to impairment of performance of active
responses while amphetamine-produced increases of CA activity facilitate
such responding. The fact that decreasing CA activity does not impair
performance of tasks with passive response requirements while amphetamine, rather than facilitating, impairs performance of such tasks, suggests that CA are not involved in learning *per se*. The results of these experiments on acquisition, especially those using β-adrenergic agonists and
blockers, lead to the interpretation that both dopaminergic and α-adre-
nergic systems are necessary for the expression of active learned behavior,
while β-adrenergic systems are involved with the suppression of this behavior. The fact that acquisition can be impaired without affecting memory
(Mason and Iversen, 1974) suggests that distinct CA systems are involved in
mediating these processes.

4.4. Memory

4.4.1. Treatments Which Decrease CA Activity

Decreased CNS NE activity immediately after training can impair
later performance, even when NE activity has returned to normal by the
time of the performance. Diethyldithiocarbamate, the active metabolite of
disulfiram, impairs later performance of a one-trial passive avoidance task
in mice when 250 mg/kg sc or 900 mg/kg (route not given) are
administered immediately or 1 hr, respectively, after the single training
trial, but does not cause impairment when administered 2 or 3 hr, respec-

tively, after the training trial (Randt *et al.*, 1971; Van Buskirk *et al.*, 1973). A dose of 1400 mg/kg ip (but not 500 mg/kg) impairs later performance of an active avoidance task when administered 1 min after the training trials, but not when given 24 hrs afterwards (Dismukes and Rake, 1972). Neither AMPT (200 mg/kg sc) nor the dopamine-β-hydroxylase inhibitor FLA-63 (20 mg/kg sc), when given 24 hr after training, has any effect on later performance of an active avoidance task in mice (Ahlenius, 1973). These results suggest that the consolidation process is impaired by decreased CNS NE levels within 1 hr of training, but that consolidation and retention at later periods are not affected. However, the effects of the diethyldithiocarbamate treatment may be due not to decreased NE levels, but rather to the production of brain seizures, which this drug causes at doses greater than 600 mg/kg (Van Buskirk *et al.*, 1973), or to retrograde state-dependency effects (Ahlenius, 1973).

Results suggesting that decreased CNS NE activity can improve memory have been reported by Merlo and Izquierdo (1971). They found that either propranolol (2 mg/kg ip) or pronethalol (10 mg/kg ip) administered immediately after each training session improved performance on an active avoidance task in rats, measured either as number of conditioned avoidance responses made or number of rats reaching a criterion of 90% avoidance for four consecutive sessions. Sessions were spaced 24 hr apart to minimize proactive effects on performance. Dismukes and Rake (1972) also found that dichloroisoproterenol (75 mg/kg sc) given 1 min after training impaired later performance of an active avoidance task in mice, while the same dose given 24 hr after training had no effect. The differences in effect between dichloroisoproterenol and other β-receptor blockers could be due to the former's possession of considerably more β-agonist effect than the others (Fitzgerald, 1969).

4.4.2. Treatments Which Increase CA Activity

Most experiments in which amphetamine is given within 4 hr after training have found an improvement in later performance, suggesting that amphetamine improves consolidation (Doty and Doty, 1966; Hall, 1969; Krivanek and McGaugh, 1969; Johnson and Waite, 1971; Evangelista and Izquierdo, 1971; Castellano, 1974). Amphetamine given after training also reverses the amnesia produced by protein synthesis inhibitors (Barondes and Cohen, 1968; Roberts *et al.*, 1970; Serota *et al.*, 1972; Bloom *et al.*, 1974) and this effect can be blocked by pentobarbital (Barondes and Cohen, 1968). NE or DA administered intraventricularly to mice immediately after training improves performance on a retention test 24 hr later (Haycock *et al.*, 1974). In rats pretreated with diethyldithiocarbamate (300 mg/kg sc), NE administered intraventricularly immediately after training almost completely reverses the diethyldithiocarbamate-induced amnesia. NE administered 2 hr after training has less of an effect, while NE administered 5 hr after training has no effect. Appropriate control experiments ruled out possible confounding effects on motor activity or state dependency (Stein *et al.*, 1975).

There is evidence that the dopaminergic nigrostriatal pathway is involved in memory. Electrical stimulation of the pars compacta of the substantia nigra during acquisition impairs later performance of a passive avoidance task in rats (Routtenberg and Holzman, 1973). Such stimulation did not affect acquisition performance, and stimulation of surrounding brain regions did not affect later performance. Electrical stimulation of the caudate–putamen complex immediately after each training trial impairs later performance of a food-motivated maze task in rats (Peeke and Herz, 1971). These effects may be mediated by an interference with normal dopaminergic activity.

4.4.3. Interpretation

The evidence on the role of CA in memory is suggestive, but many of the techniques used have problems of specificity. The studies using dopamine-β-hydroxylase inhibitors are confounded by possible retrograde state-dependency effects (Wright, 1974) and electrical seizure activity (Van Buskirk *et al.*, 1973); those using β-adrenergic blockers are confounded by membrane-stabilizing effects (Fitzgerald, 1969); and those using amphetamine are confounded by central stimulation or arousal effects (Barondes and Cohen, 1968; McGaugh, 1973). A possible explanation for amphetamine's reversal of the amnesia produced by protein synthesis inhibitors is the finding that NE administered intracranially can attenuate the protein synthesis inhibition caused by electroconvulsive shock (Essman, 1973). The major contradiction apparent in these results is the fact that both amphetamine, a stimulant, and the β-adrenergic blockers, which are sedatives (Murmann *et al.*, 1966; Bainbridge and Greenwood, 1971), facilitate memory. Future experiments using β-adrenergic blockers without membrane stabilizing properties, e.g., sotalol (Fitzgerald, 1969), or electrical stimulation of specific adrenergic systems should help clarify this issue.

4.5. Postacquisition Performance

4.5.1. Treatments Which Decrease CA Activity

Treatments which decrease CNS CA activity almost always impair postacquisition performance (e.g., Lenard *et al.*, 1972; Tanaka *et al.*, 1972).

This impairment may be due to state-dependency effects (Ahlenius, 1973), sedation (elsewhere in these volumes), or motor deficits (elsewhere in these volumes) as well as to disruption of learning. The evidence suggests that both NE and DA are necessary for maintaining active learned responding. The performance deficit in active avoidance caused by 6-OHDA can be reversed by intraventricular administration of either L-NE or DA (Lenard *et al.*, 1972; Lenard, personal communication). The dopamine-receptor blocker pimozide impairs performance of many types of active tasks (Janssen *et al.*, 1968; Carter *et al.*, 1974). Disulfiram, which decreases brain levels of NE only, can impair performance of an active avoidance response in rats (Krantz and Seiden, 1968). In studies where disulfiram has no effect on active responding (Hurwitz *et al.*, 1971), the deficit produced by decreased NE levels may be compensated for by the effects of the increased DA levels often produced by disulfiram. Phentolamine (α-adrenergic blocker) impairs performance of active learned responses (Hastings and Stutz, 1973; Wise *et al.*, 1973; Delbarre and Schmitt, 1974), while propranolol (β-adrenergic blocker) has no effect on such responses (Laverty and Taylor, 1968; Hastings and Stutz, 1973). In tasks with passive response requirements, e.g., differential reinforcement of low rates of responding (DRL), both FLA-63 (dopamine-β-hydroxylase inhibitor) (Ahlenius and Engel, 1972) and propranolol (Richardson *et al.*, 1972) disrupt performance by decreasing the ability to withhold an active response. Propranolol has the same effect when administered into the basolateral amygdala (Richardson *et al.*, 1972), and lesions of this area also disrupt performance on a DRL schedule (Pellegrino, 1968) and on passive avoidance (Coover *et al.*, 1973). Phentolamine improves performance of a task with passive response requirements (Wise *et al.*, 1973). These results suggest that α-adrenergic systems are important for the maintenance of active behavior, while β-adrenergic systems (β-receptors in the amygdala) are involved in suppression of active behavior.

4.5.2. Treatments Which Increase CA Activity

Increased CA activity in the CNS almost always results in improved postacquisition performance. Amphetamine, in doses less than 5 mg/kg, usually has this effect as long as a minimum tendency to respond exists and the baseline rate of responding is not too high (Stein and Wise, 1970). This improved performance is usually accompanied by increased spontaneous and unconditioned motor activity, which can account for the results in tasks with active response requirements. In tasks with passive or loose active response requirements, e.g., DRL or discrimination, amphetamine rarely improves performance, usually having no effect or disrupting behavior (Grossman and Sclafani, 1971; Sanger *et al.*, 1974). When the baseline rate of active responding is high, amphetamine may decrease learned responding (e.g., Rosen and La Flore, 1973). These generalizations hold even within a single session: during a fixed interval schedule of reinforcement, amphetamine can increase responding during the initial portion of the interval, when the baseline response rate is low; and decrease responding during the final portion, when the baseline rate is high (Grossman and Sclafani, 1971). At high doses, which cause stereotyped behavior by a dopaminergic mechanism (Fog, 1972; also elsewhere in these volumes), amphetamine may decrease active learned responding, probably by response competition due to the stereotyped behavior.

Experiments using secondary amine tricyclic antidepressants have reported contradictory results on performance. Several experiments using positive reinforcement have found an increase in learned responding, while experiments using negative reinforcement have found a decrease (Sigg, 1968). For example, Morpurgo (1965) found that desipramine (5 mg/kg ip) caused an 18% decrease in active avoidance responses in trained rats. The discrepancy between this impairment and the facilitation of active avoidance acquisition in mice reported by Yen *et al.* (1971) may be due to state-dependency effects present in the postacquisition paradigm.

The behavioral effects of CA given centrally depend on the site of administration. CA injected into the mesencephalic reticular formation inhibit both positively and negatively reinforced behavior, as well as causing signs of lethargy and sedation (including high amplitude, slow wave EEG) which could account for this disruption of performance (Grossman and Sclafani, 1971). NE given intraventricularly improves performance of an active avoidance response in rats (Segal and Mandell, 1970) but disrupts performance of a passive response task (Wise *et al.*, 1973). D-NE or DA do not have this effect (Wise *et al.*, 1973). The site of this effect has been localized in the amygdala by Margules (1971a,b). Direct placement of L-NE crystals in the amygdala of rats disrupted the performance of a passive response task without affecting performance on an active task. This effect was blocked by pretreatment with phentolamine, but not with a β-adrenergic blocker, LB-46 (Margules, 1971a). Further study of 49 sites in and around the amygdala localized this antisuppression effect of NE to the dorsal portion of the corticomedial division of the amygdala (Margules, 1971b). Placement of NE in the dentate gyrus of rats also has an antisuppression effect, but such treatment also increases the performance of active learned responses, so that the effect is not as specific as in the amygdala (Margules and Margules, 1973). In addition, direct application of isoproterenol in the amygdala improves performance of a passive task (Margules, 1971a). These results suggest there might exist two reciprocal adrenergic systems, one, *alpha,* which activates behavior, and one, *beta,* which suppresses behavior.

Electrical stimulation of CA neurons improves performance of active responses and can itself serve as reinforcement for learning active responses. The improved performance may be accompanied by increased motor activity (Stein, 1965), which could account for the improvement, or the improved performance may be relatively specific, i.e., unconditioned responding is not increased (Margules and Stein, 1968). Stimulation of several CA-containing brain regions can serve as reinforcement, including the lateral hypothalamus (Crow, 1972), posterior hypothalamus (Wise *et al.*, 1973; Lippa *et al.*, 1973), substantia nigra (Phillips and Fibiger, 1973) and locus coeruleus (Crow *et al.*, 1973). Pharmacological evidence suggests that this reinforcement effect is mediated by both DA and NE neurons (German and Bowden, 1974). Stimulation by electrodes in the posterior hypothalamus is blocked by low doses of haloperidol or pimozide (DA receptor blockers), but unaffected by phentolamine or FLA-63, indicating that DA neurons are involved (Lippa *et al.*, 1973; Carter *et al.*, 1974). Stimulation by electrodes in the lateral and posterior hypothalamus is facilitated by amphetamine and L-NE, but not by D-NE or DA, while such stimulation is blocked by disulfiram and phentolamine, but not by propranolol (Hastings and Stutz, 1973; Wise *et al.*, 1973). Furthermore, the blocking effect of disulfiram is overcome by L-NE (Wise and Stein, 1969). The pattern of anatomical and pharmacological results suggests that reinforcement of active responses is mediated by at least two separate CA systems: a ventral dopaminergic system with cell bodies around the interpeduncular nucleus and axons running into the pars compacta of the substantia nigra and via the medial forebrain bundle (MFB) through the posterior and lateral hypothalamus, and a dorsal α-adrenergic system with cell bodies in the locus coeruleus and axons running in the MFB (German and Bowden, 1974).

4.5.3. Interpretation

Stein (1969) has proposed a neurophysiological basis for the facilitation of learned behavior caused by treatments which increase CA activity. His theory is that there is an α-adrenergic reinforcement system with cell bodies in the midbrain area (including locus coeruleus), axons running in the MFB, and synapses in the limbic forebrain (including amygdala), hypothalamus, and neocortex. When activated, this system strengthens connections between learning experience and learned behavior, increasing the probability of occurrence of learned responses. The system works by inhibiting cholinergic neurons which normally inhibit behavior (Carlton, 1969). Thus, activation of the system would facilitate behavior by disinhibition.

There is anatomical, physiological, and pharmacological evidence for the existence of such an α-adrenergic system. Both histofluorescent (Hillarp *et al.*, 1966) and lesion techniques (Heller *et al.*, 1966) have shown that

Stein's proposed system exists anatomically. Activation of the system, either by electrical stimulation or with amphetamine, releases NE in the amygdala and hypothalamus (Stein and Wise, 1969). The pharmacological evidence mentioned in the previous section supports the idea that this system is α-adrenergic.

The behavioral evidence suggests that this is not a specific reinforcement system, but rather one which generally activates behavior. With few exceptions (Verhave, 1958; Margules and Stein, 1968), the increase in learned responding is accompanied by increases in spontaneous and unconditioned motor activity and unconditioned goal-directed behavior which could account for the improved performance (Grossman and Sclafani, 1971). In tasks with passive response requirements, activation of the system disrupts, rather than improves, performance (Grossman and Sclafani, 1971). However, Cooper *et al.* (1971) found that AMPT impaired performance of a passive response task with MFB stimulation as reinforcement. In rats trained to run down an alleyway for rewarding brain stimulation, AMPT does not alter the effects of putative reinforcement parameters, such as number and intensity of stimulating pulses, but does decrease the maximum running speed attained by the rats (Gallistel and Edmonds, 1973).

Margules and Margules (1973) have pointed out that the anatomical structure of Stein's proposed system is more in keeping with a general arousal or activating function than with a specific reinforcement function. The system is monosynaptic, without the multiple sensory input one might expect of a behaviorally selective system involved with learning. Furthermore, it has many collaterals, so that activation of the system has effects in many forebrain structures simultaneously. This makes it unlikely that one particular learned response could be selectively reinforced by activation of the system.

Thus, just as in the acquisition experiments, the data on postacquisition performance suggest that both dopaminergic and α-adrenergic systems are involved in the expression of active learned responses, while β-adrenergic systems are involved in their suppression.

5. BEHAVIOR AS INDEPENDENT VARIABLE

5.1. Problems with CA as Dependent Variable

Two main dependent variables have been looked at in experiments where behavior was the independent variable: (i) endogenous levels of CA and catabolites, (ii) turnover of CA. The latter can be studied by two methods: (i) nonisotopically, either by inhibiting CA synthesis and observing the resulting decline in CA levels, or by inhibiting CA catabolism and observing the resulting increase in CA levels; or (ii) isotopically, by administering radioactively labeled CA or precursors and observing changes in specific activity of CA (Costa and Neff, 1970). The techniques for measuring CA turnover have several methodological pitfalls. With the nonisotopic method, significant effects may be masked unless maximal inhibition is maintained throughout the experiment. With the isotopic methods, the dose of labeled CA or precursor must be small enough not to disturb the endogenous pool or alter metabolism. One must also assume that the label is taken up by the same cells and handled metabolically in the same way as endogenous CA or precursor. These assumptions are certainly not completely true for label administered iv or intraventricularly (Costa and Neff, 1970). To the extent that these methodological pitfalls are avoided, an increase in specific activity of brain CA after administration of labeled precursor indicates increased synthesis of CA, while a decrease in specific activity of brain CA after administration of labeled CA also indicates increased CA synthesis.

5.2. Negatively Reinforced Behavior

The effect of conditioned avoidance behavior on CA in rats has been studied using endogenous levels of CA and both isotopic and nonisotopic turnover methods. Fuxe and Hanson (1967) gave avoidance-trained rats either saline or AMPT before an avoidance test session. Control rats received an equivalent number of UCS's (electric shocks) after being given AMPT. Rats given saline showed an increase in the number and intensity of fluorescent NE nerve terminals throughout the brain, as compared with control rats, but no change in CA nerve cell bodies or serotonin nerve terminals. Rats given AMPT showed a decrease in number and intensity of fluorescent NE nerve terminals, especially in the prosencephalon, and a similar decrease in DA terminals in the caudate, nucleus accumbens, and tuberculum olfactorium, but not in the median eminence. These decreases were proportional to the decreases in conditioned avoidance caused by the AMPT. These results suggest that avoidance behavior, but not the stress of shocks, causes increased CA synthesis and turnover. Since motor activity varied with avoidance, these results could be due to motor processes, rather than learning.

Fulginiti and Orsingher (1971) found a similar result of increased CA synthesis during avoidance behavior using the isotopic method. They gave labeled tyrosine to naive rats and measured NE specific activity in the hypothalamus and cerebral cortex. Experimental rats were given 100 avoidance training trials and achieved 7–72% avoidance, thus receiving 93–28 UCS's (electric shocks). Control rats were kept in their home cages, receiving no stimuli or training. There was no effect of avoidance behavior on levels of endogenous NE, but there was a 24–143% increase in NE specific activity, suggesting increased synthesis of NE during avoidance. This increase in specific activity was independent of the number of UCS's received, suggesting that it was not due to increased exposure to shock among the experimental group. However, motor activity was probably greatly different between the two groups, which could account for the results.

5.3. Positively Reinforced Behavior

Experiments using positively reinforced behavior have also found an increase in CA turnover during learned behavior. Yuwiler and Olds (1973) trained rats with chronic electrodes in the hypothalamus to lever-press for self-stimulation. The rats were given a 20-min test session (during which they made 700–1000 responses per 8-min period), then killed, and their brains analyzed for CA. Three control groups were also tested: (1) rats without electrodes or training, (2) trained rats who did not receive self-stimulation during the test session, (3) trained rats who were given stimulation (480/8 min) during the test session. The experimental group had significantly lower levels of hypothalamic NE, whole brain NE, and whole brain DA than did any of the control groups. This result suggests that learned behavior caused increased CA turnover. It is unlikely to be due to increased stress due to receiving brain stimulation because control group 3 had the same increase in adrenal corticoids as did the experimental group.

Lewy and Seiden (1972) studied the effects of bar-pressing for water on levels of endogenous NE and specific activity of NE (after intraventricular administration of labeled NE) in the brain stem-diencephalon of water-deprived rats. Experimental rats were compared with water-deprived and normal controls. There was no effect of conditioning or water deprivation on levels of endogenous NE, but there was a 25% decrease in specific activity of NE in the experimental group, suggesting increased synthesis of NE. There was roughly equivalent motor activity in the experimental and water-deprived groups, but water consumption or the specific act of bar-pressing, as well as conditioning, could be responsible for the results.

5.4. Interpretation

All of these experiments, using behavior as an independent variable, had adequate controls for the dependent variable of CA turnover; all used measurement and labeling techniques which did not affect behavior or CA turnover. The reason these experiments are difficult to interpret lies in the lack of specificity of the behavioral variable. The observed increases in CA turnover could be due to behavioral processes occurring in addition to learning, e.g., water-deprivation in the Lewy and Seiden (1972) experiment or motor activity in the Fulginiti and Orsingher (1971) experiment. Many of these other behavioral processes are also accompanied by increased CA turnover (Gordon *et al.,* 1966; also elsewhere in these volumes).

6. CONCLUSIONS

Although no experiment approaches the ideals of chemical, anatomical, and behavioral specificity, the pattern of results discussed in this chapter suggests that three types of CA systems play a role in learned behavior: (i) an α-adrenergic behavioral activating system with cell bodies in the locus coeruleus, axons running in the MFB, and synapses in the limbic forebrain (including amygdala), hypothalamus, and neocortex; (ii) a dopaminergic behavioral activating system consisting of two components, one with cell bodies around the interpeduncular nucleus and axons running into the substantia nigra and via the MFB into the hypothalamus and prosencephalon, and the other with cell bodies in the substantia nigra and axons running to the striatum; (iii) a β-adrenergic behavioral inhibiting system with synapses in the basolateral amygdala. The existence of separate α- and β-adrenergic systems with opposing behavioral functions may be responsible for many of the contradictory results obtained when CNS NE activity is altered. The evidence also suggests that NE plays a role in memory consolidation.

This pattern of results, particularly the fact that the observed effects of these systems vary with the response requirements of the task involved, suggests these CA systems do not play a role in learning *per se,* but rather in the expression of active learned behavior. This mechanism is distinct from the role of NE in memory consolidation, since it can be impaired without affecting memory. It is still possible, in theory, for CA to be involved with learning *per se,* with their role masked by the effects of the CA behavioral activating systems. This assumption would explain the contradictory effects of CA on active *vs.* passive learning, but appears to be an unneeded violation of the law of parsimony.

7. REFERENCES

Ahlenius, S., 1973, Inhibition of catecholamine synthesis and conditioned avoidance acquisition, *Pharmacol. Biochem. Behav.* 1:347.

Ahlenius, S., and Engel, J., 1972, Effects of a dopamine (DA)-β-hydroxylase inhibitor on timing behaviour, *Psychopharmacologia* **24**:243.

Algeri, S., and Cerletti, C., 1974, Effects of L-dopa administration on the serotonergic system in rat brain: correlation between levels of L-dopa accumulated in the brain and depletion of serotonin and tryptophan, *European J. Pharmacol.* **27**:191.

Andén, N. E., and Strombom, U., 1974, Adrenergic receptor blocking agents: Effects on central noradrenaline and dopamine receptors and on motor activity, *Psychopharmacologia* **38**:91.

Andén, N. E., Dahlstrom, A., Fuxe, K., and Larsson, K., 1966, Functional role of the nigro-striatal dopamine neurons, *Acta Pharmacol. Toxicol.* **24**:263.

Anlezark, G. M., Crow, T. J., and Greenway, A. P., 1973, Impaired learning and decreased cortical norepinephrine after bilateral locus coeruleus lesions, *Science* **181**:682.

Azzaro, A. J., and Rutledge, C. O., 1973, Selectivity of release of norepinephrine, dopamine and 5-hydroxytryptamine by amphetamine in various regions of rat brain, *Biochem. Pharmacol.* **22**:2801.

Bainbridge, J. G., and Greenwood, D. T., 1971, Tranquillizing effects of propranolol demonstrated in rats, *Neuropharmacology* **10**:453.

Barondes, S. H., and Cohen, H. D., 1968, Arousal and the conversion of "short-term" to "long-term" memory, *Proc. Natl. Acad. Sci. (U.S.)* **61**:923.

Barrett, R. E., and Balch, T. S., 1971, Uptake of catecholamines into serotonergic nerve cells as demonstrated by fluorescence histochemistry, *Experientia* **15**:663.

Barrett, R. J., and Steranka, L. R., 1974, An analysis of *d*-amphetamine produced facilitation of avoidance acquisition in rats and performance changes subsequent to drug termination, *Life Sci.* **14**:163.

Barrett, R. J., Leith, N. J., and Ray, O. S., 1974, An analysis of the facilitation of avoidance acquisition produced by *d*-amphetamine and scopolamine, *Behav. Biol.* **11**:180.

Bartholini, G., DaPrada, M., and Pletscher, A., 1968, Decrease of cerebral 5-hydroxytryptamine by 3,4-dihydroxyphenylalanine after inhibition of extracerebral decarboxylase, *J. Pharm. Pharmacol.* **20**:228.

Bloom, A. S., Quinton, E. E., and Carr, L. A., 1974, Cycloheximide-induced amnesia: Possible involvement of brain catecholamines, *Soc. Neurosci. Prog.* (abstr.) p. 146.

Blumberg, J. B., and Sulser, F., 1974, The effect of antipsychotic drugs on the cyclic 3′,5′-adenosine monophosphate (cAMP) system on rat limbic forebrain, *Federation Proc.* **33**:286.

Bohdanecky, Z., and Jarvik, M. E., 1967, The effect of *d*-amphetamine and physostigmine upon acquisition and retrieval in a single trial learning task, *Arch. Intern. Pharmacodyn.* **170**:58.

Breese, G. R., and Traylor, T. D., 1970, Effect of 6-hydroxydopamine on brain norepinephrine and dopamine: Evidence for selective degeneration of catecholamine neurons, *J. Pharmacol. Exptl. Therap.* **174**:413.

Breese, G. R., and Traylor, T. D., 1971, Depletion of brain noradrenaline and dopamine by 6-hydroxydopamine, *Brit. J. Pharmacol.* **42**:88.

Butcher, L. L., and Engel, J., 1969, Behavioral and biochemical effects of L-dopa after peripheral decarboxylase inhibition, *Brain Res.* **15**:233.

Butcher, L. L., and Hodge, G. K., 1973, Evidence that 6-hydroxydopamine (6-OHDA) is a nonspecific neurotoxic agent when administered intracerebrally, *Soc. Neurosci. Prog.* (abstr.) p. 372.

Carlton, P. L., 1969, Brain-acetylcholine and inhibition, in: *Reinforcement and Behavior* (J. T. Tapp, ed.), pp. 286–327, Academic Press, New York.

Carter, D., Phillips, A. G., and Fibiger, H. C., 1974, Are central dopaminergic neurons substrates for intracranial self-stimulation (ICS)?, *Soc. Neurosci. Prog.* (abstr.) p. 162.

Castellano, C., 1974, Cocaine, pemoline and amphetamine on learning and retention of a discrimination test in mice, *Psychopharmacologia* **36**:63.

Cooper, B. R., Black, W. C., and Paolino, R. M., 1971, Decreased septal-forebrain and lateral hypothalamic reward after alpha methyl-*p*-tyrosine, *Physiol. Behav.* **6**:425.

Cooper, B. R., Breese, G. R., Grant, L. D., and Howard, J. L., 1973, Effects of 6-hydroxydopamine treatments on active avoidance responding: Evidence for involvement of brain dopamine, *J. Pharmacol. Exptl. Therap.* **185**:358.

Coover, G., Ursin, H., and Levine, S., 1973, Corticosterone and avoidance in rats with basolateral amygdala lesions, *J. Comp. Physiol. Psychol.* **85**:111.

Costa, E., and Neff, N. H., 1970, Estimation of turnover rates to study the metabolic regulation of the steady state level of neuronal monoamines, in: *Handbook of Neurochemistry, Vol. IV* (A. Lajtha, ed.), pp. 45–90, Plenum Press, New York.

Coyle, Jr., J. T., Wender, P., and Lipsky, A., 1973, Avoidance conditioning in different strains of rats: Neurochemical correlates, *Psychopharmacologia* **31**:25.

Crow, T. J., 1972, A map of the rat mesencephalon for electrical self-stimulation, *Brain Res.* **36**:265.

Crow, T. J., Spear, P. J., and Arbuthnott, G. W., 1972, Intracranial self-stimulation with electrodes in the locus coeruleus, *Brain Res.* **36**:275.

Delbarre, B., and Schmitt, H., 1974, Effects of clonidine and some alpha-adreno-receptor blocking agents on avoidance conditioned reflexes in rats: their interactions and antagonism by atropine, *Psychopharmacologia* **35**:195.

Dismukes, R. K., and Rake, A. V., 1972, Involvement of biogenic amines in memory formation, *Psychopharmacologia* **23**:17.

Doty, B., and Doty, L., 1966, Facilitating effects of amphetamine on avoidance conditioning in relation to age and problem difficulty, *Psychopharmacologia* **9**:234.

Essman, W. B., 1973, *Neurochemistry of Cerebral Electroshock*, Spectrum, New York.

Evangelista, A. M., and Izquierdo, I., 1971, The effect of pre- and post-trial amphetamine injections on avoidance responses of rats, *Psychopharmacologia* **20**:42.

Euler, U. S. V., 1972, Synthesis, uptake, and storage of catecholamines in adrenergic nerves, the effect of drugs, in: *Handbook of Experimental Pharmacology, Vol. 33, Catecholamines,* (H. Blaschko and E. Muscholl, eds.), pp. 186–230, Springer, New York.

Everett, G. M., and Borcherding, J. W., 1970, L-Dopa: Effect on concentrations of dopamine, norepinephrine, and serotonin in brains of mice, *Science* **168**:849.

Farnebo, L. O., 1971, Effect of *d*-amphetamine on spontaneous and stimulation-induced release of catecholamines, *Acta Physiol. Scand. Suppl.* **371**:45.

Fibiger, H. C., Phillips, A. G., and Zis, A. P., 1974, Deficits in instrumental responding after 6-hydroxydopamine lesions of the nigro-neostriatal dopaminergic projection, *Pharmacol. Biochem. Behav.* **2**:87.

Fitzgerald, J. D., 1969, Perspectives in adrenergic beta-receptor blockade, *Clin. Pharmacol. Therap.* **10**:292.

Fog, R., 1972, On stereotypy and catalepsy: Studies on the effect of amphetamines and neuroleptics in rats, *Acta Neurol. Scand. Suppl.* **50**:1.

Fulginiti, S., and Orsingher, O. A., 1971, Effects of learning, amphetamine and nicotine on the level and synthesis of brain noradrenaline in rats, *Arch. Intern. Pharmacodyn.* **190**:291

Furchgott, R. F., 1972, The classification of adrenoceptors (adrenergic receptors). An evaluation from the standpoint of receptor theory, in: *Handbook of Experimental Pharmacology Vol. 33, Catecholamines* (H. Blaschko and E. Muscholl, eds.), pp. 283–335, Springer, New York.

Fuxe, F., and Hanson, L. C. F., 1967, Central catecholamine neurons and conditioned avoidance behavior, *Psychopharmacologia* **11**:439.

Fuxe, K., and Ungerstedt, U., 1970, Histochemical, biochemical and functional studies on central monoamine neurons after acute and chronic amphetamine administration, in: *Amphetamines and Related Compounds* (E. Costa and S. Garattini, eds.), pp. 257–288. Raven, New York.

Gallistel, C. R., and Edmonds, D., 1973, Temporal summation and the neuropharmacology of the reward effect in self-stimulating rats, *Soc. Neurosci. Prog.*, (abstr.) p. 191.

German, D. C., and Bowden, D. M., 1974, Catecholamine systems as the neural substrate for intracranial self-stimulation: a hypothesis, *Brain Res.* 73:381.

Goldstein, M., 1966, Inhibition of norepinephrine biosynthesis at the dopamine-β-hydroxylation stage, *Pharmacol. Rev.* 18:77.

Goldstein, M., and Frenkel, R., 1971, Inhibition of serotonin synthesis by dopa and other catechols, *Nature (New Biol.)* 233:179.

Goldstein, M., and Nakajima, K., 1967, The effect of disulfiram on catecholamine levels in the brain, *J. Pharmacol. Exptl. Therap.* 157:96.

Gordon, R., Spector, S., Sjoerdsma, A., and Udenfriend, S., 1966, Increased synthesis of norepinephrine and epinephrine in the intact rat during exercise and exposure to cold, *J. Pharmacol. Exptl. Therap.* 153:440.

Gregory, K., 1968, The action of the drug prenylamine (segontin) on exploratory activity and aversive learning in a selected strain of rats, *Psychopharmacologia* 13:22.

Grewaal, D. S., Fibiger, H. C., and McGeer, E. G., 1974, 6-Hydroxydopamine and striatal acetylcholine levels, *Brain Res.* 73:372.

Grossman, S. P., and Sclafani, A., 1971, Sympathomimetic amines, in: *Pharmacological and Biophysical Agents and Behavior* (E. Furchtgott, ed.), pp. 269–344, Academic Press, New York.

Gupta, B. D., and Holland, H. C., 1972, An examination of the effects of stimulant and depressant drugs on escape/avoidance conditioning in strains of rats selectively bred for emotionality/non-emotionality: A multivariate analysis of the effects of drugs on conditioned avoidance responses and intertrial activity, *Neuropharmacology* 11:23.

Hall, M. E., 1969, Effects of posttrial amphetamine and strychnine on learning as a function of task difficulty, *Commun. Behav. Biol.* 4:171.

Hastings, L., and Stutz, R. M., 1973, The effect of α- and β-adrenergic antagonists on the self-stimulation phenomenon, *Life Sci.* 13:1253.

Haycock, J. W., Van Buskirk, R. B., Ryan, J. R., and McGaugh, J. L., 1974, Retrograde facilitation of inhibitory avoidance learning with posttrial intraventricular injections of norepinephrine and dopamine, *Soc. Neurosci. Prog.* (abstr.) p. 251.

Heller, A., Seiden, L. S., and Moore, R. Y., 1966, Regional effects of lateral hypothalamic lesions on brain norepinephrine in the cat, *Intern. J. Neuropharmacol.* 5:91.

Hery, F., Rouer, E., and Glowinski, J., 1973, Effect of 6-hydroxydopamine on daily variations of 5-HT synthesis in the hypothalamus of the rat, *Brain Res.* 58:135.

Hillarp, N. A., Fuxe, K., and Dahlstrom, A., 1966, Demonstration and mapping of central neurons containing dopamine, noradrenaline, and 5-hydroxy-tryptamine and their reactions to psychopharmaca, *Pharmacol. Rev.* 18:727.

Ho, A. K. S., and Loh, H. H., 1972, Evidence of adrenergic-cholinergic interaction in the central nervous system. II. Dopamine and its analogues, *European J. Pharmacol.* 19:145.

Hökfelt, T., Fuxe, K., Goldstein, M., and Johansson, O., 1974, Immunohistochemical evidence for the existence of adrenaline neurons in the rat brain, *Brain Res.* 66:235.

Howard, J. L., Grant, L. D., and Breese, G. R., 1974, Effects of intracisternal 6-hydroxydopamine treatment on acquisition and performance of rats in a double T-maze, *J. Comp. Physiol. Psychol.* 86:995.

Hurwitz, D. A., Robinson, S. M., and Barofsky, I., 1971, The influence of training and avoidance performance on disulfiram-induced changes in brain catecholamines, *Neuro-pharmacology* **10**:447.

Innes, I. R. and Nickerson, M., 1970, Drugs acting on postganglionic adrenergic nerve endings and structures innervated by them (sympathomimetic drugs), in: *The Pharmacological Basis of Therapeutics* (L. S. Goodman and A. Gilman, eds.), pp. 257–288. Macmillan, New York.

Jacks, B. R., De Champlain, J., and Cordeau, J. P., 1972, Effects of 6-hydroxydopamine on putative transmitter substances in the central nervous system, *European J. Pharmacol.* **18**:353.

Janssen, P. A. J., and Allewijn, F. T. N., 1968, Pimozide, a chemically novel, highly potent and orally long-acting neuroleptic drug, Part II: Kinetic study of the distribution of pimozide and metabolites in brain, liver and blood of the Wistar rat, *Arzneimittel-Forsch.* **18**:279.

Janssen, P. A. J., Niemegeers, C. J. E., Schellekens, K. H. L., Dresse, A., Lenaerts, F. M., Pinchard, A., Schaper, W. K. A., Nueten, J. M. V., and Verbruggen, F. J., 1968, Pimozide, a chemically novel, highly potent and orally long-acting neuroleptic drug, Part I: The comparative pharmacology of pimozide, haloperidol, and chlorpromazine, *Arzneimittel-Forsch.* **18**:261.

Johnson, F. N., and Waite, K., 1971, Apparent delayed enhancement of memory following post-trial methylamphetamine hydrochloride, *Experientia* **27**:1316.

Johnson, G. A., Kim, E. G., and Boukma, S. J., 1972, 5-Hydroxyindole levels in rat brain after inhibition of dopamine β-hydroxylase, *J. Pharmacol. Exptl. Therap.* **180**:539.

Juge, A., Sordet, F., Jouvet, M., and Pujol, J. F., 1972, Modification du metabolisme de la serotonine (5-HT) cerebrale apres 6-hydroxydopamine (6-HDA) chez le rat, *Ct. R. Acad. Sci. (Paris)* **24**:3266.

Juorio, A. V., and Vogt, M., 1965, The effect of prenylamine on the metabolism of cate-cholamines and 5-hydroxytryptamine in brain and adrenal medulla, *Brit. J. Pharmacol.* **24**:566.

Karobath, M., Diaz, J. L., and Huttunen, M. O., 1971, The effect of L-dopa on the concentra-tions of tryptophan, tyrosine and serotonin in rat brain, *European J. Pharmacol.* **14**:393.

Kebabian, J., Petzold, G., and Greengard, P., 1972, Dopamine-sensitive adenylate cyclase in caudate nucleus of rat brain, and its similarity to the "dopamine receptor," *Proc. Natl. Acad. Sci. (U.S.)* **69**:2145.

Kimble, G. A., 1961, *Hilgard and Marquis' Conditioning and Learning,* 2nd Edition, Appleton Century Crofts, New York.

Knapp, S., Mandell, A. J., and Geyer, M. A., 1974, Effects of amphetamines on regional tryp-tophan hydroxylase activity and synaptosomal conversion of tryptophan to 5-hydroxytryptamine in rat brain, *J. Pharmacol. Exptl. Therap.* **189**:676.

Koslow, S. H., and Schlumpf, M., 1974, Epinephrine concentrations in discrete brain nuclei of the rat measured by mass fragmentography, *Soc. Neurosci. Prog.* (abstr.) p. 290.

Krantz, K. D., and Seiden, L. S., 1968, Effects of diethyldithiocarbamate on the conditioned avoidance response of the rat, *J. Pharm. Pharmacol.* **20**:166.

Krivanek, J., and McGaugh, J. L., 1969, Facilitating effects of pre- and posttrial amphetamine administration on discrimination learning in mice, *Agents Actions* **1**:36.

Kulkarni, A. S., and Job, W. M., 1967, Facilitation of avoidance learning by *d*-amphetamine, *Life Sci.* **6**:1579.

Lal, H., 1969, Control of learned conditioned-avoidance responses (CAR) by amphetamine and chlorpromazine, *Psychopharmacologia* **14**:33.

Langelier, P., Roberge, A. G., Boucher, R., and Poirier, L. J., 1973, Effects of chronically administered L-dopa in normal and lesioned cats, *J. Pharmacol. Exptl. Therap.* **189**:676.

Laverty, R., and Taylor, K. M., 1968, Propranolol uptake into the central nervous system and the effect on rat behaviour and amine metabolism, *J. Pharm. Pharmacol.* **20**:605.

Lenard, L. G., Clody, D. E., and Beer, B., 1972, Long-term conditioned avoidance deficits in rat after intraventricular injection of 6-hydroxydopamine: Restoration of performance with L-norepinephrine, *Proc. Am. Psychol. Assoc.* **7(Part2)**:823.

Lewy, A. J., and Seiden, L. S., 1972, Operant behavior changes norepinephrine metabolism in rat brain, *Science* **175**:454.

Lidbrink, P., Jonsson, G., and Fuxe, K., 1971, The effect of imipramine-like drugs on uptake mechanisms in the central noradrenaline and 5-hydroxytryptamine neurons, *Neuropharmacology* **10**:521.

Lippa, A. S., Antelman, S. M., Fisher, A. E., and Canfield, D. R., 1973, Neurochemical mediation of reward: A significant role for dopamine?, *Pharmacol. Biochem. Behav.* **1**:23.

Maj, J., Grabowska, M., and Kwiek, J., 1970, The effect of disulfiram, diethyldithiocarbamate and dimethyldithiocarbamate on serotonin and 5-hydroxyindole-3-acetic acid brain levels in rats, *Biochem. Pharmacol.* **19**:2517.

Margules, D. L., 1971*a*, Alpha and beta adrenergic receptors in amygdala: Reciprocal inhibitors and facilitators of punished operant behavior, *European J. Pharmacol.* **16**:21.

Margules, D. L., 1971*b*, Localization of anti-punishment actions of norepinephrine and atropine in amygdala and entopeduncular nucleus of rats, *Brain Res.* **35**:177.

Margules, D. L., and Margules, A. S., 1973, The development of operant responses by noradrenergic activation and cholinergic suppression of movements, in: *Efferent Organization and the Integration of Behavior* (J. D. Maser, ed.), pp. 203–228, Academic Press, New York.

Margules, D. L., and Stein, L., 1968, Facilitation of Sidman avoidance behavior by positive brain stimulation, *J. Comp. Physiol. Psychol.* **66**:182.

Marley, E., and Stephenson, J. D., 1972, Central actions of catecholamines, in: *Handbook of Experimental Pharmacology, Vol. 33, Catecholamines* (H. Blaschko and E. Muscholl, eds.), pp. 463–537, Springer-Verlag, Berlin.

Mason, S. T., and Iversen, S. D., 1974, Learning impairment in rats after 6-hydroxydopamine-induced depletion of brain catecholamines, *Nature* **248**:697.

Masuoka, D., and Hansson, E., 1967, Autoradiographic distribution studies of adrenergic blocking agents. II. ^{14}C-propranolol, a β-receptor-type blocker, *Acta Pharmacol. Toxicol.* **25**:447.

Mayer, S. E., 1962, The physiological disposition of ^{3}H-dichloroisoproterenol, *J. Pharmacol. Exptl. Therap.* **135**:204.

McGaugh, J. L., 1973, Drug facilitation of learning and memory, *Ann. Rev. Pharmacol.* **13**:229.

Meek, J., Fuxe, K., and Andén, N. E., 1970, Effects of antidepressant drugs of the imipramine type on central 5-hydroxytryptamine neurotransmission, *European J. Pharmacol.* **9**:325.

Merlo, A. B., and Izquierdo, I., 1965, Effects of inhibitors of *O*-methyltransferase and of adrenergic blocking agents on conditioning and extinction in rats, *Med. Pharmacol. Expt.* **13**:217.

Merlo, A. B., and Izquierdo, I., 1967, The effect of catecholamines on learning in rats, *Med. Pharmacol. Expt.* **16**:343.

Merlo, A. B., and Izquierdo, J. A., 1971, Effect of post-trial injection of beta adrenergic blocking agents on a conditioned reflex in rats, *Psychopharmacologia* **22**:181.

Moore, K. E., and Dominic, J. A., 1971, Tyrosine hydroxylase inhibitors, *Federation Proc.* **30**:859.

Morpurgo, C., 1965, Drug-induced modifications of discriminated avoidance behavior in rats, *Psychopharmacologia* **8**:91.

Murmann, W., Almirante, L., and Saccani-Guelfi, M., 1966, Central nervous system effects of four β-adrenergic receptor blocking agents, *J. Pharm. Pharmacol.* **18**:317.

Nickerson, M., and Hollenberg, N. K., 1967, Blockade of α-adrenergic receptors in: *Physiological Pharmacology Vol. 4, The Nervous System-Part D, Autonomic Nervous System Drugs* (W. S. Root and F. G. Hofmann, eds.), pp. 243–305, Academic Press, New York.

Novick, I., and Pihl, R., 1969, Effect of amphetamine on the septal syndrome in rats, *J. Comp. Physiol. Psychol.* **68**:220.

Obianwu, H. O., 1965, The effect of prenylamine (Segontin) on the amine levels of brain, heart, and adrenal medulla in rats, *Acta Pharmacol.* **23**:383.

Osborne, R. H., and Kerkut, G. A., 1972, Inhibition of noradrenaline biosynthesis and its effects on learning in rats, *Comp. Gen. Pharmacol.* **3**:359.

Overton, D. A., 1974, Experimental methods for the study of state-dependent learning, *Federation Proc.* **33**:1800.

Peeke, H. V. S., and Herz, M. J., 1971, Caudate nucleus stimulation retroactively impairs complex maze learning in the rat, *Science* **173**:80.

Pellegrino, L., 1968, Amygdaloid lesions and behavioral inhibition in the rat, *J. Comp. Physiol. Psychol.* **65**:483.

Philippu, A., Glowinski, J., and Besson, M. J., 1974, *In vivo* release of newly synthesized catecholamines from the hypothalamus by amphetamine, *Naunyn-Schmiedebergs Arch. Pharmakol.* **282**:1.

Phillips, A. G., and Fibiger, H. C., 1973, Dopaminergic and noradrenergic substrates of positive reinforcement: Differential effects of *d*- and *l*-amphetamine, *Science* **179**:575.

Poirier, L. J., Langelier, P., Roberge, A., Boucher, R., and Kitsikis, A., 1972, Non-specific histopathological changes induced by the intracerebral injection of 6-hydroxydopamine (6-OH-DA), *J. Neurol. Sci.* **16**:401.

Rahmann, H., 1970, The influence of methamphetamine on learning, long-term memory, and transposition ability in golden hamster, in *Amphetamines and Related Compounds* (E. Costa and S. Garattini, eds.), pp. 813–817, Raven, New York.

Randt, C. T., Quartermain, D., Goldstein, M., and Anagnoste, B., 1971, Norepinephrine biosynthesis inhibition: Effects on memory in mice, *Science* **172**:498.

Rech, R. H., Borys, H. K., and Moore, K. E., 1966, Alterations in behavior and brain catecholamine levels in rats treated with α-methyltyrosine, *J. Pharmacol. Exptl. Therap.* **153**:412.

Richardson, J. S., Stacey, P. D., Russo, N. J., and Musty, R. E., 1972, Effects of systemic administration of propranolol on the timing behavior (DRL-20) of rats, *Arch. Intern. Pharmacodyn.* **197**:66.

Roberts, R. B., Flexner, J. B., and Flexner, L. B., 1970, Some evidence for the involvement of adrenergic sites in the memory trace, *Proc. Natl. Acad. Sci. (U.S.)* **66**:310.

Rosen, A. J., and La Flore, J. E., 1973, Effects of intraperitoneal and intraventricular *d*-amphetamine administration on active avoidance performance in the rat, *Life Sci.* **13**:1573.

Routtenberg, A., and Holzman, N., 1973, Memory disruption by electrical stimulation of substantia nigra, pars compacta, *Science* **181**:83.

Sanger, D. J., Key, M., and Blackman, D. E., 1974, Differential effects of chlordiazepoxide and *d*-amphetamine on responding maintained by a DRL schedule of reinforcement, *Psychopharmacologia* **38**:159.

Sansone, M., and Renze, P., 1971, Shuttle-box avoidance behavior of hamsters: A further investigation on the effects of amphetamine and methylphenidate, *Pharmacol. Res. Commun.* **3**:113.

Saper, C. B., and Sweeney, D. C., 1973, Enhanced appetitive discrimination learning in rats treated with α-methyltyrosine, *Psychopharmacologia* **30**:37.

Schubert, J., Fyro, B., Nyback, H., and Sedvall, G., 1970, Effects of cocaine and amphetamine on the metabolism of tryptophan and 5-hydroxytryptamine in mouse brain *in vivo, J. Pharm. Pharmacol.* **22**:860.

Schubert, P., Kretuzberg, G. W., Reinhold, K,, and Herz, A., 1973, Selective uptake of ^{3}H-6-hydroxydopamine by neurones of the central nervous system, *Expt. Brain Res.* **17**:539.

Segal, D. S., and Mandell, A. J., 1970, Behavioral activation of rats during intraventricular infusion of norepinephrine, *Proc. Natl. Acad. Sci. (U.S.)* **66**:289.

Serota, R. G., Roberts, R. B., and Flexner, L. B., 1972, Acetoxycycloheximide-induced transient amnesia: protective effects of adrenergic stimulants, *Proc. Natl. Acad. Sci. (U.S.,)* **69**:340.

Sigg, E. B., 1968, Tricyclic thymoleptic agents and some newer antidepressants, in: *Psychoharmacology, A Review of Progress 1957-1967,* (D. H. Efron, ed.), pp. 655–669, U.S. Government Printing Office, Washington, D.C.

Stein, L., 1965, Facilitation of avoidance behavior by positive brain stimulation, *J. Comp. Physiol. Psychol.* **60**:9.

Stein, L., 1969, Chemistry of purposive behavior, in: *Reinforcement and Behavior,* (J. T. Tapp, ed.), pp. 328–355, Academic Press, New York.

Stein, L., and Wise, C. D., 1969, Release of norepinephrine from hypothalamus and amygdala by rewarding medial forebrain bundle stimulation and amphetamine, *J. Comp. Physiol. Psychol.* **67**:189.

Stein, L., and Wise, C. D., 1970, Behavioral pharmacology of central stimulants, in: *Principles of Psychopharmacology* (W. G. Clark and J. delGiudice, eds.), pp. 313–325, Academic Press, New York.

Stein, L., Belluzzi, J. D., and Wise, C. D., 1975, Memory enhancement by central administration of norepinephrine, *Brain Res.* **84**:329.

Stjarne, L., and Lishajko, F., 1966, Drug-induced inhibition of noradrenaline synthesis *in vitro* in bovine splenic nerve tissue, *Brit. J. Pharmacol.* **27**:398.

Sulser, F., and Bass, A. D., 1968, Pharmacodynamic and biochemical considerations on the mode of action of reserpine-like drugs, in: *Psychopharmacology: A Review of Progress 1957-1967* (D. H. Efron, ed.), pp. 1065–1075, U.S. Government Printing Office, Washington, D.C.

Sulser, F., and Sanders-Bush, E., 1971, Effect of drugs on amines in the CNS, *Ann. Rev. Pharmacol.* **11**:209.

Tagliamonte, A., Tagliamonte, P., Perez-Cruet, J., Stern, S., and Gessa, G. L., 1971, Effect of psychotropic drugs on tryptophan concentration in the rat brain, *J. Pharmacol. Exptl. Therap.* **177**:475.

Tanaka, C., Yoh, Y. J., and Takaori, S., 1972, Relationship between brain monoamine levels and Sidman avoidance behavior in rats treated with tyrosine and tryptophan hydroxylase inhibitors, *Brain Res.* **45**:153.

Thoa, N. B., Weise, V. K., and Kopin, I. J., 1972, Effect of L-dihydroxyphenylalanine on methylation of ^{3}H-norepinephrine and ^{3}H-histamine, *Biochem. Pharmacol.* **21**:2345.

Thoenen, H., and Tranzer, J. P., 1973, The pharmacology of 6-hydroxydopamine, *Ann. Rev. Pharmacol.* **13**:169.

Tyce, G. M., 1971, Effect of dihydroxyphenylalanine administered with a monoamine oxidase inhibitor on glucose metabolism in rat brain, *Biochem. Pharmacol.* **20**:2371.

Van Buskirk, R., Haycock, J. W., and McGaugh, J. L., 1973, Memory deficits following inhibition of catecholamine biosynthesis in mice, *Soc. Neurosci. Prog.,* (abstr.) p. 191.

Vasquez, B. J., deGardella, N., and Izquierdo, I., 1967, Opposite and antagonistic effects of amphetamine and catecholamines in the acquisition of a trace avoidance conditioned reflex in rats, *Med. Pharmacol. Expt.* **16**:325.

Verhave, T., 1958, The effect of methamphetamine on operant level and avoidance behavior, *J. Exptl. Anal. Behav.* **1**:207.

Weissman, A., and Koe, B. K., 1965, Behavioral effects of L-α-methyltyrosine, an inhibitor of tyrosine hydroxylase, *Life Sci.* **4**:1037.

Wise, C. D., and Stein, L., 1969, Facilitation of brain self-stimulation by central administration of norepinephrine, *Science* **163**:299.

Wise, C. D., Berger, B. D., and Stein, L., 1973, Evidence of α-noradrenergic reward receptors and serotonergic punishment receptors in the rat brain, *Biol. Psychiat.* **6**:3.

Wolthuis, O. L., 1971, Experiments with UCB 6215, a drug which enhances acquisition in rats: Its effects compared with those of metamphetamine, *European J. Pharmacol.* **16**:283.

Wright, D.C., 1974, Differentiating stimulus and storage hypotheses of state-dependent learning, *Federation Proc.* **33**:1797.

Wurtman, R. J., and Romero, J. A., 1972, Effects of levodopa on nondopaminergic brain neurons, *Neurology* **22**:72.

Wurtman, R. J., Rose, C. M., Matthysse, S., Stephenson, J., and Baldessarini, R., 1970, L-Dihydroxyphenylalanine: Effect on *S*-adenosylmethionine in brain, *Science* **169**:395.

Yen, H. C. Y., Katz, M. H., and Krop, S., 1971, Effects of some psychoactive drugs on conditioned avoidance response in aggressive mice, *Arch. Intern. Pharmacodyn.* **190**:103.

Yuwiler, A., and Olds, M. E., 1973, Catecholamines and self-stimulation behavior: Effects on brain levels after stimulation and pretreatment with DL-α-methyl-*p*-tyrosine, *Brain Res.* **50**:331.

Zis, A. P., Fibiger, H. C., and Phillips, A. G., 1974, Involvement of nigro-striatal dopaminergic neurons in the acquisition of a conditioned avoidance response (CAR), *Soc. Neurosci. Prog.* (abstr.) p. 496.

Chapter 2

Stress and Catecholamines*

Eric A. Stone

Millhauser Laboratories of the Department of Psychiatry
New York University Medical Center
New York, New York

1. INTRODUCTION

In the past two decades there has been a remarkable expansion of knowledge about the effects of stress on biogenic amines of the nervous system. The present chapter will attempt to cover recent advances in this field and will concentrate primarily on the effects of stress on tissue catecholamines.

Any discussion of stress becomes controversial owing to difficulties in defining this concept (Lazarus, 1966). Some authors in fact have urged that the term "stress" be stricken from the scientific vocabulary. However, most people still use and will continue to use the concept of stress, though ill-defined, because of the simple fact that a better concept has not been advanced.

The concept of stress arose as a result of Hans Selye's observations that a large number of damaging or potentially damaging stimuli led to similar physiological reactions, including the secretion of adrenal corticosteroids and catecholamines, gastrointestinal lesions, and glandular and cardiovascular alterations. Presumably all such stimuli (stressors) in addition to their specific effects, also induced to a greater or lesser extent a similar "nonspecific" state in the organism, i.e., the state of stress. This state then gave rise to a variety of nonspecific biochemical, physiological, and behavioral responses.

* Supported in part by Research Scientist Development Award MH-24296.

The concept of stress as used above is an intervening variable. The utility of an intervening variable lies in its ability to simplify complex empirical relationships between large numbers of variables (Miller, 1959). The apparent ability of the concept of stress to perform this function has led to its widespread use and abuse. It is informative to note, however, that some of our fundamental scientific entities, the atom, the electron, and the gene were once intervening variables.

The meaning of stress will ultimately depend on whether it is in fact one variable and also if its biological characteristics can be described to make the concept less abstract. To date no one has proven that stress is a unitary variable. On the contrary, to account for the opposite behavioral responses to enjoyable stimuli, such as athletics and sex, and aversive stimuli, such as pain, both types of which are called stressful because they produce similar autonomic responses, Bernard (1968) has suggested two states of stress, "eustress" and "dystress," respectively. As far as biological approaches are concerned, the present trend is to look for some state of CNS activity produced by widely divergent types of stressful stimulation whether they be enjoyable or aversive, or whether they actually harm the organism or simply threaten harm. This approach appears to be promising: for example one of the common effects of stressful stimuli is to increase the activity of central noradrenergic neurons. It may ultimately be possible to define stress in terms of a unitary biological response or set of responses.

It is becoming clear that an important aspect of stress is the feedback that occurs between the response and the stressor (Lazarus, 1966; Glass and Singer, 1972; Weiss, 1972). "Coping with stress," if successful, refers to a negative feedback condition in which the response, usually behavioral, decreases the intensity of the stressful stimulation. The amount of stress an individual experiences is therefore dependent on both the stressor and the effects of the response. Holmes' measure of life-change units (Holmes and Rahe, 1967) appears to be an index of this interaction and is gaining acceptance as a key variable in the production of pathological states induced by stress. Frequently, however, responses to stress are inadequate or so inappropriate and inefficient that the responses fail to decrease the initial stressor, and become stressors in and of themselves. In this case a positive feedback condition occurs in which the response adds to the stress. The positive feedback condition, or so-called "vicious cycle," is often slowed down or terminated by additional responses, such as severe mental or physical illness requiring hospitalization, drug abuse, or suicide. Several authors have suggested that what we mean by "psychological stress" is closely related to the perceived feedback between response and stressor (Weiss, 1972). The degree of psychological stress is thought to be inversely related to the perceived control over the stressor.

2. TISSUE LEVELS OF NOREPINEPHRINE AND DOPAMINE

Studies of the effects of stress on tissue concentrations of nor-epinephrine (NE) and dopamine (DA) were prompted by several findings. It had been shown that levels of urinary catecholamines (CA) are elevated during stressful situations, presumably reflecting an increased secretion of these substances. Under certain conditions of severe stress in animals, the concentration of epinephrine (E) in the adrenal gland was found to be reduced. Euler (1964), Levi (1967), and Frankhenhaeuser (1971) have reviewed these findings in detail. With the discovery by von Euler in 1948 that NE is the transmitter of peripheral sympathetic nerves, several investigators sought to obtain local estimates of sympathetic nervous activity in organs during stress by measuring their content of NE. It was implicitly assumed that the production of NE was constant and that increased sympathetic activity would lead to increased release with a subsequent fall in NE levels. This research was begun in 1951 by Bengt Hökfelt and has continued to the present. Researchers have examined virtually every organ in the body for changes in NE content following a wide variety of stressors. I have summarized much of this work in Tables I, II, and III. We now know that the basic assumptions behind this work were wrong: alterations in sympathetic activity and in NE turnover can, and frequently do take place without altering levels of the neurohormone. Nevertheless, the results of this work were fruitful: many stressors were found to alter levels of NE and other catecholamines.

As can be seen in Tables I, II, and III decreases and increases in brain NE and DA levels and peripheral organ NE content can occur after diverse treatments, such as acute and chronic foot-shock, drum stress, hemorrhage, burns, and various types of psychological stimuli. The amount of change is quite variable and seems to depend on the type and severity of stress and the species used. In addition to these factors several general patterns have emerged. Generally, NE in most brain regions decreases with acute stress but either shows no change or tends to rise if the same stress is repeated several times in periods lasting more than 24 hr, or if the stress is given chronically. The same pattern appears to hold for NE in peripheral organs although there are less data in this area. Brain DA levels appear to be more resistant to change after acute stress, but as with brain NE, these values also tend to rise after chronic stress. It has been suggested that changes in NE levels in brain precede those in peripheral organs either temporally or as the severity of the stress is increased (Bliss and Ailion, 1969). However, the data concerning this notion are still inconclusive (Hift *et al.,* 1965; Ordy *et al.,* 1966).

Table I. Effect of Stress on Brain NE Level

Acute stress[a]	%Δ	Species	Reference	Chronic stress	%Δ	Species	Reference
Foot-shock	−40	Rat	Maynert and Levi, 1964	Foot-shock	+10	Rat	Nielson and Fleming, 1968
	−55	Monkey	Ordy et al., 1966		+20	Rat	Thierry et al., 1968
	−30	Rat	Moore and Lariviere, 1964		+15	Rat	Pare and Livingston, 1970
	−40	Guinea pig[b]	Paulsen and Hess, 1963		+20	Rat	Huttunen, 1971
	−20	Rat	Bliss and Zwanziger, 1966		−5	Rat	Zigmond and Harvey, 1970
	−20	Guinea pig	Bliss and Zwanziger, 1966		−10	Rat	Weiss et al., 1970
	−10	Rat	Thierry et al., 1968				
	−30	Rat	Bliss et al., 1968				
	−25	Rat	Bliss and Ailion, 1969				
	−35	Rat	Taylor and Laverty, 1969a, 1969b				
	−30	Rat	Pare and Livingston, 1970				
	−20	Rat	Zigmond and Harvey, 1970				
	−30	Rat	Fulginiti and Orsingher, 1971				
	−10	Rat	Goldberg and Salama, 1969				
	0	Rat	Barchas and Freedman, 1963				
Treadmill	−10	Rat	Barchas and Freedman, 1963	Treadmill	0	Rat	Elo and Tirri, 1972
	−15	Rat	Gordon et al., 1966				
	−30	Rat	Stone, 1971, 1973a				
	−45	Rat	Pogodaev et al., 1972				
Swim				Swim			
15°	−20	Rat	Barchas and Freedman, 1963	0°	0	Rat	Nielson and Fleming, 1968
	−20	Rat	Ruther et al., 1966a, 1966b	19°	−5	Rat	Stern et al., 1971
	−15	Rat	Stone, 1970a, 1970b				
23°	−40	Rat	Moore and Lariviere, 1964				
37°	−40	Rat	Moore and Lariviere, 1964				
	0	Rat	Bliss and Zwanziger, 1966				
	0	Rat	Stone, 1970b				

Condition	Change	Species	Reference
Burns	−20	Rat	Stoner and Elson, 1971
Limb ischemia	−30	Rat	Stoner and Elson, 1971
Hemorrhage	−70	Rabbit	Coleman and Glaviano, 1963
	−40	Dog	Hift et al., 1965
Conflict	−20	Rat	Pare and Livingston, 1970
Conflict	+30	Rat	Pare and Livingston, 1970
Anoxia	−10	Cat	Vogt, 1954
	0	Rat	Barchas and Freedman, 1963
ESB			
Reward	−20	Rat	Bliss and Zwanziger, 1966
	−10	Rat	DiCara and Stone, 1970
	0	Rat	Arbuthnott et al., 1970
Averse	−20	Rat	Bliss and Zwanziger, 1966
Rage	−40	Cat	Reis and Gunne, 1965
	−40	Cat	Gunne and Reis, 1963
Sham rage	−35	Cat	Reis and Fuxe, 1969
	−35	Cat	Reis et al., 1967
Social separation	−55	Monkey	Ordy et al., 1966
Isolation	+15	Rat	Geller et al., 1965
	+25	Mouse	Welch and Welch, 1965
	0	Mouse	Anton et al., 1968
	−10	Mouse	Welch and Welch, 1968b
Insulin	0	Guinea pig	Paulsen and Hess, 1963
	−30	Cat	Vogt, 1954
Learning			
CAR[a]	+	Rat	Fuxe and Hanson, 1967
CAR	+5	Rat	Weiss et al., 1970
CAR	0	Rat	Fulginiti and Orsingher, 1971
CAR	−5	Rat	Hurwitz et al., 1971
Learning CAR	+20	Rat	Weiss et al., 1970
Visceral	(+−)	Rat	DiCara and Stone, 1970
Appetitive	+10	Rat	Lewy and Seiden, 1972

Table I. Continued

Acute stress[a]	%Δ	Species	Reference	Chronic stress	%Δ	Species	Reference
Drum	+15	Mouse	Goldberg and Salama, 1970	Drum	+10	Rat	Riege and Morimoto, 1970
Seizures				Seizures			
ECS[e]	−25	Rat	Breitner et al., 1964	ECS	+15	Rat	Kety et al., 1967
ECS	−5	Rat	Nielson and Fleming, 1968	ECS	0	Rat	Kato et al., 1967
ECS	+120	Rat	Kato et al., 1967				
Audio[f]	−20	Rat	Breitner et al., 1964				
Metraz.[g]	−10	Rat	Breitner et al., 1964	Metraz.	−10	Rat	Kato et al., 1967
Metraz.	+80	Rat	Kato et al., 1967				
Oxygen	−50	Rat	Buckingham et al., 1966				
Oxygen	−50	Rat	Haggendal, 1967				
Oxygen	−80	Mouse	Faiman and Heble, 1966				
Oxygen	−25	Rat	Blenkarn et al., 1969				
Restraint	−20	Rat	Carr and Moore, 1968	Restraint	0	Rat	Lamprecht et al., 1972
	−15	Guinea pig	Bliss and Zwanziger, 1966				
	−10	Rat	Lidbrink et al., 1972				
	−10	Rat	Hrubes and Benes, 1969				
	−10	Rat	Corrodi et al., 1968				
	0	Mouse	Welch and Welch, 1968c				
	+5	Rat	Moore and Lavriviere, 1964				
	+10	Mouse	Welch and Welch, 1968b				
Cold	−10	Rat	Maynert and Levi, 1964	Cold	+25	Rat	Ingenito, 1968
	0	Rat	Barchas and Freedman, 1963		+20	Rat	Bhagat, 1969
	0	Rat	Corrodi et al., 1967		+10	Rat	Ingenito and Bonnycastle, 1967
	0	Rat	Gordon et al., 1966		0	Rat	Reid et al., 1968
	0	Rat	Reid et al., 1968		0	Mouse	LeBlanc et al., 1967
	0	Rat	Simmonds, 1969				

Stressor	Change	Species	Reference
	0	Rat	Ingenito and Bonnycastle, 1967
	0	Rat	Goldberg and Salama, 1969
	+5	Rat	Goldstein and Nakajima, 1966
	+5	Rat	Corrodi et al., 1970
	+10	Mouse	Welch and Welch, 1970
Heat	−20	Rat	Corrodi et al., 1967
	−15	Rat	Ingenito and Bonnycastle, 1967
	−5	Rat	Reid et al., 1968
	0	Rat	Simmonds, 1969
	+30	Rat	Menon and Dandiya, 1969
Aggregation	−20	Mouse	Bliss and Ailion, 1969
	−	Mouse	Welch and Welch, 1965
	0	Mouse	Moore, 1964
Fighting	−20	Mouse	Welch and Welch, 1969a
	−10	Mouse	Bliss and Zwanziger, 1966
	−5	Mouse	Welch and Welch, 1968c
	+45	Mouse	Welch and Welch, 1970
	−30	Mouse	Welch and Welch, 1968e
	+10	Mouse	Welch and Welch, 1969b
	(+−)	Mouse	Eleftheriou and Church, 1968
Witness[h]	+20	Rat	Salama and Goldberg, 1973
Muricide[i]	−15	Rat	Tsuchiya et al., 1969
Sleep deprivation	−10	Rat	Stone, 1971
	−35	Rat	Tsuchiya et al., 1969
	−30	Cat	Hernandez-Peon et al., 1969
	0	Rat	Bliss, 1967
	0	Rat	Pujol et al., 1968
	+10	Rat	Schildkraut and Hartmann, 1972
	+15	Rat	Stern et al., 1971
	−50 (exhaust[j])	Rat	Bliss, 1967
Shaking	−20	Rat	Rosecrans, 1969
Formalin	−20	Rat	Carr and Moore, 1968

Table I. Continued

Acute stress[a]	%Δ	Species	Reference	Chronic stress	%Δ	Species	Reference
Ether	−30	Cat	Vogt, 1954				
Noise	−10	Rat	Moore and Lariviere, 1964				
	0	Rat	Maynert and Levi, 1964	Food, H$_2$O deprivation	0	Rat	Barchas and Freedman, 1963
				Virus encephalitis	0	Mouse	Lycke et al., 1970

[a] Less than 24 hr duration.
[b] Guinea pig.
[c] Electrical stimulation of brain.
[d] Conditioned avoidance response.
[e] Electroconvulsive shock.
[f] Audiogenic.
[g] Metrazol.
[h] Witness to a fight.
[i] Mouse-killing behavior.
[j] Exhaustion occurring during sleep deprivation.

THE
UNIVERSITY OF WINNIPEG
PORTAGE & BALMORAL
WINNIPEG, MAN.   R3B 2E9
CANADA

Bliss and his colleagues (1966), noting that several stressors that reduce brain NE have strong emotional effects, have suggested that brain NE reduction during stress is the result of emotional arousal. This hypothesis however is confounded by the fact that strong emotional stimuli such as electric foot-shock also elicit high levels of muscular exertion and widespread autonomic changes. A satisfactory dissection of the effects of emotional arousal from its peripheral components on brain NE has not yet been achieved. However, several authors have attempted to do this and their results favor Bliss' interpretation. DiCara and I trained rats that were paralyzed with curare to either speed up or slow down their heart rates (DiCara and Stone, 1970). After the 2-hr training period the animals were killed for determination of NE in various brain regions. A significant decrease of brain stem NE was observed in the rats trained to slow down their hearts, despite the fact that these rats were totally incapable of skeletal muscular activity. Significantly, the rats trained to slow their hearts under curare appeared more frightened following this procedure than rats trained to speed up their hearts. Welch and Welch (1968e) have also attempted to produce an emotionally arousing condition with little muscular exertion by placing a single mouse in a cage above a second cage containing a group of fighting mice. The mouse witnessing the fighting could not fight and was relatively inactive but remained alert throughout the 75-min experiment. The authors found that the "witness" mouse had a significantly reduced level of brain stem NE. Reis and his colleagues have also dealt with this problem in their research on the rage-response in cats. These authors have shown that attack behavior in cats produced by electrical stimulation of the amygdala or hypothalamus produces a drop in brain stem NE (Reis and Gunne, 1965). They have also found a similar neurochemical response in cats who show sham rage after supracollicular decerebration (Reis *et al.,* 1967). The latter procedure produces periodic bursts of skeletal muscle activity in the form of attack-like movements and peripheral sympathetic activation, including a rise in heart rate and blood pressure. By sectioning the spinal cord, they were able to abolish both the peripheral motor and autonomic concomitants of sham rage, however, the cats still showed the same reduction in brain stem NE.

Another factor which influences the response of brain NE levels to stress is the degree of control an animal has over the stressor. Weiss and I performed an experiment in which two rats received electric shock through tail electrodes (Weiss *et al.,* 1970). The rats' tails were wired in series so that both rats, each in a separate cage, received the identical schedule and amount of tail shock. The only difference between the animals was that one was permitted to escape or avoid the shock for both animals by turning a wheel, whereas the other rat had no control over the occurrence of the

Table II. Effect of Stress on Brain DA Level[a]

Acute stress	%Δ	Species	Reference	Chronic stress	%Δ	Species	Reference
Foot-shock	−15	Rat	Moore and Lariviere, 1964	Foot-shock	+30	Rat	Nielson and Fleming, 1968
	−15	Rat	Taylor and Laverty, 1969b				
	−5	Rat	Bliss et al., 1968				
	0	Rat	Bliss and Zwanziger, 1966				
	0	Rat	Bliss and Ailion, 1971				
	0	Mouse	Bliss and Ailion, 1971				
Swim	23°,37° +5	Rat	Moore and Lariviere, 1964	Swim 0°	+55	Rat	Nielson and Fleming, 1968
ESB							
Rage	+25	Cat	Gunne and Reis, 1963				
	+25	Cat	Reis and Gunne, 1965				
Reward	0	Rat	Arbuthnott et al., 1970				
Aggregation	0	Mouse	Bliss and Ailion, 1969	Isolation	−5	Mouse	Welch and Welch, 1968b
Noise	−5	Rat	Moore and Lariviere, 1964	CAR	+5	Rat	Geller et al., 1965
CAR	0	Rat	Fuxe and Hanson, 1967				
	0	Rat	Hurwitz et al., 1971				
Cold	−20	Rat	Corrodi et al., 1967				
	−10	Rat	Corrodi et al., 1970				
	+5	Rat	Goldstein and Nakajima, 1966				
	+20	Mouse	Welch and Welch, 1970				
	+	Rat	Lichtensteiger, 1969				

Stress		Change	Species	Reference
Heat		+10	Rat	Ingenito and Bonnycastle, 1967
		0	Rat	Corrodi et al., 1967
Seizures				
	ECS	+5	Rat	Nielson and Fleming, 1968
	ECS	+10	Rat	Engel et al., 1968
	Oxygen	(+−)	Rat	Haggendal, 1967
Drum		+60	Mouse	Goldberg and Salama, 1970
Fighting		−50	Mouse	Welch and Welch, 1969a
		+30	Mouse	Welch and Welch, 1970
Restraint				
	<2 hr	+10	Mouse	Welch and Welch, 1968b,c
	<2 hr	+10	mouse	Welch and Welch, 1970
	<2 hr	+10	Rat	Carr and Moore, 1968
	>2 hr	−10	Rat	Corrodi et al., 1968
	>2 hr	−5	Rat	Hrubes and Benes, 1969
	>2 hr	−5	Rat	Moore and Lariviere, 1964
	>2 hr	0	Mouse	Bliss and Ailion, 1971
	>2 hr	+10	Rat	Lidbrink et al., 1972
Treadmill		−10	Rat	Gordon et al., 1966
Formalin		−5	Rat	Carr and Moore, 1968

Stress	Change	Species	Reference
Heat	+10	Rat	Ingenito and Bonnycastle, 1967
Drum	+5	Rat	Riege and Morimoto, 1970
Fighting	+10	Mouse	Welch and Welch, 1969b
Sleep depriv.	+240	Cat	Hernandez-Peon et al., 1969
	0	Rat	Bliss, 1967
(Exhaust)	−55	Rat	Bliss, 1967
Viral encephal.	0	Mouse	Lycke et al., 1970

[a] See footnotes to Table I.

Table III. Effect of Stress on Peripheral Levels of NE

Stress	%Δ	Species	Reference
Heart			
Acute:			
Hemorrhage	−85	Rabbit	Coleman and Glaviano, 1963
	−40	Rabbit	Zetterstrom et al., 1964b
	−40	Dog	Zetterstrom et al., 1964b
	−35	Dog	Hift et al., 1965
Heart block	−85	Dog	Chidsey et al., 1964
	−50	Dog	Kaiser et al., 1965
Endotoxin	−50	Dog	Zetterstrom et al., 1964b
Anoxia	−50	Rat	Hokfelt, 1951
Foot-shock	−55	Monkey	Ordy et al., 1966
Social separation	−50	Monkey	Ordy et al., 1966
Seizure O_2	−65	Rat	Buckingham et al., 1966
Swim 25°	(+−)	Rat	Hökfelt, 1951
Cold	−75	Rat	Chan and Johnson, 1968
	−40	Rat	Leduc, 1961
	−15	Rat	Corrodi et al., 1967
	0	Mouse	Oliverio and Stjarne, 1965
	0	Rat	Gordon et al., 1966
	0	Rat	Corrodi et al., 1970
	+5	Rat	Goldstein and Nakajima, 1966
Heat	−25	Rat	Corrodi et al., 1967
	0	Rat	Landsberg and Axelrod, 1968
Treadmill	−5	Rat	Gordon et al., 1966
Learning	(+−)	Rat	DiCara amd Stone, 1970
Aggregation	0	Mouse	Moore, 1964
	0	Mouse	Bliss and Ailion, 1969
Chronic:			
Cold	0	Rat	Leduc, 1961
Isolation	0	Mouse	Anton et al., 1968
Starvation	+	Rat	Hokfelt, 1951
Liver			
Acute:			
Hemorrhage	−70	Rabbit	Coleman and Glaviano, 1963
	−65	Dog	Zetterstrom et al., 1964b
	−25	Dog	Hift et al., 1965
Endotoxin	−45	Dog	Zetterstrom et al., 1964b
Swim 25°	−35	Rat	Hokfelt, 1951
Cold	−25	Rat	Leduc, 1961
	−50	Rat	Chan and Johnson, 1968
Anoxia	−40	Rat	Hokfelt, 1951

Table III.   Continued

Stress	%Δ	Species	Reference
Chronic:			
Cold	+65	Rat	Leduc, 1961
Starvation	+	Rat	Hokfelt, 1951
Spleen			
Acute:			
Hemorrhage	−100	Rabbit	Coleman and Glaviano, 1963
	−65	Dog	Zetterstrom *et al.*, 1964*b*
	−70	Dog	Hift *et al.*, 1965
Endotoxin	−20	Dog	Zetterstrom *et al.*, 1964*b*
Foot-shock	−50	Rat	Bliss and Ailion, 1969
Cold	−25	Rat	Chan and Johnson, 1968
	−15	Rat	Leduc, 1961
Aggregation	0	Rat	Bliss and Ailion, 1969
Chronic:			
Cold	+55	Rat	Leduc, 1961
Skeletal Muscle			
Acute:			
Hemorrhage	−50	Rabbit	Coleman and Glaviano, 1963
Cold	−40	Rat	Leduc, 1961
Chronic:			
Cold	+25	Rat	Leduc, 1961
Kidney and Intestine			
Acute:			
Hemorrhage	−50	Dog	Hift *et al.*, 1965
Lung			
Acute:			
Hemorrhage	+20	Dog	Hift *et al.*, 1965

shock. We found that the animal that could avoid or escape showed a significant elevation of brain NE compared to a third nonshocked control rat, whereas the animal without control showed a significant reduction. Electric foot-shock when given in an unavoidable and inescapable manner reliably reduces brain NE (Table I), but when the same stressor is used in conjunction with conditioned avoidance responses it produces either no change or an increase in brain NE (Table I). The factor of control over the stressor appears to be operative here and possibly with other types of stress. Other important factors seem to be the type and severity of stress, the species studied, and the duration of stress. Cold stress, for example, has little effect on brain NE levels and in this respect does not resemble most other acute stressors. One reason may be that cold is not a strong emotional stimulus. As for species, the rat, guinea pig, cat, dog, and monkey tend to show decreases in brain NE after acute stress, but mice may respond with an increase. Welch and Welch (1970) have consistently found increases in both brain NE and DA after subjecting mice to acute restraint or fighting. These authors have also systematically varied the duration of stress and have shown that restraining mice for as little as 1.25 min will significantly elevate brain amines. As the duration of the stress increases the levels of NE and DA may fall back to normal or subnormal levels. Hökfelt (1951) found a similar biphasic effect of swimming stress on heart NE content in the rat.

The changes in amine content—at least the reduction of NE levels—during acute stress are most likely the result of increased neuronal activity. Electrical stimulation of the locus coeruleus, which contains the cell bodies of noradrenergic neurons in the brain, rapidly reduces the level of NE in the cerebral cortex of rats to about 60% of control levels in about 15 min (Korf *et al*, 1973*c*). Further stimulation keeps the level at about 60%. This is similar to the effect of electric foot-shock on whole brain NE in rats where a plateau of about 65% of control is reached after approximately 45 min of stress (Maynert and Levi, 1964). Unilateral electrolytic lesions destroying the locus coeruleus immediately prior to foot-shock in rats prevents the stress-induced reduction of NE in the cerebral cortex ipsilateral to the lesion but not on the contralateral side (Korf *et al.*, 1973*b*). Similarly, denervation of the cat spleen shortly before hemorrhage prevents the reduction of splenic NE after this stress (Zetterstrom *et al.*, 1964*a*; Dahlstrom and Zetterstrom, 1965). Furthermore, barbiturates (Maynert and Levi, 1964; Lidbrink *et al.*, 1972), benzodiazepine tranquillizers (Taylor and Laverty, 1969*b*), and meprobamate (Lidbrink *et al.*, 1972) all prevent the reduction of brain NE to foot-shock or restraint stress in rats. These drugs have in common the ability to reduce elevated neuronal activity in the CNS. An increase in the firing rate of locus coeruleus units has in fact been reported during states of increased arousal (Chu and Bloom, 1973).

Currently, there are two theories to explain stress-induced changes in CNS catecholamine levels. The first, advanced by Bliss *et al.* (1968) assumes that during stress both the synthesis and utilization of NE (or DA) are increased. A reduction in amine content occurs when the rate of synthesis is elevated but cannot keep pace with an increased rate of utilization. An increase in amine content—which Bliss has never found during acute stress—would presumably be explained by a disproportionate increase in biosynthesis. In support of these notions several investigators have found increased rates of synthesis and catabolism of NE, and less consistently DA, in the brain during a variety of acute stressors (see next section). However, Welch and Welch (1970), who have usually found increased amine levels after stress, point out that it is difficult to explain these increases on the basis of increased biosynthesis because of the commonly accepted notion that increased synthesis is secondary to increased release. One current theory of the short-term regulation of NE and DA biosynthesis employs a negative feedback mechanism in which increased amine utilization depletes a small intraneuronal amine pool whose function is to partially inhibit tyrosine hydroxylase (Weiner, 1970). Thus, during states of heightened neuronal activity when more of the amine is released, the small pool is depleted and tyrosine hydroxylase is disinhibited, thereby leading to a rise in synthesis. When the elevated synthesis rate replenishes the small pool, tyrosine hydroxylase is inhibited and synthesis is slowed. If the foregoing negative feedback system is an accurate one, it should not permit levels of NE or DA to rise above normal levels. Yet these amines do increase substantially after inhibition of monoamine oxidase (MAO) or after certain types of acute stress. Therefore, in order to explain stress-induced elevations of brain NE or DA on the basis of increased biosynthesis one must assume either (i) that the negative feedback system is not as accurate as has been suggested and that considerable increases in amine levels can occur before synthesis is totally inhibited, or (ii) that the accelerated synthesis during stress is independent of amine level or utilization and is due to some other factor associated with nerve impulses.

The second theory, advanced by Welch and Welch (1970), states that under resting, nonstressful conditions the rate of ongoing synthesis greatly exceeds the rate of neuronally released CA with the excess amine being constantly removed through oxidative deamination by intraneuronal MAO. During stress there is a rapid, temporary, and partial reduction in MAO activity as a result of increased nerve impulses. The inhibition of MAO makes more amine available for release without altering the rate of synthesis. When the amount of catecholamine saved by inhibition of MAO is less than the increase in release, one observes a decreased level of the neurohormone. An increased level of amine after stress occurs when the amount saved by inhibition of MAO exceeds the amount released. According to the above authors the increased accumulation of labeled NE and DA from labeled tyrosine observed by other investigators during stress or nerve stimulation is the result of diminished MAO activity and not the result of increased biosynthesis.

Although this theory can account for the rapid stress-induced increases in brain NE and DA, it is not supported by metabolic studies of brain amines during stress. If MAO activity were partially inhibited during stress, one would expect to find less deaminated metabolites of NE and DA. The available evidence is not consistent with this prediction. 3-Methoxy-4-hydroxyphenylglycol sulfate (MOPEG-SO$_4$) is the major O-methylated deaminated metabolite of rat brain NE (Schanberg et $al.$, 1968). Rats stressed by electric foot-shock (Korf et $al.$, 1973b) or cold (Meek and Neff,

1973*a*) show elevated levels of endogenous MOPEG-SO$_4$ in their brains. Greater amounts of ^{3}H-*O*-methylated deaminated metabolites (most of which in the rat brain is ^{3}H-MOPEG-SO$_4$) have been found in the brains of rats previously labeled intracerebrally with ^{3}H-NE or ^{3}H-DA and then subjected to foot-shock (Bliss *et al.*, 1968), foot-shock with shaking stress (Ladisich and Baumann, 1971) or exhaustive running stress (Stone, 1973*a*). The ^{3}H-deaminated catechol metabolites of ^{3}H-NE, consisting of 3,4-dihydroxyphenylglycol (DOPEG) and 3,4-dihydroxymandelic acid (DOMA), do not appear to be affected by foot-shock stress (Bliss *et al.*, 1968: Ladisich and Baumann, 1971). Recently, Sugden and Eccleston (1971), Meek and Neff (1973*b*), and our group (Stone, 1973*b*) have identified conjugated DOPEG to be the major deaminated catechol metabolite of exogenous NE in rat brain. In a recent experiment we failed to find a change in levels of conjugated DOPEG after acute running stress in rats.* There has not been sufficient study of the various metabolites of brain DA during acute stress. However, Bliss and Ailion (1971) have reported that levels of homovanillic acid (HVA), the major *O*-methylated deaminated metabolite of DA, are elevated in mice and rats after footshock, restraint, swimming stress, or psychosocial stimulation. Engel *et al.* (1968) has also reported an increase in rat brain HVA after a single electroconvulsive shock (ECS). From the above studies it would appear that total MAO activity, rather than being decreased, may be somewhat increased during stress. In agreement with this, Maynert and Levi (1964) and Bliss *et al.* (1968) found that pharmacological inhibition of MAO prevents the footshock-induced reduction of rat brain NE. Pryor *et al.* (1972) have reported increases in the *in vitro* MAO activity of rat brain after chronic ECS treatments. The latter finding might reflect an adaptation to increased use of MAO during stress.

One of the weak points of Welch and Welch's theory is that it is not sufficiently specific to predict the effect of stress on stores of brain amines labeled with their radioactive isotopes. For example, it has been firmly established that foot-shock stress produces an increased rate of disappearance of tritiated NE (^{3}H-NE) from the rat's brain. Although the degree of increased loss may be to some extent dependent on which compartment of endogenous NE the ^{3}H-NE is located in, the change with stress is always in the direction of an increased loss, and this occurs regardless of whether or not total NE levels decrease or whether the ^{3}H-NE is exogenous or has been synthesized endogenously from ^{3}H-DA or ^{3}H-tyrosine (Thierry *et al.*, 1968, 1971; Bliss *et al.*, 1968; Taylor and Laverty, 1969*a*). The MAO inhibition theory can predict either no change, an increase, or a decrease in the rate of disappearance of ^{3}H-NE during stress, depending on what is assumed about

---

* This compound does increase after foot-shock. See note following references.

the location and specific radioactivity (S.A.) of the amine. If it is assumed that ^{3}H-NE in the brain is homogeneously mixed with all pools of endogenous NE, then during stress the NE protected from deamination by a reduced MAO activity and now ready for release will have the same S.A. as the NE normally released. Under these conditions, stressed and control rats should lose ^{3}H-NE at identical rates. On the other hand, if the S.A. of the NE conserved for release is greater than that of the normally released NE, the result should be a greater loss of ^{3}H-NE in the stressed animals. However, if the S.A. of the conserved NE is less than that of the normally released NE, the result would be a retarded loss of the labeled amine during stress.

We know very little about the changes in the subcellular distribution of catecholamines that underlie changes in total levels after stress. This area will probably be a fruitful one for future research. It is not known whether the reduction of brain NE observed after acute stress represents less NE per granulated vesicle, the loss of some NE storing vesicles, or the loss of NE from nonvesicular sites. It is unlikely that stress produces a loss of storage vesicles because the rate of recovery of NE levels in the brain after stress is much faster (1 to 2 hr) than the time required for synthesis and axonal transport of newly formed vesicles (Dahlstrom and Haggendal 1967). Levi and Maynert (1964) have similarly failed to find an altered distribution of particle bound and "free" NE in rat brain homogenates after footshock-induced depletion. In some of our recent experiments we have examined the ability of the rat hypothalamus, partially depleted of NE after exhaustive running stress, to take up and store intraventricularly injected ^{3}H-NE or ^{3}H-NE synthesized endogenously from injected ^{3}H-DA (Stone, 1973b). We found that the stressed rat's hypothalamus is equally efficient in accumulating exogenous ^{3}H-NE as the hypothalamus of the nonstressed control rat. In fact, the stressed animals accumulated 50% more ^{3}H-NE derived from injected ^{3}H-DA than their nonstressed counterparts. Thus despite the finding of others (Kirshner and Viveros, 1972) that catecholamine release is accompanied by losses in ATP and chromogranins, compounds necessary for NE storage, we could detect no defect in the storage ability of stress-depleted hypothalamic nerve endings. Other investigators (Smith *et al.*, 1970) have shown that the neuronal release of NE is accompanied by a release of dopamine-β-hydroxylase (DβH), presumably through a process of exocytosis during which the soluble contents of the NE storage vesicles are exuded through the cell membrane into the synaptic cleft. However, as noted above, in our experiments the stressed rats who presumably had less DβH were apparently more efficient than controls in converting ^{3}H-DA to ^{3}H-NE. We have concluded therefore that stress-depleted NE terminals in the CNS retain all the biochemical apparatus necessary for the synthesis and storage of NE. We believe that after acute stress there is less NE per vesicle and more available sites for binding NE within the vesicle but that these sites are preferentially replenished with newly synthesized NE and not through an increased uptake and binding of extraneuronal NE. A similar conclusion about the refilling of stores of brain NE depleted by electrical stimulation of the locus coeruleus was reached by Korf et al. (1973c).

Although uptake and binding of extraneuronal NE appear to play important roles in the maintenance of stores of NE in some peripheral sympathetic nerves (Chang and Chieuh, 1968; Bhatnagar and Moore, 1971; Bhagat and Friedman, 1969), it is still unclear to what extent these factors serve to maintain the bulk of stored NE in the brain during states of increased release (Rosecrans, 1969; Thierry et al., 1971; Henley et al, 1973). Thierry et al. (1971) have reported that in the rat brain newly taken up NE initially enters a labile pool from which most of it is released rather than stored. The tendency to release rather than store newly taken up NE may explain why uptake and binding do not appear to play important roles in the maintenance of stores of brain NE. Moreover, this characteristic of central noradrenergic neurons may be one factor that increases their susceptibility to lose significant amounts of stored NE during stress. If the above interpretation is correct and newly synthesized NE replenishes stress-depleted stores of brain NE, it would be important to determine how this process affects the release of NE after acute stress, since several investigators have demonstrated that the pool of NE that is released by nerve impulses—the so-called "functional pool"—is filled predominantly with newly synthesized NE (Kopin et al., 1968; Thierry et al., 1971).

A subcellular analysis of the increases in NE and DA levels after acute stress presents problems similar to those discussed above for reduced amine levels. The increased levels of amines observed after chronic or repeated stress, however, appear to represent more complex phenomena involving the induction of enzymes in the biosynthesis and metabolism of catecholamines (see next section). There is some indirect evidence suggesting that chronic stress induces morphological changes in central CA-containing neurons. Several authors have found that chronic stress increases the uptake of ^{3}H-NE in the brain (Thierry et al., 1968; Pujol et al., 1968; Bhagat, 1969) while others have failed to confirm this finding or have found decreases (Ladisich et al., 1969; Kety et al., 1967; Schildkraut and Hartmann, 1972). Henley et al. (1973) has recently examined the kinetics of ^{3}H-NE uptake in homogenates from brains of mice subjected to chronic fighting stress. These authors report an increased apparent K_m and V_{max} which they interpret respectively as a decreased affinity of individual uptake sites for NE and an increase in the total number of uptake sites. They speculate that the increase in uptake sites may be due either to ". . . de novo synthesis of new terminal branches in the catecholamine neurons of the cerebral cortex or to a physical change in the carrier protein. . . ." Bjorklund, Stenevi, and their co-workers have shown that axonal sprouting occurs in monoaminergic neurons in the rat brain after lesions or implants (Stenevi, 1971). These results suggest the intriguing hypothesis that chronic stress may induce axonal sprouting in central noradrenergic or dopaminergic neurons.

3. TURNOVER

The rate of turnover of NE or DA is equal to the synthesis or utilization of the amine when the latter two processes are at equal rates, i.e., under steady state conditions. NE turnover is considerably increased during nerve stimulation even though total levels of the amine do not change (Weiner, 1970; Arbuthnott et al., 1970). For this reason turnover is a more sensitive index of neuronal activity than is total amine content and has replaced the latter measure in studies of stress. Rates of NE and DA turnover have been estimated with a variety of techniques: an increased turnover of the CA in an organ may be reflected by an increase in (i) the loss of endogenous NE or DA after pharmacological inhibition of biosynthesis using α-methyltyrosine (AMT) and disulfiram or FLA-63 to block the enzymes tyrosine hydroxylase and dopamine-hydroxylase, respectively (Brodie et al., 1966; Goldstein and Nakajima, 1967; Corrodi et al., 1970); (ii) the loss of radioactive NE or DA administered exogenously (Montanari et al., 1963; Iversen and Glowinski, 1966) or derived endogenously from labeled precursor tyrosine, dopa, or DA (Udenfriend and Zaltzman-Nirenberg, 1963; Iversen and Glowinski, 1966); (iii) the level of major metabolites such as MOPEG-SO$_4$ for NE (Meek and Neff, 1973a) or homovanillic acid (HVA) for DA (Hornykiewicz, 1966); (iv) the rise in NE or DA levels after inhibition of MAO (Green and Erickson, 1960; Neff and Costa, 1968); (v) the rate of formation of labeled NE and DA from labeled tyrosine (Roth et al., 1966; Bapna et al., 1971); and (vi) the capture of released NE with a perfusion device such as the push-pull cannula (Stein and Wise, 1969). Although the use of such diverse methods makes comparisons between experiments difficult, it also avoids misinterpretations stemming from artifacts peculiar to any single technique.

Using these techniques most workers have found that acute stressors increase NE turnover in the brain and periphery (see Tables IV and VII). The turnover of brain DA may also increase with acute stress (Table V) but this response is less reliable. Unfortunately, the data on increased NE turnover during stress is still largely qualitative (i.e., increase, decrease, or no change; see Tables IV and VII) because most workers have either not

Table IV.   Effect of Stress on Brain NE Turnover[a]

Stress	Change	Species	Method	Reference
Acute				
Foot-shock	+	Rat	Loss of NE after AMT	Korf *et al.*, 1973*b*
	+	Rat	Loss of NE after AMT	Bliss *et al.*, 1968
	+	Rat	Loss of ^{3}H-NE	Bliss *et al.*, 1968
	+	Rat	Loss of ^{3}H-NE	Thierry *et al.*, 1968
	+	Rat	Loss of ^{3}H-NE	Thierry *et al.*, 1971
	+	Rat	Loss of ^{3}H-NE	Ladisich and Baumann, 1971
	+	Rat	Loss of ^{3}H-NE from ^{3}H-tyrosine	Thierry *et al.*, 1971
	+	Rat	Loss of ^{3}H-NE from ^{3}H-DA	Bliss *et al.*, 1968
	+	Rat	Loss of ^{3}H-NE from ^{3}H-DA	Thierry *et al.*, 1968
	+	Rat	Loss of ^{3}H-NE from ^{3}H-DA	Thierry *et al.*, 1971
	+	Rat	Loss of ^{3}H-NE from ^{3}H-DA	Taylor and Laverty, 1969*a*,*b*
	+60%	Rat	Increased MOPEG-SO$_4$	Korf *et al.*, 1973*b*
Cold	+	Rat	Loss of NE after AMT	Gordon *et al.*, 1966
	+70%	Rat	Loss of NE after AMT	Reid *et al.*, 1968
	0	Rat	Loss of NE after AMT	Corrodi *et al.*, 1967
	+75%	Rat	Loss of NE after disulfiram	Goldstein and Nakajima, 1966
	0	Rat	Loss of NE after FLA-63	Corrodi *et al.*, 1970
	+150%	Rat	Loss of ^{3}H-NE	Simmonds, 1969, 1971
	0	Mouse	Loss of ^{3}H-NE from ^{3}H-dopa	Draskoczy *et al.*, 1966
	+20%	Rat	Increased MOPEG-SO$_4$	Meek and Neff, 1973*a*
Restraint	+	Rat	Loss of NE after AMT	Corrodi *et al.*, 1968
	(+−)	Mouse	Loss of NE after AMT	Welch and Welch, 1968*b*
	+	Rat	Loss of NE after AMT	Lidbrink *et al.*, 1972

Table IV.   Continued

Stress	Change	Species	Method	Reference
	+	Rat	Loss of NE after AMT	Carr and Moore, 1968
Heat	+	Rat	Loss of NE after AMT	Corrodi et al., 1967
	+90%	Rat	Loss of NE after AMT	Reid et al., 1968
	+140%	Rat	Loss of ^{3}H-NE	Simmonds, 1969
	+110%	Rat	Loss of NE from ^{3}H-dopa	Reid et al., 1968
Treadmill	+	Rat	Loss of NE after AMT	Gordon et al., 1966
	+60%	Rat	Loss of ^{3}H-NE	Stone, 1973a
	+20%	Rat	Increased ^{3}H-MOPEG-SO$_4$ from ^{3}H-NE	Stone, 1973b
	+130%	Rat	Increased ^{14}C-NE from ^{14}C-tyrosine	Gordon et al., 1966
Fighting	0	Mouse	Loss of NE after AMT	Welch and Welch, 1968d
Aggregation	+	Mouse	Loss of NE after AMT	Bliss and Ailion, 1969
	+110%	Mouse	increase of NE after MAOI[b]	Bliss and Ailion, 1969
Shaking	+	Rat	Loss of NE after AMT	Rosecrans, 1969
ESC	+	Rat	Loss of ^{3}H-NE	Schildkraut et al., 1971
Burns	+	Rat	Loss of NE after AMT	Stoner and Elson, 1971
Limb ischemia	+	Rat	Loss of NE after AMT	Stoner and Elson, 1971
ESB reward	+	Rat	Loss of NE after AMT	Arbuthnott et al., 1970
	+	Rat	Push-pull with ^{3}H-NE	Stein and Wise, 1969
Handling	+	Rat	Push-pull with ^{3}H-NE	Winson and Gerlach, 1971
Formalin	+	Rat	Loss of NE after AMT	Carr and Moore, 1968
Learning CAR	+	Rat	Loss of NE after AMT	Fuxe and Hanson, 1967

Table IV.   Continued

Stress	Change	Species	Method	Reference
CAR	+	Rat	Loss of NE after disulfiram	Hurwitz et al., 1971
CAR	+80%	Rat	Increased^{14}C-NE from ^{14}C-tyrosine	Fulginiti and Orsingher, 1971
Extinction	+	Rat	Push-pull with ^{3}H-NE	Sparber and Tilson, 1972
Swim 15°	−	Rat	Loss of NE after AMT	Stone, 1970a
	−	Rat	Loss of ^{3}H-NE	Stone, 1970b
Chronic				
Foot-shock	+	Rat	Loss of ^{3}H-NE	Thierry et al., 1968
Treadmill	+	Rat	Increase of NE after MAOI	Elo and Tirri, 1972
Cold	+10%	Rat	Loss of NE after AMT	Reid et al., 1968
	+75%	Rat	Loss of NE after AMT	Bhagat, 1969
Sleep deprivation	+70%	Rat	Loss of ^{3}H-NE	Pujol et al., 1968
	+	Rat	Loss of ^{3}H-NE	Mark et al., 1972
	+	Rat	Loss of ^{3}H-NE	Schildkraut and Hartmann, 1972
	+	Rat	Increase of NE after MAOI	Stern et al., 1971
Viral encephalitis	+	Mouse	Increase of NE after MAOI	Lycke et al., 1970
Learning (appetitive)	+	Rat	Loss of ^{3}H-NE	Lewy and Seiden, 1972
Isolation	−	Mouse	Loss of NE after AMT	Welch and Welch, 1968a

[a] See footnotes to Table I.
[b] Inhibition of monoamine oxidase.

computed rates of turnover or have not used appropriate experimental designs to permit this. Also, a number of authors have used stressors that alter amine levels. In a strict sense the term "turnover" has no meaning when amine levels change because synthesis is not equal to utilization. When this occurs the two processes should be measured independently.

The increased turnover of NE during stress is thought to reflect an increased rate of nerve impulses in noradrenergic neurons. Most of the aforementioned measures of turnover have been shown to increase during electrical stimulation of noradrenergic neurons, and, the stress-induced

Table V. Effect of Stress on Brain DA Turnover[a]

Stress	Change	Species	Method	Reference
Acute				
Foot-shock	+	Rat	Loss of DA after AMT	Bliss et al., 1968
	+	Rat	Loss of DA after AMT	Bliss and Ailion, 1971
	+	Mouse	Loss of DA after AMT	Bliss and Ailion, 1971
	0	Rat	Loss of ^{3}H-DA	Thierry et al., 1968
	0	Rat	Loss of ^{3}H-DA	Bliss et al., 1968
	+	Rat	Loss of ^{3}H-DA	Taylor and Laverty, 1969a
	+	Rat	Loss of ^{3}H-DA	Thierry et al., 1971
	+	Rat	Loss of ^{3}H-DA from ^{3}H-tyrosine	Thierry et al., 1971
	+75%	Rat	Increased HVA	Bliss and Ailion, 1971
	+65%	Mouse	Increased HVA	Bliss and Ailion, 1971
Restraint	0	Rat	Loss of DA after AMT	Corrodi et al., 1968
	(+−)	Mouse	Loss of DA after AMT	Welch and Welch, 1968b
	0	Rat	Loss of DA after AMT	Carr and Moore, 1968
	−	Rat	Loss of DA after AMT	Lidbrink et al., 1972
	+75%	Rat	Increased HVA	Bliss and Ailion, 1971
	+35%	Mouse	Increased HVA	Bliss and Ailion, 1971
Treadmill	+20%	Rat	Increased ^{14}C-DA from ^{14}C-tyrosine	Gordon et al., 1966
Cold	0	Rat	Loss of DA after AMT	Reid et al., 1968
	0	Rat	Loss of DA after AMT	Corrodi et al., 1967
Heat	0	Rat	Loss of DA after AMT	Corrodi et al., 1967
	(?+)[b]	Rat	Loss of ^{3}H-DA from ^{3}H-dopa	Reid et al., 1968
Aggregation	0	Mouse	Loss of DA after AMT	Bliss and Ailion, 1969
	+40%	Mouse	Increased HVA	Bliss and Ailion, 1971
Swim 37°	+25%	Mouse	Increased HVA	Bliss and Ailion, 1971
Formalin	0	Rat	Loss of DA after AMT	Carr and Moore, 1968
Fighting	0	Mouse	Loss of DA after AMT	Welch and Welch, 1968d

Table V.   Continued

Stress	Change	Species	Method	Reference
Learning CAR	0	Rat	Loss of DA after AMT	Fuxe and Hanson, 1967
ECS	+55%	Rat	Increased HVA	Engel et al., 1968
	0	Dog	Increased HVA	Cooper et al., 1968
ESB reward	+	Rat	Loss of DA after AMT	Arbuthnott et al., 1970
Chronic				
Isolation	−	Mouse	Loss of DA after AMT	Welch and Welch, 1968a
Aggregation	+20%	Mouse	Increased HVA	Bliss and Ailion, 1971
ECS	+25%	Dog	Increased HVA	Cooper et al., 1968
Viral encephalitis	+300	Mouse	Increased HVA	Lycke et al., 1970

[a] See footnote for Table I.
[b] Insufficient data.

increase of NE turnover can be blocked by drugs that inhibit neuronal activity (Taylor and Laverty, 1969b; Lidbrink et al., 1972) or by lesions that destroy noradrenergic cell bodies (Korf et al., 1973b). Other factors such as storage, metabolism, reuptake, and blood flow, which may alter turnover independently of nerve impulse rate, do not appear to play major roles in increasing NE turnover during stress (Rubenson, 1969; Stone 1973a,b). It should be emphasized, however, that only tentative conclusions about impulse rate can be drawn from measures of turnover rate because the processes by which nerve impulses liberate NE are not yet fully understood. As will be discussed below, these problems become quite apparent when there is a change in the steady state level of the amine.

It is difficult at present to determine which measure of turnover is most sensitive to changes in neuronal activity, since there are no experiments comparing all of the above methods. However, as discussed previously, several investigators have shown that the small functional pool of NE is comprised mainly of newly synthesized NE. Thierry et al. (1971) have reported that ^{3}H-NE which enters this pool in the rat brain either via synthesis from labeled precursors or via the initial uptake of the exogenous amine is more rapidly released by foot-shock stress than is ^{3}H-NE located in storage pools. However, these findings have not been corroborated by Schildkraut et al. (1971), who found that a single electroconvulsive shock releases as much or more ^{3}H-NE from storage pools as from the functional pool in the rat brain.

Table VI. Persistent Effects of Stress on Brain NE and DA Turnover[a]

Stress	Change	Duration post-stress	Species	Method	Reference
Norepinephrine					
Acute					
Foot-shock	+	3 hr	Rat	Loss of NE after AMT	Goldberg and Salama, 1969
	+35%	0.25 hr	Rat	Increased ^{3}H-NE from ^{3}H-tyrosine (in vitro)	Thierry et al., 1971
Drum	+	3 hr	Rat	Loss of NE after AMT	Goldberg and Salama, 1969
	0	3 hr	Mouse	Loss of NE after AMT	Goldberg and Salama, 1970, 1972
Treadmill	+60%	6 hr	Rat	Loss of NE after AMT	Stone, 1973a
	+60%	6 hr	Rat	Loss of ^{3}H-NE	Stone, 1971, 1973a
Muricide	+95	24 hr	Rat	Loss of ^{3}H-NE	Salama and Goldberg, 1973
Swim 15°	–	2 hr	Rat	Loss of NE after AMT	Stone, 1970b
	–	2 hr	Rat	Loss of ^{3}H-NE	Stone, 1970a
Chronic					
Prenatal foot-shock	+	45 days	Rat	Loss of ^{3}H-NE	Huttunen, 1971
ECS	+50%	24 hr	Rat	Loss of ^{3}H-NE	Kety et al., 1967
ECS	+	24 hr	Rat	Loss of ^{3}H-NE	Ladisich et al., 1969
Drum	0	3 hr	Mouse	Loss of NE after AMT	Goldberg and Salama, 1972
Swim 0°	+	? hr[b]	Rat	Increase of NE after MAOI	Stern et al., 1971
Dopamine					
Acute					
Swim 15°	–	2 hr	Rat	Loss of DA after AMT	Stone, 1970b
Drum	0	3 hr	Mouse	Loss of DA after AMT	Goldberg and Salama, 1972
Chronic					
Drum	+115%	3 hr	Mouse	Loss of DA after AMT	Goldberg and Salama, 1972

[a] See footnotes to Table I.
[b] Insufficient data.

Table VII. Effect of Stress on Turnover of NE in Peripheral Organs

Stress	Change	Species	Method	Reference
Heart				
Acute				
Foot-shock	+	Rat	Loss of ^{3}H-NE	Rubenson, 1969
Cold	+50%	Mouse	Loss of ^{3}H-NE	Oliverio and Stjärne, 1965
	+	Rat	Loss of NE after AMT	Gordon et al., 1966
	+	Rat	Loss of NE after disulfiram	Goldstein and Nakajima, 1966
	+100%	Mouse	Loss of ^{3}H-NE from ^{3}H-dopa	Draskoczy et al., 1966
	+	Rat	Loss of NE after AMT	Corrodi et al., 1967
	+	Rat	Loss of ^{3}H-NE	Rubenson, 1969
	+300%	Rat	Loss of ^{3}H-NE	Bhagat and Friedman, 1969
	+	Rat	Loss of NE after FLA-63	Corrodi et al., 1970
Restraint	+	Rat	Loss of ^{3}H-NE	Rubenson, 1969
Treadmill	+	Rat	Loss of NE after AMT	Gordon et al., 1966
	+70%	Rat	Increased ^{14}C-NE from ^{14}C-tyrosine	Gordon et al., 1966
Learning (visceral)	(+−)	Rat	Loss of ^{3}H-NE	DiCara and Stone, 1970
Aggregation	0	Mouse	Loss of NE after AMT	Bliss and Ailion, 1969
Heat	−	Rat	Loss of NE after AMT	Corrodi et al., 1967
	−	Rat	Loss of ^{3}H-NE	Landsberg and Axelrod, 1968

Spleen

Acute

Treadmill	+140%	Rat	Increased ^{14}C-NE from ^{14}C-tyrosine	Gordon et al., 1966
Foot-shock	0	Rat	Loss of ^{3}H-NE	Rubenson, 1969
Cold	0	Rat	Loss of ^{3}H-NE	Rubenson, 1969
Restraint	0	Rat	Loss of ^{3}H-NE	Rubenson, 1969
Aggregation	0	Mouse	Loss of NE after AMT	Bliss and Ailion, 1969

Skeletal Muscle

Acute

Foot-shock	+	Rat	Loss of ^{3}H-NE	Rubenson, 1969
Cold	0	Rat	Loss of ^{3}H-NE	Rubenson, 1969
Restraint	0	Rat	Loss of ^{3}H-NE	Rubenson, 1969

Kidney

Acute

Foot-shock	+	Rat	Loss of ^{3}H-NE	Rubenson, 1969
Restraint	+	Rat	Loss of ^{3}H-NE	Rubenson, 1969

Brown Fat

Acute

Cold	+100%	Mouse	Loss of ^{3}H-NE from ^{3}H-dopa	Draskoczy et al., 1966

Salivary Gland

Acute

Cold	0	Rat	Loss of ^{3}H-NE	Rubenson, 1969

Skin

Acute

Cold	+	Rat	Loss of ^{3}H-NE	Rubenson, 1969

An interesting characteristic of the noradrenergic response to stress is the fact that the increased turnover apparently does not habituate to chronic stress (Table IV). In fact it can become greater when animals are exposed to stress for longer periods of time (Thierry *et al.,* 1968). Since chronic stress elevates levels of the enzymes tyrosine hydroxylase (Musacchio *et al.,* 1969), dopamine-β-hydroxylase (Roffman *et al.,* 1973), phenylethanolamine-*N*-methyltransferase (Axelrod *et al.,* 1970), and MAO (Pryor *et al.,* 1972) in the periphery and to a lesser extent in the CNS, it has been suggested that noradrenergic neurons adapt to prolonged stimulation by increasing the synthesis of biosynthetic and catabolic enzymes so as to facilitate the synthesis, release, and destruction of the amine during subsequent exposure to stress (Thoenen, 1970). As discussed previously, chronic stress may also elevate levels of NE and produce a long-lasting reduction in the reuptake of NE. The latter process is responsible for inactivation of a major fraction of released NE; a reduction in reuptake would be adaptive in the above sense, since it would facilitate the action of NE upon receptors.

From the above it appears that noradrenergic neurons are particularly susceptible to long-term biochemical and physiological changes induced by stress. This notion is further supported by experiments in which the turnover of NE has been measured after stress is terminated (Table VI). Once chronic stress is terminated, the increase in brain NE turnover persists for at least one day and possibly for as long as 45 days. This is presumably due to the persistence of high levels of biosynthetic enzymes (Lamprecht *et al.,* 1972). Acute stress also produces a persistent increase in NE turnover. We have found that hypothalamic NE turnover remains elevated in rats for at least 6 hr after termination of 3 hr of running stress (Stone, 1971; 1973*a*). Others have found that acute foot-shock, drum stress, or muricide can lead to persistent increases in brain NE turnover lasting 3 to 24 hr post-stress (Goldberg and Salama, 1969; Salama and Goldberg, 1973). These changes presumably reflect a persistent post-stress elevation in noradrenergic neuronal activity since the stressors are of too short duration for significant enzyme induction to occur (Mueller *et al.,* 1969). However, the aftereffects of a single acute stress may play a role in the induction of enzymes seen after repeated daily stress, since the aftereffect would serve to maintain heightened levels of neuronal activity in the intervals between each daily stress.

Difficulties in interpretation of the physiological meaning of turnover have arisen in experiments where levels of amines are altered by stress. Goldberg and Salama (1972) found that acute drum stress produced an increased level of brain DA but did not change the rate-constant of DA loss after administration of AMT. The decay curve of brain DA after synthesis inhibition with AMT is exponential with time, indicating that the amount of

DA lost is a proportion of the total amount of remaining DA (Costa and Neff, 1966). In the above experiment, therefore, the amount of DA lost was somewhat greater in the stressed group because of the difference in initial levels, even though the stressed and control groups had the same rate constant. If one assumes that the rate constant of DA loss after AMT is directly related to the rate of nerve impulse activity, then one must conclude that both groups had the same rate of neuronal activity but that the stressed animals lost a greater amount of DA per nerve impulse. This odd conclusion raises a number of fundamental questions, as yet unsettled, concerning the relationship between rates of turnover and the release and loss of monoamines induced by nerve impulses (Smith and Winkler, 1972). Suffice it to say that turnover rate is only an indirect measure of nerve impulse rate and, as such, must eventually be corroborated with other techniques such as direct electrophysiological recording of neuronal activity.

4. METABOLITES

Studies of the effects of stress on the metabolism of NE and DA have been helpful in measuring turnover, as discussed previously, and also in clarifying the manner in which stress increases the utilization of amines. One of the current problems facing investigators is which metabolite, if any, most accurately reflects released NE in the brain. This problem discussed below has not yet been resolved.

Levels of brain normetanephrine (NM) have been thought to be an index of neuronally released NE because catechol-O-methyltransferease is largely located outside the nerve terminal (Axelrod, 1966). NM formation should increase with stress if stress increases neuronal activity. This has been tested, but the results are not consistent. Schildkraut et al. (1971) and Thierry et al. (1968) have found that ECS or foot-shock, both of which increase brain NE turnover, produce increases in the levels of ^{3}H-NM from ^{3}H-NE in the rat brain. However, using similar types of stress Ladisich et al. (1969) and Bliss et al. (1968) have not consistently found increased NM formation, but rather have found increased levels of O-methylated deaminated metabolites. This discrepancy may be explained by the finding of Schildkraut et al. (1971) that NM levels increase during stress only when ^{3}H-NE is newly taken up and is in labile pools of NE. However, another and possibly more important factor is that NM is rapidly converted to MOPEG-SO$_4$ in the rat brain (Schanberg et al., 1968b). The fact that NM is an intermediate rather than an end product of brain NE metabolism makes the latter metabolite a less reliable index of neuronal activity.

Recent attention has been focused on MOPEG-SO$_4$, the major *O*-methylated deaminated metabolite of NE in the rat brain. Several investigators have found increases in MOPEG-SO$_4$ in rat brain after electrical stimulation of the locus coeruleus (Walter and Eccleston, 1972; Korf *et al.*, 1973*a*) or after acute stress (Meek and Neff, 1973*a*; Stone, 1973*b*, Korf *et*

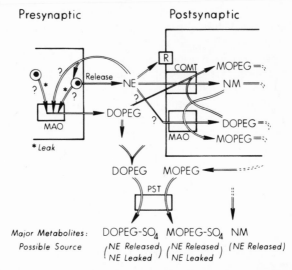

Figure 1. Schematic representation of a central noradrenergic synapse illustrating possible routes of formation of normetanephrine (NM) and the sulfate esters of dihydroxyphenylglycol (DOPEG) and methoxyhydroxyphenylglycol (MOPEG). After release from its storage vesicle by nerve impulses NE may either be recaptured by the presynaptic terminal, may activate its receptor (R), form NM via the action of catechol-*O*-methyltransferase (COMT), or be deaminated to DOPEG by monoamine oxidase (MAO) in the postsynaptic cell. With regard to postsynaptic metabolism, the resulting NM and DOPEG may be further deaminated and *O*-methylated, respectively, to form MOPEG. The latter is subsequently conjugated with sulfate by phenolsulfotransferase (PST). The location of PST is not presently known. DOPEG may be conjugated similarly to DOPEG-SO$_4$ which would prevent its conversion to MOPEG. NE that is presynaptically metabolized derives from recaptured and stored NE. The fate of NE after reuptake is uncertain: it may be bound and protected from metabolism, released again, or deaminated prior to binding or release by presynaptic MAO to form DOPEG. DOPEG may also be formed from NE that leaks from storage vesicles into the presynaptic cytoplasm and is acted upon by MAO. DOPEG formed presynaptically may diffuse into the synapse and be *O*-methylated or conjugated to form either MOPEG or DOPEG-SO$_4$, respectively. The question marks indicate metabolic steps which would cause released NE to appear as DOPEG-SO$_4$ and leaked NE as MOPEG-SO$_4$. These are the deamination and conjugation of released NE to form DOPEG-SO$_4$ either postsynaptically or presynaptically after reuptake and binding, and the *O*-methylation and conjugation of DOPEG arising from presynaptically leaked NE to form MOPEG-SO$_4$. If these pathways are shown to be of minor significance, it would be possible to conclude that MOPEG-SO$_4$ derives mainly from released NE while DOPEG-SO$_4$ results from NE deaminated presynaptically prior to release.

al., 1973*b*). However, the use of MOPEG-SO$_4$ as an index of released NE is also problematic. First, there seems to be a wide species variation in the conjugation of MOPEG in the brain (Schanberg *et al.*, 1968*a*), and, in some species, such as dogs, 3-methyoxy-4-hydroxymandelic acid (VMA) may be the predominant metabolite of brain NE (Chase *et al.*, 1971). Second, a consideration of the manner and possible sites of inactivation and metabolism of NE at the synapse leads one to suspect that MOPEG-SO$_4$ may arise in part from both presynaptically metabolized NE via DOPEG formation as well as from NE metabolized to NM following release (see Figure 1). Third, as discussed previously, several investigators have found that the deaminated catechol DOPEG, in conjugated form (presumably DOPEG-SO$_4$), may also be a major metabolite of brain NE. In our experiments using ^{3}H-NE we found that levels of DOPEG-SO$_4$ were equal to those of MOPEG-SO$_4$ in the rat hypothalamus. Together these two compounds made up 80–90% of the total metabolites of ^{3}H-NE. It is not known to what extent released NE is converted to DOPEG-SO$_4$ as an end product, but from Figure 1 it can be seen that a considerable amount may be so metabolized via reuptake of the released amine with subsequent deaminaton and conjugation. Sugden and Eccleston (1971) initially proposed that DOPEG-SO$_4$ originates primarily from presynaptic intraneuronal metabolism while MOPEG-SO$_4$ is produced from extraneuronal metabolism of released NE. In support of this notion we have found that reserpine, which promotes intraneuronal metabolism of NE produces a greater increase in DOPEG-SO$_4$ than in MOPEG-SO$_4$, whereas running stress, which presumably increases the neuronal release of NE, increases only MOPEG-SO$_4$ (Stone, 1973*b*). However, the above experiment constitutes indirect evidence. The problem of which metabolite, if any, accurately reflects released NE in the brain will ultimately be resolved by measurement of the metabolites of endogenous NE during electrical stimulation of the locus coeruleus in several species.*

5. FUNCTIONAL SIGNIFICANCE

The peripheral sympathetic nervous system constitutes one of the organism's major defensive systems against harmful agents. Animals surgically deprived of these nerves rapidly succumb to stress because of their inability to regulate autonomic functions. The central noradrenergic and dopaminergic neurons might have a similar function, since they are active during stress and are thought to regulate a variety of homeostatic processes. These include thermoregulation (Simmonds, 1969), release of pituitary hor-

---

* See note following References.

mones (Van Loon *et al.*, 1971), food intake (Miller, 1965), heart rate and blood pressure (Gagnon and Melville, 1969), arousal and general level of psychomotor activity (Geyer *et al.*, 1972; Schildkraut and Kety, 1967) among others (Stein and Wise, 1969; Kety, 1972; Randt *et al.*, 1971; Jouvet, 1969). On the basis of the above evidence one would predict that interfering with transmission in central monoaminergic neurons should leave animals without adequate physiological or behavioral responses to cope with stress. In support of this notion, Blaskowski *et al.* (1970) have found a reduced resistance to restraint stress after pharmacological depletion of central monoamines. However, the latter finding is difficult to interpret because both central and peripheral stores of NE and DA as well as serotonin were depleted. Simmonds and Uretsky (1970) and Zigmond and Stricker (1972) have used intraventricularly injected 6-hydroxydopamine to achieve selective depletions of central NE and DA in rats; these authors have found no evidence of reduced resistance to either cold or heart stress. Intracerebral 6-hydroxydopamine does, however, produce in rats a marked irritability (Nakamura and Thoenen, 1972), deficits in conditioned avoidance behavior (Taylor and Laverty, 1972), and in feeding (Zigmond and Stricker, 1972; Ungerstedt, 1971). Obviously much more work is necessary in these areas before we can understand the functional significance of the increased turnover of brain NE and DA during stress.

Another area that is the focus of current research is the possible relationship between altered amine metabolism and so called "diseases of stress" such as hypertension (Mendlowitz *et al.*, 1970) and mental depression (Schildkraut, 1973). Workers in these areas, however, are still grappling with the methodological difficulties of obtaining direct measures of brain monoamine metabolism in humans (Extein *et al.*, 1973). The development of better animal models of stress-induced disorders (McKinney and Bunney, 1969; Henry *et al.*, 1967) will facilitate future research on their biochemical etiology. In this regard we and other investigators have been studying brain amine metabolism in rats subjected to swimming in cold water (Barchas and Freedman, 1963; Ruther *et al.*, 1966a; Stone, 1970a,b. This stress is unique in that it produces a reserpinelike behavioral syndrome characterized by decreased psychomotor activity without sleep, eye closure, catalepsy, and shivering. These effects apparently result from the severe hypothermia produced by the stress but may be mediated in part through changes in monoamine metabolism. Unlike most stressors the cold-swim procedure decreases the turnover of brain NE and DA. Its behavioral and biochemical effects can be partially or completely antagonized without altering hypothermia, by systemic administration of amphetamine or tricyclic antidepressant drugs. These agents probably exert their effects by blocking the reuptake or stimulating the impaired release and synthesis of brain CA's in the stressed rats. In support of this we have recently found that intraventricular injections of microgram quantities of NE in cold-swum rats stops the shivering, opens the eyes, and restores some active exploratory behavior (Stone and Mendlinger, 1974*a*).

The above behavioral effects of hypothermia in rats have led us to speculate on possible connections between depression and body temperature. It is well known, for example, that people frequently use low temperature phrases like "the blues," "cold and lonely" or "frigid" to describe feelings of separation or rejection. Also, mother–infant separation, a potent stimulus for anaclitic depression in human and primate infants, lowers body temperature in rat pups (Hofer, 1970) and produces in infant primates a huddled posture that would, among other things, reduce body heat loss (Kaufman and Rosenblum, 1967). Hypothermia during maternal deprivation, thus, might play a role in anaclitic depression in young animals possibly by reducing the turnover of brain amines. This early experience could have lasting neurochemical (Nielson and McIver, 1966) and behavioral effects in adult life (Levine, 1962).

6. REFERENCES

Anton, A. H., Schwartz, R. P., and Kramer, S., 1968, Catecholamines and behavior in isolated and grouped mice, *J. Psychiat. Res.* **6**:211.

Arbuthnott, G. W., Crow, T. J., Fuxe, K., Olson, L., and Ungerstedt, U., 1970, Depletion of catecholamines *in vivo* induced by electrical stimulation of central monoamine pathways, *Brain Res.* **24**:471.

Axelrod, J., 1966, Methylation reactions in the formation and metabolism of catecholamines and other biogenic amines, *Pharmacol. Rev.* **18**:95.

Axelrod, J., Mueller, R. A., Henry, J. P., and Stephens, P. A., 1970, Changes in enzymes involved in the biosynthesis and metabolism of noradrenaline and adrenaline after psychosocial stimulation, *Nature* **225**:1059.

Bapna, J., Neff, N. H., and Costa, E., 1971, A method for studying norepinephrine and serotonin metabolism in small regions of rat brain: effect of ovariectomy on amine metabolism in anterior and posterior hypothalamus, *Endocrinology* **89**:1345.

Barchas, J. D., and Freedman, D. X., 1963, Brain amines: response to physiological stress, *Biochem. Pharmacol.* **12**:1232.

Bernard, J., 1968, The eudaemonists, in: *Why Man Takes Chances* (S. Z. Klausner, ed.), pp. 6–47, Doubleday, Garden City, New York.

Bhagat, B., 1969, Effect of chronic cold stress on catecholamine levels in rat brain, *Psychopharmacoligia* **16**:1.

Bhagat, B., and Friedman, E., 1969, Factors involved in maintenance of cardiac catecholamine content: relative importance of synthesis and reuptake, *Brit. J. Pharmacol.* **37**:24.

Bhatnagar, R. K., and Moore, K. E., 1971, Effects of electrical stimulation, α-methyltyrosine and desmethylimipramine on the norepinephrine contents of neuronal cell bodies and terminals, *J. Pharmacol. Exptl. Therap.* **178**:450.

Blaszkowski, T. P., DeFeo, J. J., and Guarino, A. M., 1970, Central *vs.* peripheral catecholamines in rats during adaptation to chronic restraint stress, *Pharmacology* **4**:321.

Blenkarn, G. D., Schanberg, S. M., and Saltzman, H. A., 1969, Cerebral amines and acute hyperbaric oxygen toxicity, *J. Pharmacol. Exptl. Therap.* **166**:346.

Bliss, E. L., 1967, Sleep in schizophrenia and depression—studies of sleep loss in man and animals, in: *Sleep and Altered States of Consciousness* (S. S. Kety, E. V. Evarts, and H. L. Williams, eds.), pp. 195–210, Williams and Wilkins, Baltimore.

Bliss, E., and Ailion, J., 1969, Response of neurogenic amines to aggregation and strangers, *J. Pharmacol. Exptl. Therap.* **168**:258.

Bliss, E. L., and Ailion, J., 1971, Relationship of stress and activity to brain dopamine and homovanillic acid, *Life Sci.* **10**:1161.

Bliss, E. L., and Zwanziger, J., 1966, Brain amines and emotional stress, *J. Psychiat. Res.* **4**:189.

Bliss, E. L., Wilson, V. B., and Zwanziger, J., 1966, Changes in brain norepinephrine in self-stimulating and "aversive" animals, *J. Psychiat. Res.* **4**:59.

Bliss, E. L., Ailion, J., and Zwanziger, J., 1968, Metabolism of norepinephrine, serotonin and dopamine in rat brain with stress, *J. Pharmacol. Exptl. Therap.* **164**:122.

Breitner, C., Picchioni, A., and Chin, L., 1964, Neurohormone levels in brain after CNS stimulation including electrotherapy, *J. Neuropsychiat.* **5**:153.

Brodie, B. B., Costa, E., Dlabac, A., Neff, N. H., and Smookler, H. H., 1966, Application of steady state kinetics to the estimation of synthesis rate and turnover time of tissue catecholamines, *J. Pharmacol. Exptl. Therap.* **154**:493.

Buckingham, S., Sommers, S. C., and McNary, W. F., 1966, Sympathetic activation and serotonin release as factors in pulmonary edema after hyperbaric oxygen, *Federation Proc.* **25**:566.

Carr, L. A., and Moore, K. E., 1968, Effects of reserpine and α-methyltyrosine on brain catecholamines and the pituitary–adrenal response to stress, *Neuroendocrinology* **3**:285.

Chan, W. C., and Johnson, G. E., 1968, Inluence of cold exposure on catecholamine depleting actions of hydroxylase inhibitors, *European J. Pharmacol.* **3**:40.

Chang, C. C., and Chiueh, C. C., 1968, Increased uptake of noradrenaline in the rat submaxillary gland during sympathetic nerve stimulation, *J. Pharm. Pharmacol.* **20**:157.

Chase, T. N., Breese, G. R. Gordon, E. K., and Kopin, I. J., 1971, Catecholamine metabolism in the dog: comparison of intravenously and intraventricularly administered [^{14}C] dopamine and [^{3}H] norepinephrine, *J. Neurochem.* **18**:135.

Chidsey, C. A., Kaiser, G. A., Sonnenblick, E. H., Spann, J. F., and Braunwald, E., 1964, Cardiac norepinephrine stores in experimental heart failure in the dog, *J. Clin. Invest.* **43**:2386.

Chu, N. S., and Bloom, F. E., 1973, Norepinephrine-containing neurons: changes in spontaneous discharge patterns during sleeping and waking, *Science* **179**:908.

Coleman, B., and Glaviano, V. V., 1963, Tissue levels of norepinephrine and epinephrine in hemorrhagic shock, *Science* **139**:54.

Cooper, A. J., Moir, A. T. B., and Guldberg, H. C., 1968, The effect of electroconvulsive shock on the cerebral metabolism of dopamine and 5-hydroxytryptamine, *J. Pharm. Pharmacol.* **20**:729.

Corrodi, H., Fuxe, K., and Hökfelt, T., 1967, A possible role played by central monoamine neurons in thermoregulation, *Acta Physiol. Scand.* **71**:224.

Corrodi, H., Fuxe, K., and Hökfelt, T., 1968, The effect of immobilization stress on the activity of central monoamine neurons, *Life Sci.* **7**:107.

Corrodi, H., Fuxe, K., Hamberger, B., and Ljungdahl, A., 1970, Studies on central and peripheral noradrenaline neurons using a new dopamine-β-hydroxylase inhibitor, *European J. Pharmacol.* **12**:145.

Costa, E. and Neff, N. H., 1966, Isotopic and non-isotopic measurements of the rate of catecholamine biosynthesis, in: *Biochemistry and Pharmacology of the Basal Ganglia* (E. Costa, L. J. Cote, and M. D. Yahr, eds.), pp. 141–155, Raven Press, New York.

Dahlstrom, A., and Haggendal, J., 1967, Studies on the transport and life span of amine storage granules in the adrenergic neuron system of the rabbit sciatic nerve, *Acta Physiol. Scand.* **69**:153.

Dahlstrom, A. B., and Zetterstrom, B. E. M., 1965, Noradrenergic stores in nerve terminals of the spleen: changes during hemorrhagic shock, *Science* **147**:1583.

DiCara, L. V., and Stone, E. A., 1970, Effect of instrumental heart-rate training on rat cardiac and brain catecholamines, *Psychosomat. Med.* **23**:359.

Draskoczy, P. R. Pulley, K., and Burack, W. R., 1966, The effect of cold environment on the endogenously labeled catecholamine (CA) stores, *Pharmacologist* **8**:178.

Eleftheriou, B. E., and Church, R. L., 1968, Brain levels of serotonin and norepinephrine in mice after exposure to aggression and defeat, *Physiol. Behav.* **3**:977.

Elo, H., and Tirri, R., 1972, Effect of forced motility on the noradrenaline and 5-hydroxytryptamine metabolism in different parts of the rat brain, *Psychopharmacologia* **26**:195.

Engel, J., Hanson, L. C. F., Roos, B. E., and Strombergsson, L. E., 1968, Effect of electroshock on dopamine metabolism in rat brain, *Psychopharmacologia* **13**:140.

Euler, U. S. von, 1948, Identification of the sympathometic ergone in adrenergic nerves of cattle (sympathin-N) with laevo-noradrenaline, *Acta Physiol. Scand.* **16**:63.

Euler, U. S. von, 1964, Quantitation of stress by catecholamine analysis, *Clin. Pharmacol. Therap.* **5**:398.

Extein, I., Korf, J., Roth, R. H., and Bowers, M. B. Jr., 1973, Accumulation of 3-methoxy-4-hydroxyphenyglycol-sulfate in rabbit cerebrospinal fluid following probenecid, *Brain Res.* **54**:403.

Faiman, M. D., and Helbe, A. R., 1966, The effect of hyperbaric oxygenation on cerebral amines, *Life Sci.* **5**:2225.

Frankenhaeuser, M., 1971, Experimental approaches to the study of human behavior as related to neuroendocrine functions, in: *Society, Stress and Disease, Vol. I* (L. Levi, ed.), pp. 22–35, Oxford University Press, New York.

Fulginiti, S., and Orsingher, O. A., 1971, Effects of learning, amphetamine and nicotine on the level and synthesis of brain noradrenaline in rats, *Arch. Intern. Pharmacodyn.* **190**:291.

Fuxe, K., and Hanson, L. C. F., 1967, Central catecholamine neurons and conditioned avoidance behavior, *Psychopharmacologia* **11**:439.

Gagnon, D. J., and Melville, K. I., 1969, Alteration of centrally mediated cardiovascular manifestation by intraventricular pronethalol and phentolamine, *Intern. J. Neuropharm.* **8**:587.

Geller, E., Yuwiler, A., and Zolman, J. F., 1965, Effects of environmental complexity on constituents of brain and liver, *J. Neurochem.* **12**:949.

Geyer, M. A., Segal, D. S., and Mandell, A. J., 1972, Effect of intraventricular infusion of dopamine and norepinephrine on motor activity, *Physiol. Behavior* **8**:653.

Glass, D., and Singer, J. E., 1972, Behavioral aftereffects of unpredictable and uncontrollable aversive events, *Am. Sci.* **60**:457.

Goldberg, M. E., and Salama, A. I., 1969. Amphetamine toxicity and brain monoamines in three models of stress, *Toxicol. Appl. Pharmacol.* **14**:447.

Goldberg, M. E., and Salama, A. I., 1970, Relationship of brain dopamine to stress-induced changes in seizure susceptibility, *European J. Pharmacol.* **10**:333.

Goldberg, M. E., and Salama, A. I., 1972, Tolerance to drum stress and its relationship to dopamine turnover, *European J. Pharmacol.* **17**:202.

Goldstein, M., and Nakajima, K., 1966, The effect of disulfiram on the biosynthesis of catecholamines during exposure of rats to cold, *Life Sci.* **5**:175.

Gordon, R., Spector, S., Sjoerdsma, A., and Udenfriend, S., 1966, Increased synthesis of norepinephrine and epinephrine in the intact rat during exercise and exposure to cold, *J. Pharmacol. Exptl. Therap.* **153**:440.

Green, H., and Erickson, R. W., 1960, Effect of trans-2-phenylcylopropylamine upon nor-epinephrine concentration and monoamine oxidase activity of rat brain, *J. Pharmacol. Exptl. Therap.* **129**:237.

Gunne, L. M., and Reis, D. J., 1963, Changes in brain catecholamines associated with electrical stimulation of amygdaloid nucleus, *Life Sci.* **2**:804.

Haggendal, J., 1967, The effect of high pressure air or oxygen with and without carbon dioxide added on the catecholamine levels of rat brain, *Acta Physiol. Scand.* **69**:147.

Henley, E. D., Moisset, B., and Welch, B. L., 1973, Catecholamine uptake in cerebral cortex: adaptive change induced by fighting, *Science* **180**:1050.

Henry, J. P. Meehan, J. P., and Stephens, P., 1967, The use of psychosocial stimuli to induce prolonged hypertension in mice, *Psychosomat. Med.* **29**:408.

Hernandez-Peon, R., Drucker, R. P., Ramirez del Angel, A., Chavez, B., and Serrano, P., 1969, Brain catecholamines and serotonin in rapid sleep deprivation, *Physiol. Behav.* **4**:659.

Hift, H., Halperin, M., Hegedus, S. I., and Thomas, W. O., 1965, Tissue catecholamine levels in prolonged oligemic hypotension, *Proc. Soc. Exptl. Biol. Med.* **119**:883.

Hofer, M. A., 1970, Physiological responses of infant rats to separation from their mothers, *Science* **168**:871.

Hökfelt, B., 1951, Noradrenaline and adrenaline in mammalian tissues, *Acta Physiol. Scand. Suppl.* **25**:92.

Holmes, T. H., and Rahe, R. H., 1967, The social readjustment rating scale, *J. Psychosomat. Res.* **11**:213.

Hornykiewicz, O., 1966, Dopamine (3-hydroxy-tyramine) and brain function, *Pharmacol. Rev.* **18**:925.

Hrubes, V., and Benes, V., 1969, The time course of metabolic changes during prolonged stress in rats, *J. Psychosomat. Res.* **13**:327.

Hurwitz, D. A., Robinson, S. M., and Barofsky, I., 1971, The influence of training and avoidance performance on disulfiram induced changes in brain catecholamines, *Neuropharmacology* **10**:447.

Huttunen, M. O., 1971, Persistent alteration of turnover of brain noradrenaline in the offspring of rats subjected to stress during pregnancy, *Nature* **230**:53.

Ingenito, A. J., 1968, Norepinephrine levels in various areas of rat brain during cold acclimation, *Proc. Soc. Exptl. Biol. Med.* **127**:74.

Ingenito, A. J., and Bonnycastle, D. D., 1967, The effect of exposure to heat and cold upon rat brain catecholamine and 5-hydroxtryptamine levels, *Can. J. Physiol. Pharmacol.* **45**:733.

Iversen, L. L., and Glowinski, J., 1966, Regional studies of catecholamines in the rat brain. II. Rate of turnover of catecholamines in various brain regions, *J. Neurochem.* **13**:671.

Jouvet, M., 1969, Biogenic amines and the states of sleep, *Science* **163**:32.

Kaiser, G. G., Jellinek, M., Cooper, T., and Hanlon, C. R., 1965, Experimental heart block: effect on myocardial catecholamine concentration, *Am. J. Physiol.* **208**:477.

Kato, L., Gozsy, B., Roy, P. B., and Groh, V., 1967, Histamine, serotonin, epinephrine and norepinephrine in the rat brain, following convulsions, *Intern. J. Neuropsychiat.* **3**:46.

Kaufman, I. C., and Rosenblum, L. A., 1967, The reaction to separation in infant monkeys: anaclitic depression and conservation-withdrawal, *Psychosomat. Med.* **29**:648.

Kety, S. S., 1972, Norepinephrine in the central nervous system and its correlations with behavior, in: *Brain and Human Behavior* (A. G. Karczman and J. C. Eccles, eds.), pp. 115–128, Springer-Verlag, New York.

Kety, S. S., Javoy, F., Thierry, A. M., Julou, L., and Glowinski, J., 1967, A sustained effect of electroconvulsive shock on the turnover of norepinephrine in the central nervous system of the rat, *Proc. Natl. Acad. Sci. (U.S.)* **58**:1249.

Kirshner, N., and Viveros, O. H., 1972, The secretory cycle in the adrenal medulla, *Pharmacol. Rev.* **24**:385.

Kopin, I. J., Breese, G. R., Krauss, K. R., and Weise, V. K., 1968, Selective release of newly synthesized norepinephrine from the cat spleen during sympathetic stimulation. *J. Pharmacol. Exptl. Therap.* **161**:271.

Korf, J., Aghajanian, G. K., and Roth, R. H., 1973a, Stimulation and destruction of the locus coeruleus: opposite effects on 3-methoxy-4-hydroxyphenylglycol sulfate levels in the rat cerebral cortex, *European J. Pharmacol.* **21**:305.

Korf, J., Aghajanian, G. K., and Roth, R. H., 1973b, Increased turnover of norepinephrine in the rat cerebral cortex during stress: role of the locus coeruleus, *Neuropharmacology* **12**:933.

Korf, J., Roth, R. H., and Aghajanian, G. K., 1973c, Alterations in turnover and endogenous levels of norepinephrine in cerebral cortex following stimulation and acute axotomy of cerebral noradrenergic pathways, *European J. Pharmacol.* **23**:276.

Ladisich, W., and Baumann, P., 1971, Influence of progesterone on norepinephrine metabolism of the rat brain in connection with amphetamine and stress, *Neuroendocrinology* **7**:16.

Ladisich, W., Steinhauff, N., and Matussek, N., 1969, Chronic administration of electroconvulsive shock and norepinephrine metabolism in the rat brain. II 7-^{3}H-NE metabolism after intracisternal injection with and without the influence of drugs in different brain regions, and by 7-^{3}H-NE uptake in vitro, *Psychopharmacologia* **15**:296.

Lamprecht, F., Eichelman, B., Thoa, N. B., Williams, R. B., and Kopin, I. J., 1972, Rat fighting behavior: serum dopamine-β-hydroxylase and hypothalamic tyrosine hydroxylase, *Science* **177**:1214.

Landsberg, L., and Axelrod, J., 1968, The effect of elevated temperature on the retention of ^{3}H-norepinephrine in the hearts of normal and thyroidectomized rats, *Life Sci.* **7**:1171.

Lazarus, R. S., 1966, *Psychological Stress and the Coping Process*, McGraw-Hill, New York.

LeBlanc, J., Robinson, D., Sharman, D. F., and Tousignant, P., 1967, Catecholamines and short-term adaptation to cold in mice, *Am. J. Physiol.* **213**:1419.

Leduc, J., 1961, Catecholamine production and release in exposure and acclimation to cold, *Acta Physiol. Scand. Suppl.* **53**:183.

Levi, L., 1967, Sympatho-adrenomedullary responses to emotional stimuli: methodologic, physiologic, and pathologic considerations, in: *An Introduction to Clinial Neuroendocrinology* (E. Bajusz, ed.), pp. 78–105, S. Karger, Basel.

Levi, R., and Maynert, E. W., 1964, The subcellular localization of brain-stem norepinephrine and 5-hydroxytryptamine in stressed rats, *Biochem. Pharmacol.* **13**:615.

Levine, S., 1962, The psychophysiological effect of infantile stimulation, in: *Roots of Behavior* (E. Bliss, ed.), pp. 246–253, Hoeber, New York.

Lewy, A. J., and Seiden, L. S., 1972, Operant behavior changes norepinephrine metabolism in rat brain, *Science* **175**:454.

Lichtensteiger, W., 1969, The catecholamine content of hypothalamic nerve cells after acute exposure to cold and thyroxine administration, *J. Physiol.* **203**:675.

Lidbrink, P., Corrodi, H., Fuxe, K., and Olson, L., 1972, Barbiturates and meprobamate: decreases in catecholamine turnover of central dopamine and noradrenaline neuronal systems and the influence of immobilization stress, *Brain Res.* **45**:507.

Lycke, E., Modigh, K., and Roos, B. E., 1970, The monoamine metabolism in viral encephalitides of the mouse. I. Virological and biochemical results, *Brain Res.* **23**:235.

Mark, J., Heiner, L., Mandel, P., and Godin, Y., 1969, Norepinephrine turnover in brain and stress reactions in rats during paradoxical sleep deprivation, *Life Sci.* **8**:1085.

Maynert, E. W., and Levi, R., 1964, Stress-induced release of brain norepinephrine and its inhibition by drugs, *J. Pharmacol. Exptl. Therap.* **143**:90.

McKinney, W. T., and Bunney, W. E., 1967, Animal models of depression, *Arch. Gen. Psychiat.* **21**:240.

Meek, J. L., and Neff, N. H., 1973a, The rate of formation of 3-methoxy-4-

hydroxyphenylethyleneglycol sulfate in brain as an estimate of the rate of formation of norepinephrine, *J. Pharmacol. Exptl. Therap.* **184**:570.

Meek, J. L., and Neff, N. H., 1973*b*, Biogenic amines and their metabolites as substrates for phenol sulphotransferase (EC 2.8.2.1) of brain and liver, *J. Neurochem.* **21**:1.

Mendlowitz, M., Wolf, R. L., and Gitlow, S. E., 1970, Catecholamine metabolism in essential hypertension, *Am. Heart J.* **79**:401.

Menon, M. K., and Dandiya, P. C., 1969, Behavioral and brain neurohormonal changes produced by acute heat stress in rats: influence of psychopharmacological agents, *European J. Pharmacol.* **8**:284.

Miller, N. E., 1959, Liberalization of basic S-R concepts: extensions to conflict behavior, motivation and social learning in: *Psychology: A Study of a Science, Vol. 2. General Systematic Formulations, Learning and Special Processes* (S. Koch, ed.), pp. 196–292, McGraw-Hill, New York.

Miller, N. E., 1965, Chemical coding of behavior in the brain, *Science* **148**:328.

Montanari, R., Costa, A., Beaven, M. A., and Brodie, B. B., 1963, Turnover rates of norepinephrine in hearts of intact mice, rats and guinea pigs using tritiated norepinephrine, *Life Sci.* **2**:232.

Moore, K. E., 1964, The role of endogenous norepinephrine in the toxicity of *d*-amphetamine in aggregated mice, *J. Pharmacol. Exptl. Therap.* **144**:45.

Moore, K. E., and Lariviere, E. W., 1964, Effects of stress and *d*-amphetamine on rat brain catecholamines, *Biochem. Pharmacol.* **13**:1098.

Mueller, R. A., Thoenen, H., and Axelrod, J., 1969, Increase in tyrosine hydroxylase activity after reserpine administration, *J. Pharmacol. Exptl. Therap.* **169**:74.

Musacchio, J. M., Julou, L., Kety, S. S., and Glowinski, J., 1969, Increase in rat brain tyrosine hydroxylase activity produced by electroconvulsive shock, *Proc. Natl. Acad. Sci. (U.S.)* **63**:1117.

Nakamura, K., and Thoenen, H., 1971, Hypothermia induced by intraventricular administration of 6-hydroxydopamine in rats, *European J. Pharmacol.* **16**:46.

Neff, N. H., and Costa, E., 1968, Application of steady state kinetics to the study of catecholamine turnover after monoamine oxidase inhibition or reserpine administration, *J. Pharmacol. Exptl. Therap.* **160**:40.

Nielson, H. C., and Fleming, R. M., 1968, Effect of electroconvulsive shock and prior stress on brain amine levels, *Exptl. Neurol.* **20**:21.

Nielson, H. C., and McIver, A. H., 1966, Early cold stress: II. Effects on regional distribution of brain amines in rats, *Proc. Am. Psychol. Assoc.* **1**:155.

Oliverio, A., and Stjarne, L., 1965, Acceleration of noradrenaline turnover in the mouse heart by cold exposure, *Life Sci.* **4**:2339.

Ordy, J. M., Samorajski, T., and Schroeder, D., 1966, Concurrent changes in hypothalamic and cardiac catecholamine levels after anesthetics, tranquilizers and stress in a subhuman primate, *J. Pharmacol. Exptl. Therap.* **152**:445.

Paré, W. P., and Livingston, A. Jr., 1970, Brain norepinephrine and stomach ulcers in rats exposed to chronic conflict, *Physiol. Behav.* **5**:215.

Paulsen, E. C., and Hess, S. M., 1963, The rate of synthesis of catecholamines following depletion in guinea pig brain and heart, *J. Neurochem.* **10**:453.

Pogodaev, K. I., Turova, N. F., Lebedev, V. M., and Semavin, I. E., 1972, Changes in content of catecholamines in the brain of albino rats during stress produced by running in a revolving drum, *Byul. Eksperim. Biol. Med.* **73**:43.

Pryor, G. T., Peache, S., and Scott, M. K., 1972, The effect of repeated electroconvulsive shock on avoidance conditioning and brain monoamine oxidase activity, *Physiol. Behav.* **9**:623.

Pujol, J. F., Mouret, J., Jouvet, M., and Glowinski, J., 1968, Increased turnover of cerebral norepinephrine during rebound of paradoxical sleep in the rat, *Science* **159**:112.

Randt, C. T., Quartermain, D., Goldstein, M., and Anagnoste, B., 1971, Norepinephrine biosynthesis inhibition: effects on memory in mice, *Sceince* **172**:498.

Reid, W. D., Volicer, L., Smookler, H., Beaven, M. A. and Brodie, B. B., 1966, Brain amines and temperature regulation, *Pharmacology* **1**:329.

Reis, D. J., and Fuxe, K., 1969, Brain norepinephrine: evidence that neuronal release is essential for shame rage behavior following brainstem transaction in cat, *Proc. Natl. Acad. Sci (U.S.)* **64**:108.

Reis, D. J., and Gunne, L. M., 1965, Brain catecholamines: relation to the defense reaction evoked by amygdaloid stimulation in cat, *Science* **149**:450.

Reis, D. J., Miura, M., Weinbren, M., and Gunne, L. M., 1967, Brain catecholamines: relation to defense reaction evoked by acute brainstem transaction in cat, *Science* **56**:1768.

Riege, W. H., and Morimoto, H., 1970, Effects of chronic stress and differential environments upon brain weights and biogenic amine levels in rats, *J. Comp. Physiol. Psychol.* **71**:396.

Roffman, M., Freedman, L. S., and Goldstein, M., 1973, The effect of chronic swim stress on dopamine-β-hydroxylase activity, *Life Sci.* **12**:369.

Rosecrans, J. A., 1969, Brain amine changes in stressed and normal rats pretreated with various drugs, *Arch Intern. Pharmacodyn.* **180**:460.

Roth, R. H., Stjarne, L., and Euler, U. S. von, 1966, Acceleration of noradrenaline biosynthesis by nerve stimulation, *Life Sci.* **5**:1071.

Rubenson, A., 1969, Alterations in noradrenaline turnover in the peripheral sympathetic neurons induced by stress, *J. Pharm. Pharmacol.* **21**:878.

Ruther, E., Ackenheil, M., and Matussek, N., 1966a, Amine metabolism in CNS after stress-situation, *Act. Nerv. Sup.* **8**:416.

Ruther, E., Ackenheil, M., and Matussek, N., 1966b, Beitrag zum Noradrenalin- und Serotonin-Stoffwechsel in Rattenhirn nach Stress-Zustanden, *Arzneinmittel-Forsch.* **16**:261.

Salama, A. I., and Goldberg, M. E., 1973, Temporary increase in forebrain norepinephrine turnover in mouse-killing rats, *European J. Pharmacol.* **21**:372.

Schanberg, S. M., Breese, G. R., Schildkraut, J. J., Gordon, E. K., and Kopin, I. J., 1968a, 3-Methoxy-4-hydroxyphenylglycol sulfate in brain and cerebrospinal fluid, *Biochem. Pharmacol.* **17**:2006.

Schanberg, S. M., Schildkraut, J. J., Breese, G. R., and Kopin, I. J., 1968b, Metabolism of normetanephrine-H^3 in rat brain—identification of conjugated 3-methoxy-4-hydroxyphenylglycol as the major metabolite, *Biochem. Pharmacol.* **17**:247.

Schildkraut, J. J., 1975, Depressions and biogenic amines, in: *American Handbook of Psychiatry, Vol. 6*, (D. Hamburg, H. K. H. Brodie, and, S. Arieti, eds.), Basic Books, New York (in press).

Schildkraut, J. J., and Hartmann, E., 1972, Turnover and metabolism of norepinephrine in rat brain after 72 hours on a D-deprivation island, *Psychopharmacologia* **27**:17.

Schildkraut, J. J., and Kety, S. S., 1967, Biogenic amines and emotion, *Science* **156**:21.

Schildkraut, J. J., Draskoczy, P. R., and Lo, P. S., 1971, Norepinephrine pools in rat brain: differences in turnover rates and pathways of metabolism, *Science* **172**:587.

Simmonds, M. A., 1969, Effect of environmental temperature on the turnover of noradrenaline in hypothalamus and other areas of rat brain, *J. Physiol.* **203**:199.

Simmonds, M. A., 1971, Inhibition by atropine of the increased turnover of noradrenaline in the hypothalamus of rats exposed to cold, *Brit. J. Pharmacol.* **41**:224.

Simmonds, M. A., and Uretsky, N. J., 1970, Central effects of 6-hydroxydopamine on the body temperature of the rat, *Brit. J. Pharmacol.* **40**:630.

Smith, A. D., and Winkler, H., 1972, Fundamental mechanisms in the release of catecholamines, in: *Handbook of Experimental Pharmacology, Vol. 33, Catecholamines* (H. Blaschko and E. Muscholl, eds.), pp. 538–617, Springer-Verlag, New York.

Smith, A. D., DePotter, W. P., Moerman, E. J., and DeSchaepdryver, A. F., 1970, Release of dopamine-β-hydroxylase and chromogranin upon stimulation of the splenic nerves, *Tiss. Cell.* **2**:2547.

Sparber, S. B., and Tilson, H. A., 1972, Schedule controlled and drug induced release of norepinephrine-7-³H into the lateral ventricle of rats, *Neuropharmacology* **11**:453.

Stein, L., and Wise, C. D., 1969, Release of norepinephrine from hypothalamus and amygdala by rewarding medial forebrain bundle stimulation and amphetamine. *J. Comp. Physiol. Psychol.* **67**:189.

Stenevi, U., 1971, Sprouting and plasticity of central monoamine neurons with microspectrofluorometric characterization of their intraneuronal fluorophores, *Commun. Dept. Anat. Univ. Lund (Sweden)* No. 2:1.

Stern, W. C., Miller, F. P., Cox, R. H., and Maickel, R. P., 1971, Brain norepinephrine and serotonin levels following REM sleep deprivation in the rat, *Psychopharmacologia* **22**:50.

Stone, E. A., 1970a, Swim-stress induced inactivity: relation to body temperature and brain norepinephrine, and effects of *d*-amphetamine, *Psychosomat. Med.* **32**:51.

Stone, E. A., 1970b, Behavioral and neurochemical effects of acute swim stress are due to hypothermia, *Life Sci.* **9**:877.

Stone, E. A., 1971, Hypothalamic norepinephrine after acute stress, *Brain Res.* **35**:260.

Stone, E. A., 1973a, Adrenergic activity in the rat hypothalamus following extreme muscular exertion, *Am. J. Physiol.* **224**:165.

Stone, E. A., 1973b, Accumulation and metabolism of norepinephrine in rat hypothalamus after exhaustive stress, *J. Neurochem.* **21**:589.

Stoner, H. B., and Elson, P. M., 1971, The effect of injury on monoamine concentrations in the rat hypothalamus, *J. Neurochem.* **18**:1837.

Sugden, R. F., and Eccleston, D., 1971, Glycol sulphate ester formation from [¹⁴C] noradrenaline in brain and the influence of a COMT inhibitor, *J. Neurochem.* **18**:2461.

Taylor, K. M., and Laverty, R., 1969a, The metabolism of tritiated dopamine in regions of the rat brain *in vivo*—II. The significance of the neutral metabolites of catecholamines, *J. Neurochem.* **16**:1367.

Taylor, K. M., and Laverty, R., 1969b, The effect of chlordiazepoxide, diazepam and nitrazepam on catecholamine metabolism in regions of the rat brain, *European J. Pharmacol.* **8**:296.

Taylor, K. M., and Laverty, R., 1972, The effect of drugs on the behavioral and biochemical actions of intraventricular 6-hydroxydopamine, *European J. Pharmacol.* **17**:16.

Thierry, A. M., Javoy, F., Glowinski, J., and Kety, S. S., 1968, Effects of stress on the metabolism of norepinephrine, dopamine and serotonin in the central nervous system of the rat. I. Modifications of norepinephrine turnover, *J. Pharmacol. Exptl. Therap.* **163**:163.

Thierry, A. M., Blanc, G., and Glowinski, J., 1971, Effect of stress on the disposition of catecholamines localized in various intraneuronal storage forms in the brain stem of the rat, *J. Neurochem.* **18**:449.

Thoenen, H., 1970, Induction of tyrosine hydroxylase in peripheral and central adrenergic neurons by cold exposure, *Nature* **228**:861.

Tsuchiya, K., Toru, M., and Kobayashi, T., 1969, Sleep deprivation: changes of monoamines and acetylcholine in rat brain, *Life Sci.* **8**:867.

Udenfriend, S., and Zaltzman-Nirenberg, P., 1963, Norepinephrine and 3,4-dihydroxyphenylethylamine turnover in guinea pig brain *in vivo, Science* **142**:394.

Ungerstedt, U., 1971, Adipsia and aphagia after 6-hydroxydopamine induced degeneration of the nigrostriatal dopamine system, *Acta physiol. Scand. Suppl.* **367**:95.

Van Loon, G. R., Hilger, L., King, A. B., Boryczka, A. T., and Ganong, W. F., 1971, Inhibitory effect of l-dihydroxyphenyl-alanine on the adrenal venous 17-hydroxycorticosteriod response to surgical stress in dogs, *Endocrinology* **88**:1404.

Vogt, M., 1954, The concentration of sympathin in different parts of the central nervous system under normal conditions and after the administration of drugs, *J. Physiol.* **123**:451.

Walter, D. S., and Eccleston, D., 1972, The effect of electric stimulation of the locus coeruleus on the endogenous concentration of 4-hydroxy-3-methoxyphenylethylene glycol in rat brain, *Biochem. J.,* **128**:85p.

Weiner, N., 1970, Regulation of norepinephrine biosynthesis, *Ann. Rev. Pharmacol.* **10**:273.

Weiss, J. M., 1972, Psychological factors in stress and disease, *Sci. Am.* **226**:104.

Weiss, J. M., Stone, E. A., and Harrell, N. W., 1970, Coping behavior and brain norepinephrine level in rats, *J. Comp. Physiol. Psychol.* **72**:153.

Welch, B. L., and Welch, A. S., 1965, Effect of grouping on the level of brain norepinephrine in white swiss mice, *Life Sci.* **4**:1011.

Welch, B. L., and Welch, A. S., 1968*a*, Greater lowering of brain and adrenal catecholamines in group-housed than in individually housed mice administered DL-α-methyltyrosine. *J. Pharm. Pharmacol.* **20**:244.

Welch, B. L., and Welch, A. S., 1968*b*, Differential activation by restraint stress of a mechanism to conserve brain catecholamines and serotonin in mice differing in excitability, *Nature* **218**:575.

Welch, A. S., and Welch, B. L., 1968*c*, Effect of stress and parachlorphenylalanine upon brain serotonin, 5-hydroxyindoleacetic acid and catecholamines in grouped and isolated mice, *Biochem. Pharmacol.* **17**:699.

Welch, A. S., and Welch, B. L., 1968*d*, Failure of natural stimuli to accelerate brain catecholamine depletion after biosynthesis inhibition with α-methyltyrosine, *Brain Res.* **9**:402.

Welch, A. S., and Welch, B. L., 1968*e*, Reduction of norepinephrine in the lower brainstem by psychological stimulus, *Proc. Natl. Acad. Sci. (U.S.)* **60**:478.

Welch, B. L., and Welch, A. S., 1969*a*, Fighting: preferential lowering of norepinephrine and dopamine in the brainstem, concomitant with a depletion of epinephrine from the adrenal medulla, *Commun. Behav. Biol.* **3**:125.

Welch, B. L., and Welch, A. S., 1969*b*, Sustained effects of brief daily stress (fighting) upon brain and adrenal catecholamines and adrenal, spleen, and heart weights of mice, *Proc. Natl. Acad. Sci. (U.S.)* **64**:100.

Welch, B. L., and Welch, A. S., 1970, Control of brain catecholamines and serotonin during acute stress and after *d*-amphetamine by natural inhibition of monoamine oxidase: an hypothesis, in: *Amphetamines and Related Compounds*, (E. Costa and S. Garattini, eds.), pp. 415–445, Raven Press, New York.

Winson, J., and Gerlach, J. L., 1971, Stressor-induced release of substances from the rat amygdala detected by the push-pull cannula, *Nature (New Biol.)* **230**:251.

Zetterstrom, B. E. M., Palmerio, C., and Fine, J., 1964*a*, Protection of functional and vascular integrity of the spleen in traumatic shock by denervation, *Proc. Soc. Exptl. Biol. Med.* **117**:373.

Zetterstrom, B. E. M., Palmerio, C., and Fine, J., 1964*b*, Changes in tissue catecholamines in traumatic shock, *Acta Chir. Scand.* **128**:13.

Zigmond, M. J., and Harvey, J. A., 1970, Resistance to central norepinephrine depletion and decreased mortality in rats chronically exposed to electric foot-shock, *J. Neurovisc. Relat. (wien)* **31**:373.

Zigmond, M. J., and Stricker, E. M., 1972, Deficits in feeding behavior after intraventricular injection of 6-hydroxydopamine in rats, *Science* **177**:1211.

For recent, important studies that have been published since this chapter was submitted the reader is urged to consult the following references.

Braestrup, C. and Nielsen, M., 1975, Intra- and extraneuronal formation of the two major noradrenaline metabolites in the CNS of rats, *J. Pharm. Pharmacol.* (in press).

Braestrup, C., Nielsen, M., and Scheel-Kruger, J., 1974, Accumulation and disappearance of noradrenaline and its major metabolites synthesized from intraventricularly injected ³H-dopamine in the rat brain, *J. Neurochem.* **23**:569.

Caesar, P. M., Hague, P., Sharman, D. F., and Werdinius, B., 1974, Studies on the metabolism of catecholamines in the central nervous system of the mouse, *Br. J. Pharmacol.* **51**:187.

Harlow, H. F., Plubell, P. E., and Baysinger, C. M., 1973, Induction of psychological death in rhesus monkeys, *J. Autism Child, Schiz.* **3**:299.

Hendley, E. D., and Welch, B. L., 1975, Electroconvulsive shock: sustained decrease in norepinephrine uptake affinity in a reserpine model of depression, *Life Sci.* **16**:45.

Langer, S. Z., 1974, Presynaptic regulation of catecholamine release, *Biochem. Pharmacol.* **23**:1793.

Reite, M., Kaufman, I. C., Pauley, J. D., and Stynes, A. J., 1974, Depression in infant monkeys: physiological correlates, *Psychosom. Med.* **36**:363.

Roth, R. H., Walters, J. R. and Aghajanian, G. K., 1973, Effect of impulse flow on the release and synthesis of dopamine in the rat striatum, in: *Frontiers in Catecholamine Research.* (E. Usdin and S. Synder, eds.), pp. 567–574, Pergamon Press, New York.

Shopsin, B., Wilk, S., Sathananthan, G., Gershon, S., and Davis, K., 1974, Catecholamines and affective disorders revised: a critical assessment, *J. Nerv. Ment. Dis.* **158**:369.

Stolk, J. M., Conner, R. L., Levine, S., and Barchas, J. D., 1974, Brain norepinephrine metabolism and shock-induced fighting behavior in rats: differential effects of shock and fighting on the neurochemical response to a common footshock stimulus, *J. Pharmacol. Exptl. Therap.* **190**:193.

Stone, E. A., 1975, Effect of stress on sulfated glycol metabolites of brain norepinephrine, *Life Sci.* (in press).

Stone, E. A., and Mendlinger, S., 1974a, Effect of intraventricular amines on motor activity in hypothermic rats, *Res. Comm. Chem. Pathol. Pharmacol.* **7**:549.

Stone, E. A., and Mendlinger, S., 1974b, Separation of conjugated glycol metabolites of ³H-norepinephrine in the rat brain, *Anal. Biochem.* **62**:592.

Walter, D. S., and Eccleston, S., 1973, Increase of noradrenaline metabolism following electrical stimulation of the locus coeruleus in the rat, *J. Neurochem.* **21**:281.

Weiss, J. M., Glazer, H. I., and Pohorecky, L. A., 1975, Coping behavior and neurochemical changes: an alternative explanation for the original "learned helplessness" experiments, in: *Relevance of the Psychopathological Animal Model to the Human* (A. Kling and G. Serban, eds.) Plenum Press, New York (in press).

Williams, B. J., and Pirch, J. H., 1974, Correlation between brain adenyl cyclase activity and spontaneous motor activity in rats after chronic reserpine treatment, *Brain Res.* **68**:277.

Young, L. D., McKinney, W. T., Lewis, J. L., Breese, G. R., Smith, R., Mueller, A., Howard, A. J., Prange, A. J., and Lipton, M. A., 1973, Induction of adrenal catecholamine synthesizing enzymes following mother–infant separation, *Nature* **246**:94.

Chapter 3

The Catecholamines: Possible Role in Affect, Mood, and Emotional Behavior in Man and Animals

Dennis L. Murphy and D. E. Redmond, Jr.

Laboratory of Clinical Science
National Institute of Mental Health
Bethesda, Maryland

1. INTRODUCTION

Catecholamines have been considered a physiologic component of emotional behavior since Cannon (1915) suggested that increased adrenaline secretion occurred during the "flight or fight response" to a variety of stimuli. A large body of evidence has subsequently been accumulated verifying that peripheral and central nervous system catecholamines may be altered by emotionally arousing experiences. Conversely, pharmacologic and physical manipulation of catecholamine-related metabolic pathways or structures has been demonstrated to modify the expression of emotional behavior in animals, and of affect, mood, and emotional behavior in man.

While the broad outlines of the hypotheses relating catecholamines to emotional behavior and affect are generally accepted, recent data have indicated that revision and reinterpretation of some of the more circumstantial evidence are required, particularly with regard to the application of this evidence to the formulation of hypotheses regarding the affective disorders, depression and mania (Schildkraut and Kety, 1967).

This chapter will consider some of the methodological issues and limitations in the attempts to relate catecholamines to affect, mood, and emotional behavioral regulation. It will first focus on the biological strategies utilized. Second, it will review incompletely resolved problems in the assessment of affect, mood, and emotional behavior in man and animals. The information available on the nature of the catecholamine–emotional behavior relationship in man and animals will then be surveyed from the viewpoint of the methodologic limitations in the direct study of man and in the study of relevant animal models. This will include an examination of the evidence for changes in catecholamine metabolism during affect-related behavior, and of the indirect evidence from changes in behavior which occur during the administration of catecholamine-affecting drugs. A reformulation emphasizing the importance of catecholamines in the regulation of affective arousal and the expression of emotional behavior (but perhaps not in the determination of specific affects) will be presented.

2. CATECHOLAMINES AND AFFECT: HISTORICAL PERSPECTIVES

Affects such as pleasure, happiness and joy, or pain, loss, and estrangement are among the major motivating forces in human behavior. Their existence has prompted intensive study from the time of the earliest Greek philosophers. However, the origin and exact psychological and biological phenomenology of moods, affects, and emotions remain elusive. As largely subjective states, affects such as sadness, anger, contentment, and elation are difficult, it not impossible, to approach for objective quantification, the prerequisite for scientific study.

2.1. Affects, Mood, and Emotional States as Objects of Scientific Study

Affects or moods have historically been regarded in literature, philosophy, and science as central states of mind (or, originally, of "heart") which are composed of feelings or motivating dispositions rather than cognitive phenomena alone. Although the differentiation is not regularly used, affects have sometimes been considered as relatively short-lived compared to longer-enduring mood states. Emotions have more often been considered as encompassing both the central feeling state and its physiological and behavioral expression. However, because these terms are commonly used interchangeably, the more general term "affect" will be used here.

James (1884) and Lange (1885) first questioned the traditional assumptions of affects as central feeling states and suggested that the basis for emotional experience was to be found in peripheral physiologic sensations, such as those resulting from increased pulse and blood pressure, and from visceral and skeletal muscle contractions. James suggested that "bodily changes follow directly the perception of the exciting fact, and . . . our feeling of the same changes as they occur *is* the emotion" (James, 1890).

Cannon (1927) criticized this thesis on the basis of a series of experiments demonstrating that the visceral changes described by James were nonspecific accompaniments of many different emotional and nonemotional states. He reinstated a central theory suggesting that emotions are mental events which depend upon stimulus-initiated changes in the thalamus. Some subsequent neuroanatomic views of emotion have continued to relegate the central mechanism of emotion to the relatively primitive parts of the brain including the reticular formation (Lindsley, 1951), the hypothalamus (Bard, 1950) and, more specifically, the hypothalamic nuclei involved in eating, sex, and aggression (Gellhorn and Lofbourrow, 1963), and the limbic system or "visceral brain" (Papez, 1937; MacLean, 1949). More recently, the involvement of the cerebral cortex and of cortical memory and learning in emotion has been advocated by Hebb (1966) and Pribram (1967). The importance of a high level of centrally mediated activation or arousal as a characteristic of all emotion has been emphasized by both Lindsley (1951) and Hebb (1966).

Freud and some other psychoanalytic theorists have generally described emotions and affects as either instinctive, biologically based discharge states (e.g., aggression, love) or as states arising from immediate threats or conflicts between libidinal drives (e.g., anxiety, guilt) (Freud, 1925; Federn, 1936). Freud also suggested that, under some circumstances, emotions might not be felt at all, but might be confined to the realm of the unconscious, and only revealed in body movement, slips of the tongue, free associations, and dreams.

Arnold (1970) has pointed out how many theories of emotion reflect the bias of categorizing thinking (and perhaps acting) and feeling as separate states. Other theorists such as Piaget (1954, 1973), Engel (1963), and Krueger (1928) have argued that all thinking and activity emerge from a background of feeling, which they suggest is a matrix connecting other experiences, indispensable for every activity, and both involving and contributing to perception, thought, imagination, memory, learning, motivation, communication, and action. Bleuler (1932) has taken a similar theoretical position in regard to psychopathology:

> Just as those abnormalities which we call psychopathies are practically nothing but thymopathies (disturbances of affects), so affective influences play such a dominant role in psychopathology in general that practically everything else is merely incidental. Only the feeblemindednesses, the confusions and most delirious states are predominantly disturbances of intellect. But even these are colored by affective mechanisms and often in both their practical and theoretical significance are determined by affective factors.

Emotions thus have been considered as both disorganizing, disruptive forces in some circumstances, and as organizing, motivational, and communicational forces in others (Young, 1961; Leeper, 1948; Lazarus, 1966; Engel, 1963).

In the last decade, it has been suggested that the varieties of emotional experience represent a combination of nonspecific activation or arousal of varying intensity, with specification of the emotion depending upon approach or avoidance direction (Malmo, 1959; Duffy, 1962) or upon situational and social cues (Schachter and Singer, 1962). For example, Schachter and Singer (1962) administered parenteral epinephrine to subjects who variously interpreted the resulting physiologic state as widely varying "emotions" ranging from anger to anxiety and from amusement to euphoria, depending upon the immediate social cues of the epinephrine administration situation. Somewhat similarly, the wide range of affective and behavioral responses to L-dopa have been regarded as resulting from psychomotor activation or arousal mediated by catecholamines interacting with preexisting individual differences in both personality structure and current psychobiologic state (Murphy, 1972a, 1973).

2.2. Specification of the Catecholamines and of Catecholamine-Related Anatomical Sites Involved in Affect-Related Behavior

While peripherally released adrenaline (epinephrine) was early implicated as a hormone which mediated the physiologic and the emotional responses to fear and rage-inducing stimuli, most of the current interest in the biologic factors mediating affects and affect-related behavior has focused more on biogenic amine neurotransmitters, particularly norepinephrine and dopamine, in the central nervous system. Early studies demonstrating the localization of norepinephrine to the hypothalamus and portions of the limbic system (von Euler, 1956) fit well with the development of interest in these areas as the possible brain "centers" for emotion.

Recent studies using microassay and histofluorescence techniques (Fuxe et al., 1970; Hillarp et al., 1966; Ungerstedt, 1971a) have indicated that most of the cell bodies of noradrenergic and dopaminergic neurons are present in the brain stem, i.e., the medulla, pons, and mesencephalon, while their terminals extend to almost all parts of the brain and spinal cord. The most prominent noradrenergic neuronal fibers are derived from cell bodies in the locus coeruleus in the pons and the reticular formation in the medulla and ascend through the median forebrain bundle (along with some dopaminergic fibers) to terminate in widely distributed parts of the hypothalamus, most areas of the forebrain limbic system (the septal area), the preoptic area, the amygdaloid cortex, the cingulate gyrus, the nucleus interstitialis striae terminalis, and the neocortex. Major dopaminergic pathways include the large nigro-neostriatal tract and three smaller fiber bundles extending to (i) the hypophyseal capillary portal area, (ii) the tuberculum olfactorum, nucleus accumbens, and nucleus interstitialis striae terminalis, and (iii) the neocortex.

Brain lesion and electrode stimulation studies in animals have most explicitly related some noradrenergic areas, such as the septum, to alterations in exploratory activity, rage responses, and reward mechanisms (Brady and Nauta, 1953; Fried, 1972; McCleary, 1966; Stein, 1961). Other catecholamine-related brain areas possibly relevant to affects and emotional behavior include the various noradrenergic areas in the limbic and reticular activating systems which are well known for their role in arousal mechanisms (Olds, 1962; Routtenberg, 1968), and the dopaminergic meso-limbic and corpus striatum areas; lesions of the latter produce slowed psychomotor activity and Parkinsonian-type symptoms in animals and man (Hornykiewicz, 1966; 1970).

3. CATECHOLAMINES AND AFFECT: METHODOLOGIC ISSUES IN HUMAN AND ANIMAL STUDIES

The suggested relationship between catecholamines and affects, mood, and emotional behavior has proved resistant to quantitative validation because of several major methodological problems. These include (i) the apparent lack of direct linkage between one affect and one behavioral manifestation of that specific affect, (ii) the subjectivity of affective states, and (iii) the lack of simple, direct, and specific means to alter brain cate-cholamines under controlled experimental conditions.

3.1. Problems in the Assessment of Affects and Affect-Related Behavior in Man

Affects have been assessed by individual self-reports of inner feeling states or by inference from observer-scored behavior. There are major disadvantages to both types of approach. The reliability of subjective self-analysis is not directly testable, and is undoubtedly diminished by such factors as intercurrent environmental cues, by differences in the wide range of developmental experience which each person possesses, and by many other factors, including psychologic defense mechanisms and biologic variation.

Furthermore, it is well known that mixed affective states are common, and "pure," unambivalent affective states rare. It is also known that the behavioral manifestations accompanying clinical "depression" may range from slowed (retarded) speech and activity to agitated states with marked hyperactivity and anxiety; similarly, one can be "frozen" and immobile with fear or running rapidly with fright.

Nonetheless, there have been a variety of approaches to the quantitation of subjective mood and affect. Most systematic assessments of affect have relied upon pencil and paper questionnaires. Some well-known examples include the mood adjective checklist devised by Nowlis and Nowlis (1956) and Nowlis (1965), the derivative Clyde Mood Scale (1963), the MMPI (in part) (Hathaway and McKinley, 1951), and a number of other similar protocols aimed at more specific dimensions of affect. For example, depressive affect has been assessed by the inventories described by Beck *et al.* (1961), Zung (1965), and Lubin (1965; 1966). Gottschalk *et al.* (1963) have developed a systematic assessment of some affects on the basis of standardized ratings of 5-min samples of free speech.

From human subjective experience evaluated systematically in terms of the language by which 50 people described 50 different emotional states, Davitz (1969) obtained 12 affective clusters which could be grouped into four major dimensions (Table I). He suggests that all four dimensions are involved in emotional experience and may represent more primary emotions than some commonly conceived constructs for emotions, such as anxiety, depression, happiness, and anger. Whether or not these particular factors are really more appropriate than those traditionally used in our languages is not as important as the point that the construct validity of the affective dimensions commonly used has seldom been questioned or tested.

Table I.   Twelve Clusters of Human Affect Derived from Free Descriptions of Emotional Experiences

	Clusters		
Dimension[a]	Positive	Negative: type 1	Negative: type 2
Activation	Activation	Hypoactivation	Hyperactivation
Relatedness	Moving toward	Moving away	Moving against
Hedonic tone	Comfort	Discomfort	Tension
Competence	Enhancement	Incompetence: dissatisfaction	Inadequacy

[a] All four dimensions are suggested to be involved in emotional experience, and are hypothesized by Davitz (1969) to possibly represent more primary emotions than the commonly conceived constructs for emotions such as anxiety, depression, happiness and anger (reprinted by permission).

Behavioral assessment of human affective states has been most developed in relation to the study of the clinical syndromes of depression and mania. Global behavioral ratings of total clinical symptomatology are often used to describe "depression," while the contribution of the specific affects of sadness or depression relative to components of altered behavior (such as locomotor changes, guilt, etc.) may not be explicit. Multi-item scales, i.e., affect items which can be rated separately, including depression, anxiety, anger, etc., have been used in studies of psychoactive drugs. In some instances, correlations have been established between the observer-rated items and self-ratings on some of the scales listed above (Fogel et al., 1966; Zuckerman et al., 1965; Murphy et al., 1974).

An early attempt at an objective study of affects is found in Darwin's (1872) descriptions of the apparent continuity of many emotional expressions in animals and man. In this work and in later ethologic investigations, expressions of certain presumed emotions have been observed under similar circumstances in different species and appear to be manifested in similar behavioral forms. One example of this approach to the study of emotional states is Plutchik's (1962) construction of an approximation of human subjective emotional states with suggested behavioral counterparts for objective evaluation in both animals and man. Similarly, the MRC Brain Metabolism Unit Report (1972) described some examples of manifestations of behavioral categories derived from animal studies (e.g., exploratory behavior, stereotypies) in patients with mania and depression, and pointed out the appropriateness of reapplying to man not only biochemical, but also objective behavioral analyses in such studies.

3.2. Problems in the Utilization of Animal Behavioral Models for the Study of Affect-Related Behavior

Many of the inferences concerning biological contributions to affect come from studies of animals, principally rodents. Unfortunately, the animal behaviors which are easily controlled and quantified in the laboratory (Table II) are fewer in number and far less differentiated than the available human subjective interpretations drawn from a more complex human behavioral repertoire. This, of course, allows many interpretations for each of the limited animal behaviors. For example, a decrease in food-reinforced lever-pressing might be inferred to represent loss of appetite, motor retardation, general psychomotor retardation, or impairment of reward–punishment mechanisms. On the basis of analogous symptoms seen in psychiatric disorders in humans, these might be interpreted as "depression," yet might instead represent "fear," or might result from some competing behavior. "Freezing" in rats has led to the description "cata-

Table II. Animal Behaviors Utilized in the Assessment of Catecholamine-Affecting Drugs

I.   Motor activity:
    A. Locomotor or "exploratory behavior" (measured by movement in geography).
    B. Movement in place (usually measured by strain gauges).
    C. Coordination (e.g., rotarod walking).
II. Conditioned avoidance responses (passive or active).
III. Operant-appetitive behavior (lever pressing to earn food or liquid rewards).
IV. Self-stimulation behavior (electrodes implanted in brain areas).
V.   Social behavior:
    A. Fighting.
    B. Positive behavior (e.g., huddling, grooming, and play).
    C. Sexual behaviors.

tonia," carrying with it, of course, the connotation of the whole range of human behaviors described as schizophrenia. It is primarily the limited number of animal behaviors subject to outside scrutiny, and the 200 million years of evolutionary separation, which weaken these data as a direct support for catecholamine involvement in such human subjective phenomena as affects and moods.

Some of the pitfalls in evaluating the several animal models of affective states are illustrated by the minimal efficacy of L-dopa in the treatment of depressed patients. The retardation produced in rodents by catecholamine-depleting drugs had been interpreted as a model for depression, and its reversal by L-dopa was thought to implicate the catecholamines in depression, and to predict its possible clinical efficacy as an antidepressant. It was disappointing when L-dopa was tried clinically in depressed humans and was found to produce effects similar to those in mice—it "activated" them quite consistently, but it had "antidepressant" effects in only a small number of patients. This result might have been predicted if higher species and more behaviors had been examined. Cautious analysis of the changes in social behaviors in catecholamine-depleted monkeys later given L-dopa would have predicted its failure as an antidepressant, since in spite of the "activation" and increased aggression produced by L-dopa in some of the animals, none showed a reversal of the deficits in social behaviors produced by catecholamine depletion (Redmond and Maas, 1971).

A number of other approaches to the discovery of animal models for depression have been investigated. At this point, little evidence has been obtained to implicate catecholamine alterations as a mediating mechanism in these models. Following an old idea that separations are somehow etiologic in depression, the consequences of social separation, particularly of infant and young animals from their mothers, have been noted to be similar to some aspects of human depression (Seay *et al.,* 1962; Seay and Harlow, 1965; Jensen and Tolman, 1962; Hinde *et al.,* 1966; Kaufman and Rosenblum, 1967*a,b*). The closest analogies, however, appear to be with "anaclitic depression"—with infant monkeys showing stages of protest, despair, and detachment which are similar to those described in human infants by Robertson and Bowlby (1952) and Bowlby (1961). Since the syndromes both in animals and infant humans are descriptive and behavioral, the analogies are quite good. Whether there is any connection between these syndromes in human infants or monkeys and adult depression in man is not known; the differences are numerous.

Some have looked upon depression as a learned phenomenon and have called depression a state of "learned helplessness" on the basis of animal experiments showing long-term "conditioned" effects produced by an experimental situation beyond the individual's control (Overmier and Seligman, 1967; Seligman and Maier, 1967; Seligman *et al.,* 1968). Yet the behavioral evidence for this interpretation—failure to escape subsequent shock—might be explained equally well by fear or even fatigue (Brown and Jacobs, 1949; Mullin and Mogenson, 1963; Seligmen *et al.,* 1968). It is known that when people perform shock-avoidance tasks, many factors may interfere with their performance, and depression has seldom even been suggested as an explanation.

The behavioral consequences of stress also bear some similarities to depression. Besides electrical shock, other stresses such as immobilization (Richter, 1957), forced swimming (McCulloch and Bruner, 1939; Braud *et al.,* 1969), tumbling (Anderson and Paden, 1966), and defeat in combat (Ewing, 1967; Kahn, 1951) have been studied in several species, with many of these stresses producing changes in brain catecholamines (Bliss and Zwanziger, 1966). The ability to control an electrical shock by turning it off has been shown to be effective in preventing most of the consequences of an identical, but uncontrollable shock in paired monkeys (Redmond *et al.,* 1973*b*). The behavioral consequences of this uncontrollable psychologic stress in monkeys are similar to those produced by some of the catecholamine-depleting drugs, and changes in brain catecholamines in several animal species appear to be determined by the same variables. The other environmental manipulation models might also be interpreted as stresses to the subject, with separation, failure to cope with a noxious stimulus, or loss of social rank or position all being likely to produce some stress effects.

The basic approaches to an animal model—pharmacologic, traumatic separation, conditioning or learning, and stress—all may provide additional further useful leads to understanding affects and moods in humans. The power of the inferences drawn from these models may be increased by several considerations: (i) using multiple and higher species, (ii) using multiple measures of behavior, (iii) noting the effects of experimental manipulations on natural behaviors when possible, (iv) comparing the effects of drugs demonstrated to produce affective changes in humans with the specific behavioral effect in the species being studied, and finally, (iv) studying the effect in humans of drugs or treatments known to be effective in reversing the animal behavior in question.

3.3. Problems in the Experimental Manipulation of Catecholamine Metabolism

Catecholamines do not cross the blood–brain barrier, although there is some evidence that certain brain areas (e.g., the hypothalamus and area postrema) are partially permeable to circulating catecholamines (Weil-Malherbe, 1960). Generally, however, peripherally administered catecholamines have primarily peripheral effects, and central nervous system catecholamines can be altered most directly by intraventricular or parenchymal injections of catecholamines or, more physiologically, by the systemic administration of precursor substances (e.g., L-dopa) which cross the blood–brain barrier and can be metabolized to yield increased brain catecholamines. Alternatively, CNS catecholamines can be altered by giving drugs which affect catecholamine metabolism in the brain, although in most instances these same drugs also affect catecholamine metabolism in the periphery. However, recent studies indicate that even natural catecholamine precursor substances like L-dopa have non-catecholamine-related effects, for example, on serotonin metabolism and brain methyl group metabolism (Calne and Sandler, 1970; Ng et al., 1971). Most other drugs affecting catecholamines have even more complex effects, and the simple demonstration of a catecholamine change following a drug cannot be interpreted as demonstrating a causal connection between a behavioral change and the drug-produced alteration in catecholamine metabolism. However, some degree of confidence in assessing drug effects can be achieved through overlapping evidence from the combined effects of different drugs on the same system, or by the correlation of structure–activity relationships among drugs of the same class. For example, reserpine is a drug which depletes brain catecholamines and also depletes brain serotonin and histamine. However, as some of the behavioral effects of reserpine can be reversed by L-dopa and not by the corresponding precursor of brain serotonin, 5-

hydroxytryptophan, firmer evidence is provided to implicate catecholamines in the behavioral effects of reserpine (Carlsson, 1966).

Similar problems in assessing specificity occur in studies using stereotaxic lesioning, electrical stimulation, or microinjection of catecholamine in brain areas rich in catecholamine-containing nerve cell bodies or processes. All of these methods may affect other fibers which merely traverse the area as well as those which terminate there. It is doubtful whether electrical stimulation can selectively activate nuclei, since axons have a lower electrical threshold than do cell bodies. Techniques based on tissue destruction basically study the functional capacity of those parts left intact; it is an assumption that the destroyed area originally performed the altered function. Amine injection into the cerebrospinal fluid or brain parenchyma has sometimes been assumed to affect synaptic activity in much the same way as does the endogenous amine. However, the artificial flooding of small areas of brain may not mimic the effects of the minute quantities of catecholamines normally released. Furthermore, one cannot be certain that the response to the injected catecholamine results from an action on the pathways normally involved in the function being observed, or even whether the injected amine acts only at synapses where catecholamines are the physiologic "neuromediators."

An additional variable which seems especially crucial in determining the affective and behavioral effects of drugs affecting catecholamines, is the preexisting state of the person or organism. For example, the administration of tricyclic antidepressants to depressed patients is associated with a quite consistent pattern of sustained overall clinical improvement beginning after 1–3 weeks of treatment in over 75% of most depressive patient populations (Klein and Davis, 1969). In spite of this, these drugs have seldom been reported to have euphoriant effects in normal subjects, but rather only produce irritability or a few nonspecific side effects in nondepressed, normal control subjects. Other data from depressed and nondepressed subjects receiving imipramine and MAO-inhibiting drugs indicate that clinical improvement or other behavioral changes during drug treatment with these agents may not necessarily be accompanied by reductions in self-ratings of such items as "unhappy" or "depression" despite marked changes in social and work functioning (Friedman et al., 1966; Evans and Kline, 1969; Efron, 1968). It may be that a "clinical antidepressant effect" of a drug is only indirectly associated with affect-regulating mechanisms in brain. It would seem that a reexamination is required of the reductionistic association made between central biogenic amine-affecting drugs with therapeutic actions in the so-called affective disorders and an assumed direct effect of these drugs on affect.

4. AFFECT-RELATED BEHAVIOR RESULTING FROM THE ADMINISTRATION OF CATECHOLAMINES AND CATECHOLAMINE-ALTERING DRUGS

4.1. Effects of Directly Administered Catecholamines

It is of some interest in regard to the original peripherally based James–Lange theory of emotion that intravenous or subcutaneous injections of epinephrine have the capacity to alter self-rated affect states in man. Similarly administered norepinephrine and dopamine do not appear to produce such changes.

In early studies (Maranon, 1924; Cantril and Hunt, 1932; Landis and Hunt 1932; Pollin and Goldin, 1962) subjective impressions accompanying epinephrine injections were categorized. Most individuals described physical symptoms, including increased arousal; approximately one-third of the subjects also reported emotional responses, especially anxiety. However, many of these emotional responses were described as only similar to other emotional experiences ("cold," "as if" emotions) and were considered different from normal emotional experiences.

Suspecting that cognitive factors in the interpretation of the epinephrine injection experience might be responsible for the "as if" quality of the responses, Schachter and Singer (1962) designed a series of experiments combining epinephrine injections with varying social cueing situations. During the course of performing tests to purportedly measure the effects of a drug (actually epinephrine or placebo) on visual performance, subjects were exposed to social stimuli designed to elicit either anger or euphoria. Behavioral ratings indicated that epinephrine injections were associated with a twofold intensification of the anger-related, observed behavior elicited when compared to placebo injections; self-ratings suggested similar differences, but were not statistically significant. The difference in behavioral ratings was even greater when the responses of the subjects who were completely blind to the nature of the injections were compared to those who had been told to expect to feel the physiologic effects of epinephrine, such as heart pounding and flushing. Similar differences were observed in the euphoria-inducing situation between the informed and uninformed epinephrine subjects, although in this situation the placebo-treated subjects responded nearly as much to the social cues as did the uninformed subjects.

A replication study by Schachter and Wheeler (1962) using a comedy movie as the cue situation revealed that amusement responses were greatest in epinephrine-treated subjects, less in those receiving a placebo injection, and even less in those receiving an injection of 25 mg of chlorpromazine.

This evidence suggests, at a minimum, that in a given social situation, the degree of emotional responsivity can be influenced by peripheral autonomic arousal produced by circulating epinephrine. Furthermore, this evidence is compatible with other suggestions that affect and emotional behavior may consist of two principal ingredients, a state of heightened sympathetic activation or arousal, and a specific cognitive state dependent upon external cues or internal frames of reference which qualifies how the affect or emotion is labeled, i.e., whether it is felt as elation, anxiety, anger, or some other affective state (Hunt *et al.,* 1958; Schachter and Singer, 1962). As a corollary it should be noted that high levels of arousal *per se* need not be associated with subjective change in affect or change in emotional behavior. Data from a study demonstrating a decrease in self-reported emotionality of all types in direct proportion to higher levels of spinal cord injury would seem to support this two-factor hypothesis, since higher level lesions result in proportionately less intact sympathetic innervation in body areas (Hohman, 1966). Although there are some studies which indicate some differentiation in the physiological accompaniments of different emotional states, these differences are generally slight and have high subject-to-subject variability (Ax, 1953; Schachter, 1957; Frankenhaeuser *et al.,* 1968).

4.2. Effects of Catecholamine Precursors and Catecholamine Synthesis-Inhibiting Drugs

4.2.1. L-*Dopa*

As the precursor of dopamine and norepinephrine, this amino acid has been given to Parkinsonian patients, depressed patients, and some other groups of individuals, including normal controls. Little detailed information concerning changes in affect or emotional behavior is available from the studies of normals, although most studies have concluded that this drug in moderate doses has relatively minimal effects on normal individuals (Barbeau, 1969; Ansel and Markham, 1970; Klawans *et al.,* 1972).

In Parkinsonian patients, changes in some self-rating and other psychological test instruments have regularly been found to accompany treatment with L-dopa. However, the separation of a direct drug effect on affect from the psychosocial consequences of improved motor functioning is a formidable task in patients with a chronic disorder. Thus, decreased depression ratings (O'Brien *et al.,* 1971) may represent a primary drug effect, or may only reflect the global clinical improvement produced by the drug or a combination of both. However, there have been some indications that a general alerting or awakening effect associated with increased interest in the environment may occur prior to motor improvement, and that this may represent a separable phenomenon from peripheral motor effects of the drug (Murphy, 1972a, 1973). Other possible affect-related behavioral changes which have been observed in Parkinsonian patients during L-dopa treatment include anger, irritability, anxiety, agitation, depression, hostility, paranoid ideation, hypersexuality, and hypomania (Murphy, 1973).

Depressed patients have received L-dopa in short-term studies utilizing intraveneous doses of the drug which occasionally led to brief remissions of depressive symptomatology (Degwitz et al., 1960; Klerman et al., 1963; Matussek et al., 1966; Turner and Merlis, 1964). In one longer-term, oral dosage, double-blind study (Goodwin et al., 1970), a small proportion of patients hospitalized for depression (25%) improved during L-dopa administration. A few suffered relapses during placebo substitution. The other patients remained depressed despite L-dopa doses as high as 12 g/day. Unimproved depressed patients developed increased anger and psychosis ratings on a quantitative behavioral scale, although the increased psychotic behavior occurred only in individuals who had pretreatment evidence of psychosis. Of nine depressed patients with histories of mania (bipolar patients), eight developed brief hypomanic episodes during L-dopa treatment (Murphy et al., 1971). In contrast, unipolar depressed patients (those without a history of mania) did not develop hypomania during treatment with equal doses of L-dopa. The occurrence of hypomania was dose-related and was associated with relatively greater urinary dopamine excretion in bipolar compared to the unipolar patients (Murphy et al., 1973). Unfortunately, mood self-ratings were not available in this study.

Large doses of L-dopa given to animals generally produce enhanced motor activity and conditioned avoidance responding, as well as stereotyped movements and compulsive gnawing behavior (Everett and Wiegand, 1962; Randrup and Munkvad, 1966a; Scheckel et al., 1969.). L-Dopa in combination with peripheral decarboxylase inhibitors or inhibitors of monoamine oxidase yields increased motor activity, sometimes accompanied by increased aggressiveness and rage in the case of L-dopa-MAOI combinations (Butcher and Engel, 1969; Reis et al., 1970). Biogenic amine depletion by reserpine, α-methyl-p-tyrosine and p-chlorophenylalanine appear to sensitize the animal to behavioral stimulation by L-dopa (Everett and Wiegand, 1962, Scheckel et al., 1969; Scheel-Kruger and Randrup, 1967). Tricyclic antidepressants also potentiate some behavioral effects of L-dopa, including aggressiveness and irritability, while phenothiazines and the butyrophenones antagonize the stimulant effects of L-dopa, most likely by a direct dopamine receptor-blocking effect (Carlsson, 1959; Carlsson and Lindqvist, 1963).

L-Dopa administration in animals leads to marked elevations of brain dopamine, with much smaller and variable changes in norepinephrine (Everett and Wiegand, 1962; Butcher and Engel, 1969). However, it appears that a good share of dopamine formed from L-dopa is synthesized in nondopaminergic neurons (as evidenced, for example, by the displacement and loss of serotonin from serotonin-containing neurons) (Ng *et al.*, 1971). Thus, while the prevailing view remains that the antiparkinsonian effects of L-dopa are directly related to dopamine replacement (Hornykiewicz, 1970), and, correspondingly, that the behavioral effects of L-dopa in man and animals are the consequence of increased dopaminergic tract activity, it is also possible that some behavioral effects of L-dopa result from other mechanisms. Interference with cholinergic, serotonergic, and noradrenergic as well as other mechanisms, or changes in the balance between catecholaminergic and other neurotransmitter systems may result from L-dopa administration (Scheckel *et al.*, 1969; Calne and Sandler, 1970; Wurtman *et al.*, 1970; Weintraub and van Woert, 1971). It is noteworthy that L-dopa increases locomotor activity in rats even after the majority of catecholaminergic neurons have been selectively destroyed by 6-hydroxydopamine (Uretsky and Schoenfeld, 1971). Denervation-type receptor hypersensitivity to L-dopa, and also to apomorphine and norepinephrine, develops after 6-hydroxydopamine treatment (Ungerstedt, 1971*a*, 1971*b*, 1971*c*; Haeusler *et al.*, 1969), and may well be present in patients with Parkinson's disease.

4.2.2. α-Methyl-p-Tyrosine (AMPT)

This drug is a potent and specific inhibitor of tyrosine hydroxylase, the rate-limiting enzyme in the biosynthesis of dopamine and norepinephrine (Spector *et al.*, 1965). In studies in man, AMPT has been administered to nonpsychiatric patients with pheochromocytoma, essential hypertension, and other medical diagnoses, in oral doses of 11–73 mg/kg per day, producing CNS effects, predominantly sedation and fatigue, in 44 of 46 patients (Engelman *et al.*, 1968). In this study, three of six patients who had a previous history of "psychic depression" required discontinuation of the drug due to "agitated depression." In another study, nine schizophrenic patients with a mean maximum dose of 16 mg/kg showed no consistent changes in psychiatric ratings: only daytime sedation effects were reported, with no additional comment about affective or mood changes (Gershon *et al.*, 1967). In another study, 17 "mentally ill" patients (mostly schizophrenics) received AMPT (30 mg/kg for 33 to 42 days); half became "worse," and sedation was the principal side effect (Charalampous and Brown, 1967). In a study in manic-depressive patients treated with 30–60 mg/kg AMPT, five of the seven manic patients became less manic; all three depressed patients became more depressed, with increased agitation, anxiety, and increased psychomotor activity (Brodie *et al.*, 1971).

In animals, AMPT reduces spontaneous locomotor activity, rotarod performance, and conditioned avoidance responses (Weissman and Koe, 1965; Corrodi and Hanson, 1966; Hanson, 1965; Moore, 1966; Rech *et al.*, 1966, 1968). These effects are reversed by pretreatment with monoamine oxidase-inhibiting drugs (Moore and Rech, 1967) and L-dopa (Corrodi and Hanson, 1966; Hanson, 1967*a*). The central alerting effects of amphetamine (Dominic and Moore, 1969; Weissman *et al.*, 1966; Rech and Moore, 1968; Menon *et al.*, 1967; Stolk and Rech, 1970), morphine (Menon *et al.*, 1967), LSD (Horita and Hamilton, 1969), alcohol (Menon *et al.*, 1967), mescaline (Menon *et al.*, 1967), cocaine (Menon *et al.*, 1967), and desipramine (Menon *et al.*, 1967) are also reduced by AMPT; this evidence has been suggested to implicate the catecholamines in the mechanisms of action of this diverse group of affect-altering drugs. In nonhuman primates, AMPT (200 mg/kg) produces a decrease in all types of social behaviors, both hostile–aggressive and positive (Redmond *et al.*, 1971*a,b*). The animals typically sit huddled in a corner with their heads directed downward and their eyes drooping, showing responses to, but diminished interest in, their social surroundings. Their faces are blank and masklike, and their motor movements are generally retarded. L-Dopa in large doses (100 mg/kg iv) produces a striking activation of animals concurrently treated with AMPT, but does not return their social behavior or appearance to normal (Redmond and Maas, 1971). They pace rapidly, scan, and alert to nonapparent, environmental cues, and make continuous chewing and gnawing movements. Similarly, oral treatment with L-dopa (400 mg/kg) is unsuccessful in restoring normal social behavior, although small doses of the MAO inhibitor, tranylcypromine, are effective in returning these AMPT-treated monkeys to apparently normal behavioral patterns (Redmond, 1975).

4.3. Effects of Other Drugs Which Alter Catecholamine Metabolism

4.3.1. 6-Hydroxydopamine

This drug is a catecholamine analog which selectively destroys catecholamine nerve terminals (Bloom *et al.*, 1969; Uretsky and Iversen, 1970; Laverty and Taylor, 1970; Breese and Traylor, 1970, 1971; Heikkila and Cohen, 1971). Intraventricular administration of 6-hydroxydopamine in rodents causes appetite disruptions and motor dysfunction, and reduces conditioned avoidance responses, depending on the site of administration (Ungerstedt, 1971*a,b*). Monkeys treated with it show very similar behavioral effects to those treated with AMPT, even though the neuronal lesions are strictly in the CNS instead of in the whole body, as is the case after systemic AMPT administration (Redmond *et al.*, 1972, 1973*b*; Maas *et al.*, 1972*a*, 1973).

4.3.2. α-Methyl-Dopa

α-Methyl-dopa is a weak aromatic amino acid decarboxylase inhibitor which appears to exert its effects in decreasing blood pressure by the formation of α-methylated amine metabolites (Sjoerdsma *et al.*, 1963). It also produces a depletion of brain amines, but much less than that produced by AMPT (Hess *et al.*, 1961; Sourkes *et al.*, 1961). In man, "depression" is said to be a possible side effect, but occurs as a clinical syndrome only uncommonly at the dose ranges (10–20 mg/kg per day) which are effective in reducing blood pressure (Dubach, 1963; Fullerton and Morton-Jenkins, 1963; Hamilton and Kopelman 1963, Smirk, 1963; McKinney and Kane, 1967). At much larger doses in animals (120 mg/kg per day, or more) it produces many of the same effects as AMPT (Ray and Bivens, 1965*a*; 1965*b*).

4.3.3. Amphetamine

This drug affects the release, uptake, and metabolism of catecholamines; it also has some direct effects on catecholamine receptors (Randup and Munkvad, 1966*b*; Hanson, 1967*b*; Goodman and Gilman, 1965). Serotonin receptors may also be affected (Innes, 1963). However, its actions appear to depend upon the presence of newly synthesized catecholamines, and it remains an important drug in the evaluation of the behavioral effects of the catecholamines. Its well-documented multiple effects, not only on emotional behavior and mood, but also on locomotor activity, learning, and food and water intake, illustrate another issue in the evaluation of catecholamines on mood, i.e., drug effects on other forms of motivated behavior may well interact in the production of affect- and emotion-related behavioral changes.

In man, oral or intravenous amphetamines produce increased activation, euphoria, variable changes in intellectual performance, and, in psychiatric patients, short-lived antidepressant effects. A period of fatigue sometimes accompanied by dysphoria, often follows the period of stimulation (Weiss and Laties, 1962). Amphetamines are not successfully used in the treatment of clinical depression because of their lack of sustained efficacy during continued administration (Ban, 1969). However, individual differences in response to amphetamine may have predictive value for tricyclic antidepressant drug treatment, with a positive correlation reported between amphetamine and imipramine responses in a small group of depressed patients (Fawcett and Siomopoulos, 1971). As with the tricyclic antidepressants (Schou, 1963), there exist reports of antimanic efficacy of the drug (Kulscar, 1966). The euphoriant and activating effects in man are blocked by α-methyl-p-tyrosine (Jonsson et al., 1971) and lithium carbonate (van Kammen and Murphy, 1974).

While the amphetamines are commonly categorized as stimulants and euphoriants, it is noteworthy that their subjective effects are quite variable and range from stimulation and euphoria to sedation and dysphoria (Lasagna et al., 1955; Felsinger et al., 1955). In particular, discrepancies have frequently been noted between the subjective effects of amphetamine and its behavioral effects as rated by observers (Lasagna et al., 1955; Smith and Beecher, 1964). Correct classification of amphetamine sulfate ("a stimulant") compared to secobarbital ("a depressant") and placebo ranged from only 28% to 50% in some large studies of normals (Lasagna et al., 1955; Hurst et al., 1973). In a study in prisoners, subjective assessments of being "relaxed" was the most prevalent response to amphetamine, exceeding by far other responses relating to "drive" or "nervousness" (Martin et al. 1971). The effectiveness of the amphetamines in calming hyperactive children remains an incompletely understood phenomenon, despite some more extensive advances in the last several years (Sroufe and Stewart, 1973; Arnold et al., 1973).

4.3.4. The Tricyclic Antidepressants

Imipramine, amitriptyline, and related drugs constitute one of the cornerstones of the evidence implicating biogenic amines in depression and mania. Their common biochemical effect is the inhibition of monoamine reuptake mechanisms, and their status as the most effective group of clinical antidepressant drugs has most often been explained in terms of an increase in the effective concentration of amine neurotransmitters in the synaptic cleft.

However, this direct link between behavioral–clinical effects and a biochemical mechanism has been confounded by a number of issues: (i) biochemically, these agents inhibit indoleamine as well as catecholamine reuptake; this fact provides support equal to the advocacy of an indoleamine hypothesis of the affective disorders (Lapin and Oxenkrug, 1969); (ii) they also possess some anticholinergic activity, and recently it has been suggested again that this effect contributes to their antidepressant efficacy (Janowsky et al., 1972); (iii) like the phenothiazine drugs, which they resemble in chemical structure, the tricyclics also possess receptor-blocking properties (iv) structure–activity relationships do not demonstrate a close correlation of antidepressant efficacy with uptake-inhibiting properties (Lahti and Maickel, 1971); (v) their ability to inhibit amine uptake is an immediate effect, while clinical antidepressant effects often require 2–3 weeks time; (vi) in normals, the tricyclic drugs have no euphoriant properties; in particular, their infrequent acute effects in normals are predominantly sedative and dysphoriant; (vii) in depressed patients, it is noteworthy that the small amount of data from subjective mood checklists do not indicate that these drugs have more than a slight effect on mood, despite their marked beneficial effects on the clinical syndrome of depression (Friedman *et al.*, 1966).

4.3.5. Reserpine

Pharmacological observations concerning reserpine and iproniazid in the late 1950's originally led to the hypotheses relating catecholamines and the affective disorders. Reserpine, used as an antihypertensive agent and as a tranquilizer in excited psychoses, was reported to cause depression in some patients (Muller *et al.*, 1955; Lemieux *et al.*, 1956; Harris, 1957) and to lead to depletion of norepinephrine and serotonin. Many subsequent reports of depressive symptomatology have followed these initial observations, although the authenticity of the milder "depressions" has been questioned (Ayd, 1958; Bernstein and Kaufman, 1960), and it has been suggested that clinically significant depressions occur predominantly in individuals with previous, spontaneous depressive episodes (Goodwin *et al.*, 1971).

In rodents, reserpine leads to reduced locomotor activity and reduced conditioned avoidance responding (Carlsson *et al.*, 1957; Graeff *et al.*, 1965; McGer *et al.*, 1963; Wada *et al.*, 1963; Brodie, 1965), a sedated state which has been suggested as an animal model of human depression. L-Dopa reverses many of the behavioral effects of reserpine, whereas the serotonin precursor, 5-hydroxytryptophan restores motor activity less effectively (Carlsson, 1966; Graeff *et al.*, 1965; McGer *et al.*, 1963; Wada *et al.*, 1963). This fact led to the conclusion that reserpine-induced behavioral changes were related more to catecholamines than to serotonin, and reserpine reversal was used for the screening of drugs as potential antidepressant agents. Animals pretreated with monoamine oxidase inhibitors and tricyclic antidepressants manifest behavioral excitation on reserpine administration, thought to result from the acute release of catecholamines onto receptors (Scheckel and Boff, 1964; Sulser *et al.*, 1964).

4.3.6. Monoamine Oxidase-Inhibiting Drugs

A heterogeneous group of drugs inhibit this degradatory enzyme for monoamines, and also possess other actions, such as uptake inhibition and possible direct receptor stimulation effects. MAO inhibition itself results in multiple secondary effects, including alterations in the balance between neurotransmitters and "false transmitter" amines in tissues, as well as alterations in amine synthesis, so that it is quite difficult to allocate the behavioral and mood effects of any MAO inhibitor to a specific change in catecholamines (Costa and Sandler, 1972).

In man, the MAO inhibitors are variably effective in depressed patients, and certainly do not possess as broad a spectrum of efficacy as the tricyclic antidepressants (Cole and Davis, 1967; Klein and Davis, 1969). In studies of medical patients with tuberculosis and hypertension as well as in some studies of psychiatric patients, a fairly high incidence of behavioral toxicity has been reported, with dominant effects including excess stimulation, insomnia, and, in some instances, the precipitation of hypomania, mania, or psychosis. In a study of female depressed patients which utilized mood self-ratings, the MAO-inhibiting drug iproniazid resulted in increased "energetic" and "friendly" ratings, decreased MMPI depression and psychasthenia (anxiety) ratings, and increased motor or verbal activity with increased reaction time, in comparison to placebo (Wittenborn, 1961). Interestingly, a study with imipramine carried out in a similar patient group by the same investigator did not reveal similar behavioral and mood effects (Wittenborn, 1962).

4.3.7. Phenothiazines, Butyrophenones, and Propranolol

These drugs are catecholamine receptor-blocking drugs, although their many other cellular actions (especially in the case of the phenothiazines) have been investigated for possible relevance to their behavioral effects. The phenothiazines and butyrophenones have predominantly sedative effects in animals, and block a large number of stimulant drug effects (Brucke *et al.*, 1969). Besides their status as the most effective antipsychotic agents in man, which has been suggested to correlate best with their dopamine receptor-blocking properties (Snyder and Banerjee, 1973), they have been demonstrated to be effective in mania and, recently, in depression. Although the initial studies in depressed patients were in a limited and somewhat atypical patient group, other studies have since suggested that thioridazine and chlorpromazine may equal the tricyclic drugs in antidepressant efficacy (Hollister, 1973). In contrast to the phenothiazines and butyrophenones, which have predominant α-adrenergic receptor and dopamine receptor-blocking properties, propranolol is a β-adrenergic receptor-blocking agent. Propranolol has been reported to possess sedative properties in animals, and antianxiety effects in man (Wheatley, 1969).

4.3.8. Lithium Carbonate

Lithium has diverse biochemical effects. It decreases catecholamine release, inhibits reuptake, alters catecholamine metabolism, and possesses α-adrenergic receptor-blocking properties in animals and man (Schildkraut, 1973b; Murphy et al., 1973). However, it has equal, if not more prominent effects, on serotonin metabolism. It also directly blocks the effects of many hormones, and alters other metabolic processes via its effects on electrolyte metabolism (Shopsin and Gershon, 1973). Behaviorally, lithium has profound antimanic effects, as well as moderate antidepressant and marked stabilizing, prophylactic effects in bipolar patients with recurrent manic and depressive cycles (Schou, 1968; Shopsin and Gershon, 1973).

Lithium does not affect spontaneous motor activity in animals (Ljungberg and Paalzow, 1969), or self-stimulation behavior in rats with electrodes implanted in the median forebrain bundle (Ramsey et al., 1972). However, lithium shares some characteristics with antidepressant drugs in partially antagonizing the hypothermic effect of reserpine and the "depression" in motor activity produced by tetrabenazine (Perkinson et al., 1969). Lithium also antagonizes foot-shock-induced aggression in rats (Sheard, 1970), and the biogenic amine-mediated excitatory state produced by tetrabenazine combined with desipramine (Matussek and Linsmayer, 1968) as well as the excitation produced by morphine (Carroll and Sharp, 1971).

However, lithium has minimal effects on emotional behavior and mood in individuals without "affective disorders." Although decreased self-rated anger and observer-rated aggressive behavior was recorded in one study of male prisoners (Sheard, 1971), lithium has generally been found to lack sedative properties in normals and antipsychotic properties in psychotic patients (Schou, 1968). In studies of normal students and psychiatric investigators treated with 25 mEq/day, self-rated mood (including depression, elation, irritability, enthusiasm–apathy, and energy–tiredness dimensions) only tiredness was more prominently scored during lithium treatment, while mood level and emotional range were unaffected. However, with larger dosage (50 mEq/day) some subjective indifference, passivity and a "feeling of being at a distance" were noted, although no objective behavioral changes occurred (Schou, 1968).

5. ALTERATIONS IN CATECHOLAMINE METABOLISM RESULTING FROM AFFECT-RELATED BEHAVIOR

Many experiments have demonstrated that urinary catecholamine excretion in man and in animals may be altered by physically and psychologically stressful situations. In addition, some experiments have suggested that different kinds of stress may be correlated with relative differences in the amounts of norepinephrine *vs.* epinephrine excreted (Mason *et al.*, 1960; Silverman *et al.*, 1961; Levi, 1965). The most extensive body of catecholamine-related data are from studies of patients with the so-called affective disorders, depression and mania. These studies have been reviewed in detail elsewhere (Schildkraut and Kety, 1967; Weil-Malherbe and Szara, 1971; Davis, 1970; Schildkraut, 1973*b*; Goodwin and Murphy, 1974) and can only be summarized here.

Some effects of environmental manipulations thought to be associated with changes in affect have been demonstrated to be related to changes in catecholamines. Mice housed in group cages and thus exposed to social stimulation have higher levels of brain norepinephrine than isolated mice (Axelrod *et al.*, 1970; Welch and Welch, 1971). Operant conditioning tasks lead to increased brain catecholamines (Lewy and Seiden, 1972), while inescapable shock or stress leads to decreased catecholamine levels (Weiss *et al.*, 1970). It has been suggested from studies of nonhuman primates that similar manipulations affecting brain catecholamines may lead to social behavioral changes which represent an essential component of depression–withdrawal states in animals and perhaps in humans (Redmond *et al.*, 1973*a*).

5.1. Direct Measurement of Catecholamines in Depression

The combined information from many studies of depressed and cycling manic-depressive patients can be summarized as follows: Depressed patients may have either decreased, normal, or increased urinary norepinephrine, epinephrine, normetanephrine, metanephrine, and 3-methoxy-4-hydroxy mandelic acid (VMA) excretion during their depressed periods in comparison to normals or patients studied while in remission or when manic. More studies have found increased rather than decreased urinary catecholamines and their metabolites in depressed patients (Bergsman, 1959; Bond *et al.*, 1972; Campanini *et al.*, 1970; Curtis *et al.*, 1960; Greenspan *et al.*, 1969, 1970; Rubin *et al.*, 1968; Sloane *et al.*, 1966; Takahashi *et al.*, 1968; Weil-Malherbe, 1967; Maas *et al.*, 1968, 1972*b*; Schildkraut, 1973; Schildkraut *et al.*, 1971). However, in studies of patients described as "manic-depressive" (that is a group including, often, more bipolar than unipolar patients, and generally more "endogenous" depressed patients), relatively lower catecholamine excretion has been reported during depressed periods compared to periods of remission or manic periods (Bond *et al.*, 1972; Bunney *et al.*, 1970; Greenspan *et al.*, 1969; Shinfuku *et al.*, 1961;

Shinfuku, 1965; Sloane et al., 1966; Strom-Olsen and Weil-Malherbe, 1958; Takahashi et al., 1968).

Increased catecholamines during depression are frequently suggested to be associated with the presence of agitation, anxiety, and psychosis (Bunney et al., 1967; Greenspan et al., 1970; Nelson et al., 1966; Schildkraut et al., 1965; Sloane et al., 1966; Weil-Malherbe, 1967). It is noteworthy that psychomotor retardation during depression is more characteristic of bipolar than unipolar patients, raising the possibility that variations in physical activity, as well as anxious, stressful concomitants associated with the depressed state may be contributory to some of the differing catecholamine excretion results found in studies of heterogeneous groups of depressed patients. Further evidence of the possible contribution of anxiety to altered catecholamines in depressed patients can be found in the first investigation of plasma catecholamines in depressed patients accomplished with a sensitive method adequate to measure accurately the small concentrations of amines in blood. In this study, depressed and anxious patients were found to have elevated plasma catecholamines compared to normals, and catecholamine concentrations correlated more closely with anxiety ratings than with depression ratings (Wyatt et al., 1971).

A major problem in the interpretation of the meaning of these changes in urinary and plasma catecholamines in depressed patients is that they primarily reflect changes in the peripheral sympathetic nervous system and the adrenal medulla. However, among the different catecholamine metabolites found in urine, 3-methoxy-4-hydroxyphenylglycol (MHPG) has been suggested to be preferentially formed in brain and capable of being transported into the periphery. It is not unlikely, then, that measurement of the urinary excretion of MHPG, up to 50% of which is possibly derived from brain, provides a better index of central catecholamine metabolism, although not all of the evidence is in full agreement (Chase et al., 1971; Maas et al., 1972a, 1973; Maas and Landis, 1968; Schanberg et al., 1968a,b).

Urinary excretion of MHPG has been found more uniformly decreased in some groups of depressed patients than is the case with other catecholamine metabolites (Bond et al., 1972; Greenspan et al., 1970; Maas et al., 1968; 1972b; Prange et al., 1972; Schildkraut et al., 1971; Jones et al., 1973). It has also been suggested that pretreatment urinary MHPG excretion may be predictive of tricyclic antidepressant drug responses (Maas et al., 1972b; Schildkraut et al., 1971). However, low levels of MHPG were found predictive of responses to imipramine or desipramine in one study (Maas et al., 1972b), while higher levels of MHPG correlated with an antidepressant response to amitriptyline (a tricyclic) in another study (Schildkraut et al., 1971). The basis for these apparently differing results is not yet clear, although there are some biochemical data indicating that different tricyclic antidepressants vary in their relative inhibiting effects on norepinephrine versus serotonin uptake and in their receptor-blocking properties (Carlsson *et al.*, 1969). Moreover, it appears that amitriptyline has relatively greater clinical sedative effects than imipramine, a difference which appears to be correlated with EEG response differences (Saletu *et al.*, 1973).

Cerebrospinal fluid MHPG levels have been reported as reduced in depressed patients (Gordon and Oliver, 1971; Post *et al.*, 1973), although a smaller study demonstrated no differences (Wilk *et al.*, 1972). Several studies have found reduced levels of homovanillic acid (HVA), the major metabolite of dopamine, in cerebrospinal fluid of depressed patients (Roos and Sjostrom, 1969; Papeschi and McClure, 1971; Goodwin and Sack, 1973), although in one study this alteration was found only in patients with psychomotor retardation (van Praag and Korf, 1971).

5.2. Direct Measurement of Catecholamines in Mania

Evidence concerning drugs capable of altering behavior and mood has led to the suggestion that mania is related to excess activity of central norepinephrine neurons (Schildkraut, 1965; Schildkraut and Kety, 1967). Early investigations of urinary catecholamines had generally indicated elevated norepinephrine and epinephrine excretion in hypomanic and manic patients, especially when manic and depressed phases were compared in cycling patients (Greenspan *et al.*, 1969, 1970; Rubin *et al.*, 1970; Schildkraut *et al.*, 1965; Schildkraut and Durrell, 1971; Shinfuku *et al.*, 1961; Strom-Olsen and Weil-Malherbe, 1958; Takahashi *et al.*, 1968). However, interpretation of these results is confounded by the preponderant contribution of the peripheral autonomic nervous system and the adrenal gland (as opposed to brain) to urinary catecholamines and catecholamine metabolites. Moreover, marked alterations in physical activity regularly accompany manic behavior, and physical activity itself can elevate urinary and even cerebrospinal fluid amines and their metabolites. However, the relevance of these observations can by no means be dismissed, since catecholamine excretion in disproportionate excess to pedometer-measurement motor activity has been observed in some studies of mania (Takahashi *et al.*, 1968), and, as noted above, one catecholamine metabolite, MHPG, has been suggested to yield an estimate of central nervous system catecholamine activity (Maas *et al.*, 1972*b*).

The period of transition between depression and mania (the "switch period") or the period between depression and normality has been found to be accompanied by an increased excretion of catecholamines and their metabolites (Bond *et al.*, 1972; Bunney *et al.*, 1970 1972*b,c* Shinfuku, 1965; Axelrod, 1966; Kopin and Gordon, 1962, 1963; Maas *et al.*, 1972*b*; Prange *et al.*, 1972; Greenspan *et al.*, 1969). In some instances, these changes have preceded the complete behavioral change, although drug effects, sleep variations, and early behavioral changes may have contributed to the catecholamine alterations observed in these studies.

More recently, increased urinary dopamine excretion has also been reported in manic patients (Messiha, 1970; Sloane *et al.*, 1966; Strom-Olsen and Weil-Malherbe, 1958). While it is suggested that dopamine excretion in urine is little affected by muscular work (Haggendal and Werdinius, 1966), no confirmatory evidence of increased brain dopamine release in manics was obtained from studies of the principal metabolite of dopamine, homovanillic acid (HVA), in the cerebrospinal fluid; HVA levels have not generally been found to be any higher in manic patients compared to depressed patients or controls (Roos and Sjostrom, 1969). However, one more recent study observed higher cerebrospinal fluid HVA levels during mania, although these levels were not as high as those found to be associated with increased physical and mental activity (Post *et al.*, 1973). MHPG was not regularly elevated in the cerebrospinal fluid of manic patients, although a few patients had high levels (Post *et al.*, 1973; Wilk *et al.*, 1972). It was also demonstrated that physical activity and "simulated mania" could yield cerebrospinal fluid MHPG elevations (Post *et al.*, 1973; Post and Goodwin, 1973), further indicating the difficulties in evaluating catecholamine changes in this disorder.

5.3. Nonspecific Factors Including Physical Activity as Variables in the Study of Catecholamines in Man

Physical activity as well as stress may contribute to altered catecholamine metabolism and to increased catecholamine levels in urine and cerebrospinal fluid (Rubin *et al.*, 1968; Karki, 1956). However, it has been noted in several studies that casual comparisons of agitated versus retarded depressed patient groups did not suggest differences in catecholamine excretion in these groups. One attempt to correlate pedometer-assessed motor activity with urinary catecholamine metabolite excretion in a cycling manic-depressive patient did not reveal a close correspondence between these two variables (Takahashi *et al.*, 1968). Furthermore, evidence from a study in which agitated depressed patients had reduced MHPG excretion but elevated levels of norepinephrine and other catecholamine metabolites suggests that MHPG, at least, may be relatively less affected by conditions producing increased peripheral autonomic activity (Greenspan *et al.*, 1970).

However, stress and anxiety as well as motor activity changes in short-term experimental situations have clearly been shown to affect urinary MHPG excretion to some extent (Maas *et al.*, 1971; Rubin *et al.*, 1970).

Other nonspecific factors which variably accompany depression in different individuals include (i) alterations in food and water intake, sometimes leading to marked weight changes, (ii) sleep disturbances, and (iii) hormone alterations (Weil-Malherbe and Szara, 1971). The effects of these factors on catecholamine metabolism have not yet been studied systematically or in sufficient detail to permit evaluation of their possible contribution to biogenic amine changes in depression.

5.4. Studies of Catecholamine-Related Enzymes in Patients with Depression and Mania

Monoamine oxidase (MAO), catechol-O-methyltransferase, and dopamine-β-hydroxylase are involved in the synthesis or metabolism of biogenic amines in neuronal tissues. These enzymes (or closely related isoenzymes) are also found in accessible peripheral tissues and have therefore been studied in patients with psychiatric disorders.

A form of MAO, quite similar to one form (Type B) of mitochondrial MAO from brain, exists in blood platelets and appears to be a stable, genetically regulated characteristic of the individual (Nies *et al.*, 1973; Murphy, 1973). The occurrence of higher platelet and plasma MAO activity in a mixed group of depressed patients (Nies *et al.*, 1971), and higher MAO levels in women and in older individuals (Robinson *et al.*, 1972) was interpreted as suggesting a possible relationship between MAO activity and the higher incidence of depression in females and in older individuals. Patients with bipolar depression have lower activities of platelet MAO compared to unipolar patients and normal controls (Murphy and Weiss, 1972). As biogenic amine synthesis may be suppressed and alternative biogenic amine neurotransmitterlike substances, such as octopamine, may accumulate in situations in which monoamine oxidase activity is reduced (Kopin, 1968), the possibility of false neurotransmitter effects has been suggested as yet another potential catecholamine alteration capable of contributing to depressive behavior (Murphy, 1972*b*).

Catechol-O-methyltransferase (COMT), the enzyme responsible for the extraneuronal methylation of the catecholamines and their derivitives (Axelrod and Tomchick, 1958), is found in many peripheral tissues including the red blood cell (Axelrod and Cohn, 1971). Erythrocyte COMT has been reported as reduced in female depressed patients compared to normal females or to female controls with other psychiatric or neurological diagnoses (Cohn *et al.*, 1970). Furthermore, it was noted that among the depressed females, red cell COMT was significantly lower in the unipolar as compared to the bipolar group (Dunner *et al.*, 1971).

Dopamine-β-hydroxylase (DBH), the enzyme responsible for the conversion of dopamine to norepinephrine in noradrenergic neurons and in the adrenal medulla, is measurable in plasma (Weinshilboum and Axelrod, 1971). Release of DBH from sympathetic nerves follows nerve stimulation (Weinshilboum and Axelrod, 1971), and the level of DBH in plasma has been suggested to reflect peripheral sympathetic activity, as well as genetically based individual differences (Wooten and Cardon, 1973, Wetterberg *et al.*, 1972; Lamprecht *et al.*, 1973; Weinshilboum *et al.*, 1973). Two independent studies of plasma DBH in patients with depression and mania have failed to find any difference from controls (Shopsin *et al.*, 1972; Dunner *et al.*, 1973).

6. INTERRELATIONSHIPS BETWEEN AFFECTS AND PSYCHOMOTOR ACTIVATION: A REEVALUATION OF THE ROLE OF CATECHOLAMINES IN AFFECT-RELATED BEHAVIOR

The evidence reviewed above, although mixed, suggests the existence of some connection between catecholamines and affects, mood, and emotion-related behavior. In the following discussion, we will seek to draw some more explicit conclusions concerning the nature of this relationship.

6.1. Affects and the "Affective Disorders"

It first seems necessary to draw a clear distinction between affects and the so-called "affective disorders" in deriving conclusions about the role of catecholamines in affect-related behavior. The clinical "affective disorders" are behavioral and psychological syndromes whose manifestations include a much larger range of phenomena than the affective dimension alone. This is exemplified, for example, by the major role played by the activation-retardation dimension in the clinical symptomatology of mania and bipolar depression. In fact, in some individuals diagnosed as "depressed," sadness and other forms of depressive affect are not prominent clinical features of the disorder, and may not be elicited on psychological inventories, or, at least, are present in much diminished form disproportionate to other psychological and behavioral concomitants of the clinical syndrome of "depression" (Beigel and Murphy, 1971*b*; Donnelly and Murphy, 1973). Similarly, mania does not uniformly seem to be manifested by an opposite ("bipolar") affective state from depression (Beigel and Murphy, 1971*a*; Kotin and Goodwin, 1972; Murphy *et al.*, 1974). Rather, the manic individual exhibits heightened expression of many different affects, including anger and depression as well as euphoria. Evidence suggesting that the affective elements of mania are not closely linked with the disorder, but rather seem to be manifested in relation to independent personality factors and environmental situations, has been presented in greater detail elsewhere (Murphy *et al.* 1975).

Corresponding to this view of the clinical phenomena, our current interpretation of the clinical syndromes of depression and mania places as much emphasis on nonaffective elements, such as psychomotor activity, sleep and appetitive disturbances, and cognitive dysfunction as the substrata relevant to the therapeutic effects of drugs like the tricyclic antidepressants, phenothiazines, and lithium. In part, this view is derived from the minimal effects these drugs possess on affect in normal individuals and patients, despite their profoundly beneficial effects on the clinical syndromes. However, this view does not deny that the precipitants of the syndromes may be affect-altering events, such as losses, threats to self-esteem or coping abilities, as is also observed in milder states of sadness and grief, but rather emphasizes that in the full-blown clinical syndrome, other nonaffective elements may become predominant.

6.2. Affects and Catecholamines

On the basis of the evidence reviewed above, we would propose a more limited view of the relationship between affect and catecholamines. It would seem that peripherally administered epinephrine may contribute to affect-related behavior by amplifying affective expression. Similarly, from studies of L-dopa, amphetamine, α-methyl-*p*-tyrosine, and other drugs affecting central catecholamine availability, it would seem that a similar role in enhancing arousal, psychomotor activation, and affective expression may constitute one basic affect-related action of brain catecholamines.

There is, in addition, a general trend for some drugs which increase functional brain catecholamines to be associated with euphoria and elation—a response best exemplified by the amphetamines. Similarly, some drugs which diminish catecholamine effects (e.g., α-methyl-*p*-tyrosine and reserpine) may yield depressive affect, a response which is more variable in different individuals. However, it seems significant that with catecholamine-altering drug treatment, elation seldom occurs without activation, and depression is often accompanied by retardation. (However, activation can be associated with depressive thought content and with dysphoric affect as part of both the clinical depressive and manic syndromes.) Whether these varying responses are directly biologically linked or are contributed to, in part, by behavioral and psychological reinforcement for activity or inactivity, is not yet clear. Correspondingly, it seems that the determination of a particular affect experienced and expressed (e.g., anger, amusement) may not be a single function of catecholamine-related effects, but may rather be primarily derivative from environmental cues, current psychological orientation, past experiences stored in the form of affect-specific, state-dependent memories (Henry *et al.*, 1973), as well as from psychomotor activation level and other biologic factors. This model would encompass some of the apparently conflicting data found with catecholamines and catecholamine-affecting drugs, such as epinephrine, amphetamine, and L-dopa, where diverse patterns of affect and affect-related behavior follow drug administration, and where the component common to all events seems to be primarily the activation dimension. It would also encompass the "affective disorder" phenomena, where, for example, in mania, diverse affects, including anger, irritability, depression, and euphoria are expressed in an exaggerated flow of emotional expression and psychomotor activity, and, in depression, where affective expression may be diminished—for example, the frequent complaint from depressed patients of an inability "to feel or to cry."

This model is admittedly limited in scope and represents only one part of a hypothetical psychobiology of affect. It neglects many other phenomena woven into the richness and detail of human feeling states, even as quantitated in other areas of psychological study. It seeks only to frame the available evidence on catecholamines, brain function, psychoactive drugs, and psychological–behavioral phenomena into a broadly outlined coherent schema.

6.3. Catecholamines and the Present Status of the Biogenic Amine Hypotheses for Mania and Depression

In regard to the present status of depression and mania as possible disorders of catecholamine metabolism, definitive evidence is not yet available to do more than to continue to suggest that these states may be mediated in some way by catecholamine alterations. The evidence reviewed here, and in greater detail elsewhere (Murphy *et al.*, 1975), seems more conclusive and complete in the case of catecholamine involvement in mania. In particular, the precipitation of hypomania by L-dopa and the prominence of psychomotor activation in mania suggest that enhanced dopamine-related neural function may be involved in this syndrome, perhaps to an even greater extent than norepinephrine (Murphy, 1972*a*). Depression seems to be a more heterogeneous state, with greater variety in the clinical symptoms. It does seem, however, that depression in bipolar patients, which is almost uniformly characterized by retardation, and by relatively less expressed sadness, anxiety, hypochondria, and other common accompaniments of depression in unipolar patients (Beigel and Murphy, 1971*b*; Donnelly and Murphy, 1973), may represent a state resulting from diminished function in dopamine and possibly norepinephrine-mediated systems. In contrast, the unipolar depressed patient presenting in an agitated, anxious, hand-wringing state, seeking reassurance from surrounding persons, manifests many other psychophysiologic and biochemical phenomena (including increased urinary and plasma catecholamines) which fit with an evident clinical state of increased activation accompanied by painful depressive affect.

7. SUMMARY

An attempt to summarize present information on the interrelationships between clinical phenomena in the major subgroupings of the "affective

Table III. A Comparison of Mania and Two Major Clinical Subtypes of Depression in Terms of Apparent Psychologic Status and Postulated Neuromediator Alterations

Psychobiologic status	Mania	Type I depression ("endogenous" depression, as in bipolar and some unipolar patients)	Type II depression (anxious, agitated depressions, as in many unipolar patients)
Activation and affective expression	↑	↓	↑
Social relatedness	↑	↓	↑
Hedonic tone	↑ or ↓	↓	↓
Self-estimated competence	↑	↓	↓
Postulated neuromediator alteration			
Dopamine	↑	↓	↑
Norepinephrine	↑ or ↓	− or ↓	↓
Epinephrine	↑	−	↑
Serotonin	↓	↓	↓
Acetylcholine	? − or ↓	?↑	?↑

disorders" and the evidence implicating catecholamines and other neuro-mediator substances is presented in Table III. It appears that some of the discrepancies in the original attempts to relate biogenic amines to affective states are partially resolved by recognition of the differences in the clinical manifestations of the two major types of depressive syndromes, especially in relation to the psychomotor activation dimension. It seems especially interesting that these two depressive syndromes have characteristics which, as presented in Table III, are very similar to the factor-derived clusters of affect-related phenomena found by Davitz in studies of normal individuals (see Table I).

The postulated alterations in catecholamines, indoleamines, and acetylcholine suggested in Table III have been obtained from a combination of the data reviewed or alluded to above. In attempting to integrate both the apparent heterogeneity of the clinical states of depression and advancing knowledge of biogenic amine-related brain functions, more complex mechanisms have been suggested by which catecholamines or other neuro-mediators might be altered in depression. Thus, current hypotheses include not only simple amine depletion as in the reserpine or stress models of depression (Schildkraut, 1965; Bunney and Davis, 1965; Bliss *et al.*, 1968, Weiss *et al.*, 1970) but also altered amine transmitter transport (Bunney *et al.*, 1972a), altered amine metabolism (Schildkraut, 1973b)—perhaps result-ing from changes in amine-related enzymes (Dunner and Goodwin, 1972; Murphy and Weiss, 1972) and perhaps leading to the formation of faulty amine transmitters (Murphy, 1972b)—as well as altered amine receptor function (Prange *et al.*, 1972). All of these mechanisms, alone or acting together, might produce either increased or diminished effective concentra-tions of the neuromediator substances at specific synapses. Changes in the interrelationships ("balance") between catecholamines, indoleamines, and acetylcholine in brain may also contribute to the clinical phenomena (Janowsky *et al.*, 1972; Prange *et al.*, 1972; Murphy, 1972b).

In addition, growing emphasis has been placed on the regulatory mechanisms involved in brain amine neurotransmitter function. It has been suggested by Mandell (1973), for instance, that there are redundant com-pensatory and regulatory mechanisms in the amine metabolic pathways such that a sustained alteration in function would seem unlikely unless a regulatory mechanism, such as an enzyme, were altered, *in addition to* the occurrence of a basic change, such as amine depletion, or excess synthesis of brain amines. While much of the pharmacologic data supporting the biogenic amine hypotheses of the affective disorders came from short-term, *in vitro* studies of psychoactive drugs, recently heed has been paid to the fact that tricyclic antidepressants, monoamine oxidase inhibitors, and lith-ium require up to several weeks of administration before they reach full ef-fectiveness. Since different biochemical mechanisms appear to be involved under these conditions (Mandell *et al.*, 1972; Mandell, 1973), the hypotheses linking amines to behavior must now be reconsidered in terms of secondary changes in enzymes, neurotransmitter synthesis, receptor sensitivity changes, and the like.

An inverse biogenic amine hypothesis for depression has been tentatively suggested on the basis of some of the evidence reviewed above indicating that some depressed patients demonstrate increased urinary and plasma catecholamine levels (Bunney *et al.*, 1967; Wyatt *et al.*, 1971). Evidence supporting this view also comes from clinical studies indicating that phenothiazines, such as thioridazine and chlorpromazine, are equally effective antidepressants as the tricyclic drugs, but have relatively greater adrenergic receptor-blocking effects and lesser amine uptake inhibiting effects, and hence might be acting as antagonists of excess catecholamines in depression (Murphy and Kopin, 1972; Hollister, 1973). The antidepressant effects of some other drugs which are not uptake inhibitors or MAO inhibitors (Rickels *et al.*, 1973; Ross *et al.*, 1971) and the lack of efficacy of L-dopa as an antidepressant (Goodwin *et al.*, 1970), may also be of relevance to this hypothesis. However, the failure of α-methyl-*p*-tyrosine to reverse depressive symptomatology appears to be inconsistent with this formulation (Brodie *et al.*, 1971). Certainly, the overall view of this "inverse" hypothesis would be most appropriately applied to the Type II depression syndrome (Table III).

As is evident from this review, the question of the possible role of the catecholamines in affect, emotional behavior, and the clinical syndromes of depression and mania remains in turmoil. While many lines of evidence link catecholamines and affect-related behavior, many details of the linkage remain highly controversial, and devolve upon the methodologic problems discussed above. Furthermore, the role of catecholamines in affect is certainly intertwined with other factors—biological, psychological, and environmental—which affect the individual.

8. REFERENCES

Anderson, D. C., and Paden, P., 1966, Passive avoidance response learning as a function of prior tumbling trauma, *Psychonomic Sci.* 4:129.

Ansel, R. D., and Markham, C. H., 1970, Effects of L-dopa in normal humans, in: L-*Dopa and Parkinsonism* (A. Barbeau and F. H. McDowell, eds.), pp. 69–71, F. A. Davis Company, Philadelphia.

Arnold, M. B., 1970, Perennial problems in the field of emotion, in: *Feelings and Emotions,* pp. 169–185, Academic Press, New York.

Arnold, L. E., Kirilcuk, V., Corson, S. A., and Corson, E. O'L., 1973, Levoamphetamine and dextroamphetamine: Differential effect on aggression and hyperkinesis in children and dogs, *Am. J. Psychiat.* **130**:165.

Ax, A. F., 1953, Fear and anger in humans, *Psychosomat. Med.* **15**:433.

Axelrod, J., 1966, Methylation reactions in the formation and metabolism of catecholamines and other biogenic amines, *Pharmacol. Rev.* **18**:95.

Axelrod, J., and Cohn, C. K., 1971, Methyltransferase enzymes in red blood cells, *J. Pharmacol. Exptl. Therap.* **176**:650.

Axelrod, J., and Tomchick, R. 1958, Enzymatic O-methylation of epinephrine and other catechols, *J. Biol. Chem.* **233**: 702.

Axelrod, J., Mueller, R. A., Henry, J. P., and Stephens, P. M., 1970, Changes in enzymes involved in the biosynthesis and metabolism of noradrenaline and adrenaline after psychosocial stimulation, *Nature* **255**:1059.

Ayd, F. J., Jr., 1958, Drug-induced depression—Fact or fallacy, *N.Y. J. Med.* **58**:354.

Ban, T. A., 1969, The use of the amphetamines in adult psychiatry, *Sem. Psychiat.* **1**:129.

Barbeau, A., 1969, L-Dopa therapy in Parkinson's disease: a critical review of nine years' experience, *Can. Med. Assoc. J.* **101**:791.

Bard, P., 1950, Central nervous mechanisms for the expression of anger in animals, in: *Feelings and Emotions: The Mooseheart Symposium* (M. L. Reymert, ed.), McGraw-Hill, New York.

Beck, A. T., Ward, C. H., Mendelson, M., Mock, J., and Erbaugh, J., 1961, An inventory for measuring depression, *Arch. Gen. Psychiat.* **4**:561.

Beigel, A., and Murphy, D. L., 1971*a*, Assessing clinical characteristics of the manic state, *Am. J. Psychiat.* **128**:688.

Beigel, A., and Murphy, D. L., 1971*b*, Unipolar and bipolar affective illness: differences in clinical characteristics accompanying depression, *Arch. Gen. Psychiat.* **24**:215.

Bergsman, A., 1959, Urinary excretion of adrenaline and noradrenaline in some mental diseases: clinical and experimental study, *Acta Psychiat. Neurol. Scand. Suppl.* **133**:5.

Berstein, S., and Kaufman, M. R., 1960, A psychological analysis of apparent depression following rauwolfia therapy, *J. Mt. Sinai Hosp. N.Y.* **27**:525.

Bleuler, Eugen, 1932, *Naturgeschichte der Seele, Zweite Auflage,* S., 185., Julius Springer, Berlin.

Bliss, E. L., and Zwanziger, J., 1966, Brain amines and emotional stress, *J. Psychiat. Res.* **4**:189.

Bliss, E. L., Ailion, J., and Zwanziger, J., 1968, Metabolism of norepinephrine, serotonin and dopamine in rat brain with stress, *J. Pharmacol. Exptl. Therap.* **164**:122.

Bloom, F. E., Algeri, S., Groppetti, A., Revuelta, A. and Costa, E., 1969, Lesions of central norepinephrine terminals with 6-OH-dopamine: biochemistry and fine structure, *Science* **166**:1284.

Bond, P. A., Jenner, F. A., and Sampson, G. A., 1972, Daily variations of the urine content of 3-methyoxy-4-hydroxyphenylglycol in two manic-depressive patients, *Psychol. Med.* **2**:81.

Bowlby, J., 1961, Processes of mourning, *Intern. J. Psychoanal.* **42**:317.

Brady, J. V., and Nauta, W. J., 1953, Subcortical mechanisms in emotional behavior: affective changes following septal forebrain lesions in the albino rat, *J. Comp. Physiol. Psychol.* **46**:339.

Braud, W., Wepmann, B., and Russo, D., 1969, Task and species generality of the "helplessness" phenomenon, *Psychonomic Sci.* **16**:154.

Breese, G. and Traylor, T. D., 1970, Effect of 6-hydroxydopamine on brain norepinephrine and dopamine: evidence of selective degeneration of catecholamine neurons, *J. Pharmacol. Exptl Therap.* **174**:413.

Breese, G., and Traylor, T. D., 1971, Depletion of brain noradrenaline and dopamine by 6-hydroxydopamine, *Brit. J. Pharmacol.* **42**:88.

Brodie, B. B., 1965, Some ideas on the mode of action of imipramine-type antidepressants, in: *The Scientific Basis of Drug Therapy in Psychiatry* (J. Marks and C. M. B. Pare, eds.), p. 127, Pergamon Press, Oxford.

Brodie, H. K. H., Murphy, D. L., Goodwin, F. K., and Bunney, W. E., Jr., 1971, Catecholamines and mania: the effect of α-methyl-*p*-tyrosine on manic behavior and catecholamine metabolism, *Clin. Pharmacol. Therap.* **12**:218.

Brown, J., and Jacobs, A., 1949, The role of fear in the motivation and acquisition of responses, *J. Exptl. Psychol.* **39**:747.

Brucke, F. T., Hornykiewicz, O., and Sigg, E. B., 1969, *The Pharmacology of Psychotherapeutic Drugs,* Springer-Verlag, New York.

Bunney, W. E., Jr., and Davis, J. M., 1965, Norepinephrine in depressive reactions: Review, *Arch. Gen. Psychiat.* **13**:483.

Bunney, W. E. Jr., Davis, J. M., Weil-Malherbe, H., and Smith, E. R. B., 1967, Biochemical changes in psychotic depression: high norepinephrine levels in psychotic *vs.* neurotic depression, *Arch. Gen. Psychiat.* **16**:448.

Bunney, W. E., Jr., Murphy, D. L., and Goodwin, F. K., 1970, The switch process from depression to mania: relationship to drugs which alter brain amines, *Lancet* **1**:1022.

Bunney, W. E., Jr., Goodwin, F. K., and Murphy, D. L., 1972*a*, The switch process in manic-depressive illness. III. Theoretical implications, *Arch. Gen. Psychiat.* **27**:312.

Bunney, W. E., Jr., Murphy, D. L., Goodwin, F. K., and Borge, G. K., 1972*b*, The "switch process" in manic-depressive illness. I. A systematic study of sequential behavior changes, *Arch. Gen. Psychiat.* **27**:295.

Bunney, W. E., Jr., Goodwin, F. K., Murphy, D. L., and House, K. M., 1972*c*, The "switch process" in manic-depressive illness. II. Relationship to catecholamines, REM sleep and drugs, *Arch. Gen. Psychiat.* **27**:304.

Butcher, L. L., and Engel, J., 1969, Behavioral and biochemical effects of L-dopa after peripheral decarboxylase inhibition, *Brain Res.* **15**:233.

Calne, D. B., and Sandler, M., 1970, L-dopa and Parkinsonism, *Nature* **226**:21.

Campanini, T., Catalano, A., Derisio, C., and Mardighian, G., 1970, Vanilmandelic aciduria in the different clinical phases of manic-depressive psychoses, *Brit. J. Psychiat.* **116**:435.

Cannon, W. B., 1915, *Bodily Changes in Pain, Fear and Rage,* Appleton, New York.

Cannon, W. B., 1927, The James–Lange theory of emotions: a critical examination and an alternative theory, *Am. J. Psychol.* **39**:106.

Cantril, H., and Hunt, W. A., 1932, Emotional effects produced by the injection of adrenalin, *Am. J. Psychol.* **44**:300.

Carlsson, A., 1959, the occurrence, distribution and physiological role of catecholamines in the nervous system, *Pharmacol. Rev.* **11**:490.

Carlsson, A., 1966, Drugs which block the storage of 5-hydroxytryptamine and related amines, in: *Handbuch der Experimentellen Pharmakologie,* vol. 19 (V. Erspamer, ed.), p. 529.

Carlsson, A., and Lindqvist, M., 1963, *Acta Pharmacol. Toxicol.* **20**:140.

Carlsson, A., Lindqvist, M., and Magnusson, T., 1957, 3,4-Dihydroxy-phenylalanine and 5-hydroxytryptophan as reserpine antagonists, *Nature* **180**:1200.

Carlsson, A., Corrodi, H., Fuxe, K., and Hökfelt, T., 1969, Effects of antidepressant drugs on the depletion of intraneuronal brain 5-hydroxytryptamine stores caused by 4-methyl-α-ethyl-*m*-tyramine, *European J. Pharmacol.* **5**:357.

Carroll, B. J., and Sharp, P. T., 1971, Rubidium and lithium: opposite effects on amine-mediated excitement, *Science* **172**:1355.

Charalampous, K. D., and Brown, S., 1967, A Clinical trial of α-methyl-para-tyrosine in mentally ill patients, *Psychopharmacologia* **11**:422.

Chase, T. N., Breese, G. R., Gordon, E. K., and Kopin, I. J., 1971, Catecholamine metabolism in the dog: comparison of intravenously and intraventricularly administered (^{14}C) dopamine and (^{3}H) norepinephrine, *J. Neurochem.* **18**:135.

Clyde, D. J., 1963, *Manual for the Clyde Mood Scale,* Biometric Laboratory, Miami, Fla.

Cohn, C. K., Dunner, D. L., and Axelrod, J., 1970, Reduced catechol-*O*-methyltransferase activity in red blood cells of women with primary affective disorder, *Science* **170**:1323.

Cole, J. O., and Davis, J. M., 1967, Antidepressant drugs, in: *Comprehensive Textbook of Psychiatry* (A. M. Freedman and H. I. Kaplan, eds.), pp. 1263–1275, Williams and Wilkins, Baltimore.

Corrodi, H., and Hanson, L. C. F., 1966, Central effects of an inhibitor of tyrosine hydroxylation, *Psychopharmacologia* **10**:116.

Costa, E., and Sandler, M., 1972, Monoamine oxidases—new vistas, in: *Advances in Biochemical Psychopharmacology, Vol. 5,* Raven Press, New York.

Curtis, G. C., Cleghorn, R. A., and Sourkes, T. L., 1960, Relationship between affect and excretion of adrenaline, noradrenaline and 17-hydroxycortico-steroids, *J. Psychosomat. Res.* **4**:176.

Darwin, C., 1872, *The Expression of Emotions in Man and Animals,* Philosophical Library, New York, (reprint 1955).

Davis, J. M., 1970, Theories of the biological etiology of affective disorders, *Intern. Rev. Neurobiol.* **12**:145.

Davitz, J. R., 1969, *The Language of Emotion,* Academic Press, New York.

Degwitz, R., Frowein, R., Kulenkampff, C., and Mohs, V., 1960, Uber die Wirkungen des L-Dopa beim Menschen und deren Beeinflussing durch Reserpin, Chlorpromazin, Iproniazid und Vitamine B6, *Klin. Wochschr.* **38**:120.

Dominic, J. A., and Moore, K. E., 1969, Acute effects of α-methyltyrosine on brain catecholamine levels and on spontaneous and amphetamine-stimulated motor activity in mice, *Arch. Intern. Pharmacodyn.* **178**:166.

Donnelly, E. F., and Murphy, D. L., 1973, Primary affective disorder: MMPI differences between unipolar and bipolar depressed subjects, *J. Clin. Psychol.* **29**:303.

Dubach, W. C., 1963, Methyl dopa and depression, *Brit. Med. J.* **1**:261.

Duffy, E., 1962, *Activation and Behavior,* Wiley, New York.

Dunner, D. L., and Goodwin, F. K., 1972, The effect of L-tryptophan on brain serotonin metabolism in depressed patients, *Arch. Gen. Psychiat.* **26**:364.

Dunner, D. L., Cohn, C. K., Gershon, E. S., and Goodwin, F. K., 1971, Differential catechol-*O*-methyltransferase activity in unipolar and bipolar affective illness, *Arch. Gen. Psychiat.* **25**:348.

Dunner, D. L., Cohn, C. K., Weinshilboum, R. M., and Wyatt, R. J., 1973, The activity of dopamine-β-hydroxylase and methionine-activating enzyme in blood of schizophrenic patients, *Biol. Psychiat.* **6**:215.

Efron, D. H. (ed.), 1968, *Psychopharmacology,* Public Health Service Publication, Washington, D.C.

Engel, G. L., 1963, Towards a classification of affects, in: *Expression of the Emotions in Man* (P. H. Knapp, ed.), International Universities Press, New York.

Engelman, K., Horwitz, D., Jequier, E., and Sjoerdsma, A., 1968, Biochemical and pharmacologic effects of α-methyltyrosine in man, *J. Clin. Invest.* **47**:577.

Euler, U. S. von, 1956, *Noradrenaline,* C. C. Thomas, Springfield.

Evans, W. O., and Kline, N. S., 1969, *The Psychopharmacology of the Normal Human,* C. C. Thomas, Springfield.

Everett, G. M., and Wiegand, R. G., 1962, Central amines and behavioral states: a critique and new data, *Proc. First Intern. Congr. Pharmacol.* **8**:85.

Ewing, L. S., 1967, Fighting and death from stress in a cockroach, *Science* **155**:1035.

Fawcett, J., and Siomopoulos, V., 1971, Dextroamphetamine response as a possible predictor of improvement with tricyclic therapy in depression, *Arch. Gen. Psychiat.* **25**:247.

Federn, P., 1936, On the distinction between health and pathological narcissism, in: *Ego Psychology and the Psychoses,* pp. 323–364, Basic Books, New York.

Felsinger, J. M. von, Lasagna, I., and Beecher, H. K., 1955, Drug-induced mood changes in man: (2) personality and reactions to drugs, *J. Am. Med. Assoc.* **157**:1113.

Fogel, M. L., Curtis, G. C., Kordasz, F., and Smith, W. G., 1966, Judges' ratings, self-ratings and checklist reports of affects, *Psychol. Rep.* **19**:299.

Frankenhaeuser, M., Mellis, I., Rissler, A., Bjorkvall, C., and Patkal, P., 1968, Catecholamine excretion as related to cognitive and emotional reaction patterns. *Psychosomat. Med.* **30**:109.

Freud, S., 1925, The unconscious, in: *Collected Papers, Vol. IV.,* The Hogarth Press Ltd., London.

Fried, P. A., 1972, Septum and behavior: A review, *Psychol. Bull.* **78**:292.

Friedman, A. S., Granick, S., Cotten, H. W., and Cowitz, B., 1966, Imipramine (tofranil) *vs.* placebo in hospitalized psychotic depressives, *J. Psychiat. Res.* **4**:13.

Fullerton, A. G., and Morton-Jenkins, D., 1963, Methyldopa and depression, *Brit. Med. J.* **1**:538.

Fuxe, K., Hokfelt, T., and Ungerstedt, U., 1970, Central monoaminergic tracts, in: *Principles of Psychopharmacology* (W. G. Clark, and J. del Giudice, eds.), Academic Press, New York.

Gellhorn, E., and Lofbourrow, G. N., 1963, *Emotions and Emotional Disorders,* Hoeber, New York.

Gershon, S., Hekimian, J., Floyd, A., Jr., and Hollister, L. E., 1967, α-Methyl-*p*-tyrosine (AMT) in schizophrenia, *Psychopharmacologia* **11**:189.

Goodman, L. S., and Gilman, A., 1965, *The Pharmacological Basis of Therapeutics,* The Macmillan Company, New York.

Goodwin, F. K., and Murphy, D. L., (1974), Biological factors in the affective disorders and schizophrenia, in: *Psychopharmacological Agents, Vol. III,* (M. Gordon, ed.), Academic Press, New York.

Goodwin, F. K., and Sack, R., 1973, Affective disorders: the catecholamine hypothesis revisited, in: *Frontiers in Catecholamine Research* (E. Usdin and S. Snyder, eds.), Pergamon Press, New York.

Goodwin, F. K., Murphy, D. L., Brodie, H. K. H., and Bunney, W. E., Jr., 1970, L-Dopa, catecholamines and behavior: a clinical and biochemical study in depressed patients, *Biol. Psychiat.* **2**:341.

Goodwin, F. K., Ebert, M. H., and Bunney, W. E., Jr., 1971, Mental effects of reserpine in man, in: *Complications of Medical Drugs* (R. I. Shader, ed.), Raven Press, New York.

Gordon, E. K., and Oliver, J., 1971, 3-Methoxy-4-hydroxyphenylethylene glycol in human cerebrospinal fluid, *Clin. Chem. Acta* **35**:145.

Gottschalk, L., Gleser, G., and Springer, K., 1963, Three hostility scales applicable to verbal samples, *Arch. Gen. Psychiat.* **9**:254.

Graeff, F. G., Leme, J. G., and Roch e Silva, M., 1965, Role played by catechol and indoleamines in the central actions of reserpine after monoamine oxidase inhibition, *Intern. J. Neuropharmacol.* **4**:17.

Greenspan, K., Schildkraut, J. J., Gordon, E. K., Levy, B., and Durell, J., 1969, Catecholamine metabolism in affective disorders II. Norepinephrine, normetanephrine, epinephrine, metanephrine and VMA excretion in hypomanic patients, *Arch. Gen. Psychiat.* **21**:710.

Greenspan, K., Schildkraut, J. J., Gordon, E. K., Baer, L., Aranoff, M. S., and Durell, J., 1970, Catecholamine metabolism in affective disorders III. MHPG and other catecholamine metabolites in patients treated with lithium carbonate, *J. Psychiat. Res.* 7:171.

Haggendal, J., and Werdinius, B., 1966, Dopamine in human urine during muscular work, *Acta Physiol. Scand.* 66:223.

Hamilton, M., 1960, A rating scale for depression, *J. Neurol. Neurosurg. Psychiat.* 3:56.

Hamilton, M., and Kopelman, H., 1963, Treatment of severe hypertension with methyl dopa, *Brit. Med. J.* 1:151.

Hanson, L. C. F., 1965, The disruption of conditioned avoidance response following selective depletion of brain catecholamines, *Psychopharmacologia* 8:100.

Hanson, L. C. F., 1967a, Biochemical and behavioral effects of tyrosine hydroxylase inhibition, *Psychopharmacologia* 11:8.

Hanson, L. C. F., 1967b, Evidence that the central action of (+) amphetamine is mediated via catecholamines, *Psychopharmacologia* 10:289.

Harris, T. H., 1957, Depression induced by rauwolfia compounds, *Am. J. Psychiat.* 113:950.

Hathaway, S. R., and McKinley, J. C., 1951, *Minnesota Multiphasic Personality Inventory: Manual*, Psychological Corporation, New York.

Hauesler, G., Haeffely, W., and Thoenen, H., 1969, Chemical sympathectomy of the cat with 6-hydroxydopamine, *J. Pharmacol. Exptl. Therap.* 170:50.

Hebb, D. O., 1966, *A Textbook of Psychology* (2nd ed.), W. B. Saunders, Philadelphia.

Heikkila, R., and Cohen, G., 1971, Inhibition of biogenic amine uptake by hydrogen peroxide: a mechanism for toxic effects of 6-hydroxydopamine, *Science* 172:1257.

Henry, G. M., Weingartner, H., and Murphy, D. L., 1973, Influence of affective states and psychoactive drugs on verbal learning and memory, *Am. J. Psychiat.* 130:966.

Hess, S. M., Connamacher, R. H., Ozaki, M., and Udenfriend, S., 1961, The effects of α-methyl-dopa and α-methyl-m-tyrosine on the metabolism of norepinephrine and serotonin *in vivo*, *J. Pharmacol. Exptl. Therap.* 134:129.

Hillarp, N. A., Fuxe, A., and Dahlstrom, A., 1966, Demonstration and mapping of central neurons containing dopamine, noradrenaline, and 5-hydroxytryptamine and their reactions to psychopharmaca, *Pharmacol. Rev.* 18:727.

Hinde, R., Spencer-Booth, Y., and Bruce, M., 1966, Effects of 6-day maternal deprivation on rhesus monkey infants, *Nature* 210:1021.

Hohman, G. W., 1966, Some effects of spinal cord lesions on experienced emotional feelings, *Psychophysiology* 3:143.

Hollister, L. E., 1973, *Clinical Use of Psychotherapeutic Drugs*, Charles C. Thomas, Springfield.

Horita, A., and Hamilton, A. E., 1969, Lysergic Acid diethylamide: dissociation of its behavioral and hyperthermic actions by DL-α-methyl-p-tyrosine, *Science* 164:78.

Hornykiewicz, O., 1966, Dopamine (3-hydroxytyramine) and brain function, *Pharmacol. Rev.* 18:925.

Hornykiewicz, O., 1970, Dopamine: its physiology, pharmacology and pathological neurochemistry, in: *Biogenic Amines and Physiological Membranes in Drug Therapy* (J. H. Biel and G. Abood, eds.), Marcel Dekker, New York.

Hunt, J. McV., Cole, M. W., and Reis, E. E., 1958, Situational cues distinguishing anger, fear, and sorrow, *Am. J. Psychol.* 71:136.

Hurst, P. M., Weidner, M. F., Radlow, R., and Voss, S., 1973, Drugs and placebos: drug guessing by normal volunteers, *Psychol. Rep.* 33:683.

Innes, I. R., 1963, Action of dexamphetamine on 5-hydroxytryptamine receptors, *Brit. J. Pharmacol.* 21:427.

James, W., 1884, What is an emotion?, *Mind* 9:188.

James. W., 1890, *The Principles of Psychology*, Hold, New York.

Janowsky, D. S., Davis, J. M., El Yousef, M. K., and Sekerke, H. J., 1972, A cholinergic-adrenergic hypothesis of mania and depression, *Lancet* **2**-632.

Jensen, G., and Tolman, C., 1962, Mother-infant relationship in the monkey, *Macaca nemestrina*: the effect of brief separation and mother-infant specificity, *J. Comp. Physiol. Psychol.* **55**:131.

Jones, F. D., Maas, J. W., Dekirmenjian, H., and Fawcett, J. A., 1973, Urinary catecholamine metabolites during behavioral changes in a patient with manic-depressive cycles, *Science* **179**:300.

Jonsson, L-E., Anggard, E., and Gunne, L-M., 1971, Blockade of intravenous amphetamine euphoria in man, *Clin. Pharmacol. Therap.* **12**:889.

Kahn, M. W., 1951, The effect of severe defeat at various age levels on the aggressive behavior of mice, *J. Genet. Psychol.* **79**:117.

Karki, N. T., 1956, Urinary excretion of noradrenaline and adrenaline in different age groups, its diurnal variation and effect of muscular work on it, *Acta Physiol. Scand. Suppl.* **132**:5.

Kaufman, I., and Rosenblum, L., 1967a, Depression in infant monkeys separated from their mothers, *Science* **155**:1030.

Kaufman, I., and Rosenblum, L., 1967b, The reaction to separation in infant monkeys: anaclitic depression and conservation-withdrawal, *Psychosomat. Med.* **29**:648.

Klawans, H. L., Jr., Paulson, G. W., Ringel, S. P., Barbeau, A., 1972, Use of L-dopa in the detection of presymptomatic Huntington's Chorea, *New Engl. J. Med.* **286**:1332.

Klein, D. F., and Davis, J. M., 1969, *Diagnosis and Drug Treatment of Psychiatric Disorders*, Williams and Wilkins Co., Baltimore.

Klerman, G. L., Schildkraut, J. J., Hasenbush, L. L., Greenblatt, M., and Friend, D. G., 1963, Clinical experience with dihydroxyphenylalanine (dopa) in depression, *J. Psychiat. Res.* **1**:289.

Kopin, I. J., 1968, False adrenergic transmitters, *Ann. Rev. Pharmacol.* **10**:377.

Kopin, I. J., and Gordon, E. K., 1962, Metabolism of norepinephrine-^{3}H released by tyramine and reserpine, *J. Pharmacol. Exptl. Therap.* **138**:351.

Kopin, I. J., and Gordon, E. K., 1963, Metabolism of administered and drug-released norepinephrine-7-^{3}H in rat, *J. Pharmacol. Exptl. Therap.* **140**:207.

Kotin, J., and Goodwin, F. K., 1972, Depression during mania: clinical observations and theoretical implications, *Am. J. Psychiat.* **129**:679.

Krueger, F., 1928, The essence of feeling, trans. M. B. Arnold, "The Nature of Emotion" (Arnold, M. G., ed.), in: *Selected Readings*, Penguin, Baltimore (1968).

Kulscar, I. S., 1966, Amphetamine sulfate in mania, *Lancet* **1**:1164.

Lahti, R. A., and Maickel, R. P., 1971, The tricyclic antidepressants—inhibition of norepinephrine uptake as related to potentiation of norepinephrine and clinical efficacy, *Biochem. Pharmacol.* **20**:482.

Lamprecht, F., Wyatt, R. J., Belmaker, R., Murphy, D. L., and Pollin, W., 1973, Plasma dopamine-β-hydroxylase in identical twins discordant for schizophrenia, in: *Frontiers in Catecholamine Research* (E. Usdin and S. Snyder, eds.), Pergamon Press, New York.

Landis, C., and Hunt, W. A., 1932, Adrenaline and emotion, *Psychol. Rev.* **39**:467.

Lange, C., 1885, *The Emotions* (1885 German trans. Dr. Kurella; 1887, Engl. trans.), Williams and Wilkins, Baltimore (1922).

Lapin, I. P., and Oxenkrug, G. F., 1969, Intensification of the central serotonergic processes as a possible determinant of the thymoleptic effect, *Lancet* **1**:132.

Lasagna, L., von Felsinger, J. M., and Beecher, H. K., 1955, Drug induced mood changes in man: (1) observations on healthy subjects, chronically ill patients and post addicts, *J. Am. Med. Assoc.* **157**:1006.

Laverty, R., and Taylor, K. M., 1970, Effects of intraventricular 2,4,5-

trihydroxyphenylethylamine on the storage and release of noradrenaline, *Brit. J. Pharmacol.* **40**:836.

Lazarus, R. S., 1966, *Psychological Stress and the Coping Process,* McGraw-Hill, New York.

Leeper, R. W., 1948, A motivational theory of emotion, *Psychol. Rev.* **55**:5.

Lemieux, G., Davignon, A., and Genest, J., 1956, Depressive states during rauwolfia therapy for arterial hypertension: A report of 30 cases, *Can. Med. Assoc. J.* **74**:522.

Levi, L., 1965, The urinary output of adrenaline and noradrenaline during pleasant and unpleasant emotional states, *Psychosomat. Med.* **27**:80.

Lewy, A. J. and Seiden, L. S., 1972, Operant behavior changes norepinephrine metabolism in rat brain, *Science* **175**:454.

Lindsley, D. B., 1951, Emotion, in: *Handbook of Experimental Psychology* (S. S. Stevens, ed.), p. 473, Wiley, New York.

Ljungberg, S., and Paalzow, L., 1969, Some pharmacological properties of lithium, *Acta Psychiat. Scand. Suppl.* **207**:68.

Lubin, B., 1965, Adjective checklists for measurement of depression, *Arch. Gen. Psychiat.* **12**:57.

Lubin, B., 1966, Fourteen brief depression adjective checklists, *Arch. Gen. Psychiat.* **15**:205.

Maas, J. W., and Landis, D. H., 1968, *In vivo* studies of metabolism of norepinephrine in central nervous system, *J. Pharmacol. Exptl. Therap.* **163**:147.

Maas, J. W., Fawcett, J. A., and Dekirmenjian, H., 1968, 3-Methoxy-4-hydroxyphenylglycol (MHPG) excretion in depressive states: pilot study, *Arch. Gen. Psychiat.* **19**:129.

Maas, J. W., Dekirmenjian, H., and Fawcett, J. A., 1971, Catecholamine metabolism, depression and stress, *Nature* **230**:330.

Maas, J. W., Dekirmenjian, H., Garver, D., Redmond, D. E., Jr., and Landis, D. H., 1972*a,* Catecholamine metabolite excretion following intraventricular injection of 6-OH-dopamine, *Brain Res.* **41**:507.

Maas, J. W., Fawcett, J. A., and Dekirmenjian, H., 1972*b,* Catecholamine metabolism, depressive illness and drug response, *Arch. Gen. Psychiat.* **26**:252.

Maas, J. W., Dekirmenjian, H. Garver, D., Redmond, D. E., Jr., and Landis, D. H., 1973, Excretion of catecholamine metabolites following intraventricular injection of 6-hydroxydopamine in the *Macacaspeciosa, European J. Pharmacol.* **23**:121.

MacLean, P. D., 1949, Psychosomatic disease and the "visceral brain," recent developments bearing on the Papez theory of emotion, *Psychosomat. Med.* **11**:338.

Malmo, R. B., 1959, Activation: A neuropsychological dimension, *Psychol. Rev.* **66**:367.

Mandell, A. J., 1973, *New Concepts in Neurotransmitter Regulation,* Plenum Press, New York.

Mandell, A. J., Segal, D. S., Kuczenski, R. T., and Knapp, S., 1972, Some macromolecular mechanisms in CNS neurotransmitter pharmacology and their physiological organizations, in: *The Chemistry of Mood, Motivation, and Memory* (J. McGaugh, ed.), pp. 105–148, Plenum Press, New York.

Maranon, G., 1924, Contribution a l'etude de l'action emotive de l'adrenaline, *Rev. Franc. Endocrinol.* **2**:301.

Martin, W. R., Sloan, J. W., Sapira, J. D., and Jasinski, D. R., 1971, Physiologic, subjective, and behavioral effects of amphetamine, metamphetamine, ephedrine, phenmetrazine, and methylphenidate, in man, *Clin. Pharmacol. Therp.* **12**:245.

Mason, J. W., Mangan, G., Brady, J. V., Conrad, D., Rioch, D. M., 1960, Concurrent plasma epinephrine, norepinephrine and 17-hydroxycorticosteroid levels during conditioned emotional disturbances in monkeys, *Psychosomat. Med.* **23**:344.

Matussek, N., and Linsmayer, M., 1968, The effect of lithium and amphetamine on desmethylimipramine-Ro 4-1284 induced motor hyperactivity, *Life Sci.* **7**:371.

Matussek, N., Pohlmeier, H., and Ruther, E., 1966, Die Wirkung von Dopa auf gehemmte Depressionen, *Klin. Wochschr.* **44**:727.

McCleary, R. A., 1966, Response-modulating functions of the limbic system: Initiation and suppression, in: *Progress in Physiological Psychology,* Vol. 1, (E. Stellar and J. M. Sprague, eds.), Academic Press, New York.

McCulloch, T. L., and Bruner, J. S., 1939, The effect of electric shock upon subsequent learning in the rat, *J. Psychol.* **7**:333.

McGeer, P. L., McGeer, E. G., and Wada, J. A., 1963, Central aromatic amine levels in behavior. II. Serotonin and catecholamine levels in various cat brain areas following administration of psychoactive drugs or amine precursors, *Arch. Neurol.* **99**:81.

McKinney, W. T., Jr., and Kane, F. J., Jr., 1967, Depression with the use of α-methyldopa, *Am. J. Psychiat.* **124**:1.

Menon, M. K., Dandiya, P. C., and Bapna, J. S., 1967, Modification of the effect of some central stimulants in mice pretreated with α-methyl-p-tyrosine, *Psychopharmacologia* **10**:437.

Messiha, F. S., Agallianos, D., and Clower, C., 1970, Dopamine excretion in affective states and following Li_2CO_3 therapy, *Nature* **225**:868.

Moore, K. E., 1966, Effects of α-methyltyrosine on brain catecholamines and conditioned behavior in guinea pigs, *Life Sci.* **5**:55.

Moore, K. E., and Rech, R. H., 1967, Antagonism by monoamine oxidase inhibitors of α-methyltyrosine-induced catecholamine depletion and behavioral depression, *J. Pharmacol. Exptl. Therap.* **156**:70.

MRC Brain Metabolism Unit Report, 1972, Modified amine hypothesis for the etiology of affective disorders, *Lancet* **2**:253.

Muller, J. C., Pryer, W. W., Gibbons, J. E., and Orgain, E. S., 1955, Depression and anxiety occurring during rauwolfia therapy, *J. Am. Med. Assoc.* **159**:836.

Mullin, A. D., and Mogenson, G. J., 1963, Effects of fear conditioning on avoidance learning, *Psychol. Rep.* **13**:707.

Murphy, D. L., 1972a, L-Dopa, behavioral activation and psychopathology, in "Neurotransmitters," *Res. Publ. Assoc. Res. Nervous Mental Disease* **50**:472.

Murphy, D. L., 1972b, Amine precursors, amines and false neurotransmitters in depressed patients, *Am. J. Psychiat.* **129**:141.

Murphy, D. L., 1973, Mental effects of L-dopa, *Ann. Rev. Med.* **24**:209.

Murphy, D. L., and Kopin, I. J., 1972, The transport of biogenic animes, in: *Metabolic Transport* (L. E. Hokin, ed.), p. 503, Academic Press, New York.

Murphy, D. L., and Weiss, R., 1972, Reduced monamine oxidase activity in blood platelets from bipolar depressed patients, *Am. J. Psychiat.* **128**:1351.

Murphy, D. L., Brodie, H. K. H., Goodwin, F. K., and Bunney, W. E., Jr., 1971, L-Dopa: regular induction of hypomania in "bipolar" manic-depressive patients, *Nature* **229**:135.

Murphy, D. L., Goodwin, F. K., Brodie, H. K. H., and Bunney, W. E., Jr., 1973, L-Dopa, dopamine and hypomania, *Am. J. Psychiat.* **130**:79.

Murphy, D. L., Goodwin, F. K., and Bunney, W. E., Jr., in press, The psychobiology of mania, in: *American Handbook of Psychiatry.* Vol. VI, (D. Hamburg, ed.), Basic Books, New York.

Nelson, G. N., Masuda, M., and Holmes, T. H., 1966, Correlation of behavior and catecholamine metabolite excretion, *Psychosomat. Med.* **28**:216.

Ng, K. Y., Chase, T. N., Colburn, R. W., and Kopin, I. J., 1971, L-Dopa-induced release of cerebral monoamines, *Science* **170**:76.

Nies, A., Robinson, D. S., Ravaris, C. L., and Davis, J. M., 1971, Amines and monoamine oxidase in relation to aging and depression in man, *Psychosomat. Med.* **33**:470.

Nies, A., Robinson, D. S., Lamborn, K. R., and Lampert, R. P., 1973, Genetic control of platelet and plasma monoamine oxidase activity, *Arch. Gen. Psychiat.* **28**:834.

Nowlis, V., 1965, Research with the mood adjective checklist, in: *Affect, Cognition and Personality* (S. S. Tomkins and C. E. Izard, eds.), Springer, New York.

Nowlis, V., and Nowlis, H. H., 1956, The analysis of mood, *N.Y. Acad. Sci.* **65**:345.

O'Brien, C. P., DiCiacomo, J. N., Fahn, S., and Schwarz, G. A., 1971, Mental effects of high-dosage levodopa, *Arch. Gen. Psychiat.* **24**:61.

Olds, J., 1962, Hypothalamic substrates of reward, *Psychol. Rev.* **42**:554.

Overmier, J. B., and Seligman, M. E. P., 1967, Effects of inescapable shock upon subsequent escape and avoidance responding, *J. Comp. Physiol. Psychol.* **63**:28.

Papeschi, R., and McClure, D. J., 1971, Homovanillic and 5-hydroxy-indoleacetic acid in cerebrospinal fluid of depressed patients, *Arch. Gen. Psychiat.* **25**:354.

Papez, J. W., 1937, A proposed mechanism of emotion, *Arch. Neurol. Psychiat.* **38**:725.

Perkinson, E., Ruckart, R., and DaVanzo, J. P., 1968, Pharmacological and biochemical comparison of lithium and reference antidepressants, *Proc. Soc. Exptl. Biol. Med.* **131**:685.

Piaget, J., 1954, *Les Relations Entre L'affectivite et L'intelligence dans le Developpement Mental de L'enfant,* Centre de Documentation Universitaire, Paris.

Piaget, J., 1973, The affective unconscious and the cognitive unconscious, *J. Am. Psychoanalyt. Assoc.* **21**:249.

Plutchik, R., 1962, *The Emotions: Facts, Theories and a New Model,* Random House, New York.

Pollin, W., and Goldin, S., 1962, The physiological and psychological effects of intravenously administered epinephrine and its metabolism in normal and schizophrenic men—II. Psychiatric observations, *J. Psychiat. Res.* **1**:50.

Post, R. M., and Goodwin, F. K., 1973, Simulated behavior states: an approach to specificity in psychobiological research, *Biol. Psychiat.* **7**:237.

Post, R. M., Kotin, J. K., Goodwin, F. K., and Gordon, E. K., 1973, Psychomotor activity and cerebrospinal fluid amine metabolites in affective illness, *Am. J. Psychiat.* **130**:67.

Prange, A. J., Jr., Wilson, I. C., Knox, A. E., McClane, T. K., Breese, G. R., Martin, B. R., Alltop, L. B., and Lipton, M. A., 1972, Thyroid-imipramine clinical and chemical interaction: evidence for a receptor deficit in depression, *J. Psychiat. Res.* **9**:187.

Pribram, K. H., 1967, The new neurology and the biology of emotion: a structural approach, *Am. Psychol.* **22**:830.

Ramsey, T. A., Mendels, J., Hamilton, C., and Frazer, A., 1972, The effect of lithium carbonate on self-stimulating behavior in the rat, *Life Sci.* **11**:773.

Randrup, A., and Munkvad, I., 1966*a,* Dopa and other naturally occurring substances as causes of stereotypy and rage in rats, *Acta Psychiat. Scand. Suppl.* **191**:193.

Randrup, A., and Munkvad, J., 1966*b,* Role of catecholamines in the amphetamine excitatory response, *Nature,* **211**:540.

Ray, O. S., and Bivens, L. W., 1965*a,* Behavioral effects of L-α-methyl-dopa, *Life Sci.* **4**:823.

Ray, O. S., and Bivens, L. W., 1965*b,* Effects of L-α-methyl-dopa on discrete trial behavior, *Life Sci.* **4**:1185.

Rech, R. H., and Moore, K. E., 1968, Interactions between *d*-amphetamine and α-methyltyrosine in rat shuttle-box behavior, *Brain Res.* **8**:398.

Rech, R. H., Borys, H. K., and Moore, K. E., 1966, Alterations in behavior and brain catecholamine levels in rats treated with alpha-methyltyrosine, *J. Pharmacol. Expt. Therap.* **153**:512.

Rech, R. H., Carr, L. A., and Moore, K. E., 1968, Behavioral effects of α-methyltyrosine after prior depletion of brain catecholamines, *J. Pharmacol. Exptl. Therap.* **160**:326.

Redmond, D. E., Jr., and Maas, J. W., 1971, Moods, monkeys and monoamines, Presented to the Psychiatric Research Society, Boston, Massachusetts.

Redmond, D. E., Jr., Mass, J. W., Kling, A., and Dekirmenjian, H., 1971a, Changes in primate social behavior after treatment with α-methyl-p-tyrosine, *Psychosomat. Med.* **33**:97.

Redmond, D. E., Jr., Maas, J. W., Kling, A., Graham, C. W., and Dekirmenjian, H., 1971b, Social behavior of monkeys selectively depleted of monoamines, *Science* **174**:428.

Redmond, D. E., Jr., Garver, D. L., Hinrichs, R. L., and Maas, J. W., 1972, Social behavior of nonhuman primates after intraventricular 6-hydroxydopamine, Presented at American Psychiatric Association Meeting, Dallas, Texas.

Redmond, D. E., Jr., Hinrichs, R. L., Maas, J. W., and Kling, A., 1973a, Behavior of free-ranging macaques after intraventricular 6-hydroxydopamine, *Science* **181**:1256.

Redmond, D. E., Jr., Schlemmer, F., and Maas, J. W., 1973b, Changes in social behavior in monkeys after inescapable shock, Presented at the American Psychosomatic Society, Denver, Colorado.

Reis, D. J., Moorhead, D. T., and Merlino, N., 1970, Dopa-induced excitement in the cat, *Arch. Neurol.* **22**:31.

Richter, C., 1957, On the phenomenon of sudden death in animals and man, *Psychosomat. Med.* **19**:191.

Rickels, K., Chung, H. R., Gsanalosi, I., Sablosky, L., and Simon, J. H., 1973, Iprindole and imipramine in nonpsychotic depressed outpatients, *Brit. J. Psychiat.* **123**:329.

Robertson, J., and Bowlby, J., 1952, Responses of young children to separation from their mothers, *Cours du Centre International de l'Enfance* **2**:131.

Robinson, D. S., Davis, J. M., Nies, A., Colburn, R. W., Davis, J. N., Bourne, H. R., Bunney, W. E., Jr., Shaw, D. M., and Coppen, A. J., 1972, Ageing, monoamines, and monoamine-oxidase levels, *Lancet* **1**:290.

Roos, E.-E., and Sjostrom, R., 1969, 5-Hydroxyindoleacetic acid and homovanillic acid levels in the cerebrospinal fluid after probenecid application in patients with manic-depressive psychosis, *Pharmacol. Clin.* **1**:153.

Ross, S. B., Renyi, A. L., and Ogren, S. O., 1971, A comparison of the inhibitory activities of iprindole and imipramine on the uptake of 5-hydroxytryptamine and noradrenaline in brain slices, *Life Sci.* **10**:1267.

Routtenberg, A., 1968, The two-arousal hypothesis: reticular formation and limbic system, *Psychol. Rev.* **75**:51.

Rubin, R. T., Young, W. M., and Clark, B. R., 1968, 17-Hydroxycorticosteroid and vanillylmandelic acid excretion in a rapidly cycling manic-depressive, *Psychosomat. Med.* **32**:589.

Rubin, R. T., Miller, R. G., Clar, B. R., Poland, R. E., and Arthur, R. J., 1970, *Psychosomat. Med.* **32**:589.

Saletu, B., Saletu, M., and Itil, T. M., 1973, Effect of tricyclic antidepressants on the somatosensory evoked potential in man, *Psychopharmacologia* **29**:1.

Schachter, J., 1957, Pain, fear, and anger in hypertensives and normotensives: a psychophysiologic study, *Psychosomat. Med.* **19**:17.

Schachter, S., and Singer, J. E., 1962, Cognitive, social, and physiological determinants of emotional state, *Psychol. Rev.* **69**:379.

Schachter, S., and Wheeler, L., 1962, Epinephrine, chlorpromazine, and amusement, *J. Abnorm. Soc. Psychol.* **65**:121.

Schanberg, S. M., Breese, G. R., Schildkraut, J. J., Gordon, E. K., and Kopin, I. J., 1968a, 3-Methoxy-4-hydroxyphenylglycol sulfate in brain and cerebrospinal fluid, *Biochem. Pharmacol.* **17**:2006.

Schanberg, S. M., Schildkraut, J. J., Breese, G. R., and Kopin, I. J., 1968b, Metabolism of normetanephrine-³H in rat brain identification of conjugated 3-methoxy-4-hydroxyphenylglycol as major metabolite, *Biochem. Pharmacol.* **17**:247.

Scheckel, C. L., and Boff, E., 1964, Behavioral effects of interacting imipramine and other drugs with d-amphetamine, cocaine and tetrabenazine, *Psychopharmacologia* **5**:198.

Scheckel, C. L., Boff, E., and Pazery, L. M., 1969, Hyperactive states related to the metabolism of norepinephrine and similar biochemicals, *Ann. N.Y. Acad. Sci.* **159**:939.

Scheel-Kruger, J., and Randrup, A., 1967, Stereotype hyperactive behavior produced by dopamine in the absence of noradrenaline, *Life Sci.* **6**:1389.

Schildkraut, J. J., 1965, The catecholamine hypothesis of affective disorders: A review of supporting evidence, *Am. J. Psychiat.* **122**:509.

Schildkraut, J. J., (in press), Depressions and biogenic amines, in: *American Handbook of Psychiatry* (D. Hamburg, ed.), Basic Books, New York.

Schildkraut, J. J., 1973a, Pharmacology—The effects of lithium on biogenic amines, in: *Lithium, Its Role in Psychiatric Research and Treatment* (S. Gershon and B. Shopsin, eds.), pp. 51–74, Plenum Press, New York.

Schildkraut, J. J., 1973b, Neuropharmacology of the affective disorders, *Ann. Rev. Pharmacol.* **13**:427.

Schildkraut, J. J., and Durell, J., 1967, Noradrenergic activity during the transition from depression to mania, *Lancet* **1**:653.

Schildkraut, J. J., and Kety, S. S., 1967, Biogenic amines and emotion, *Science* **156**:21.

Schildkraut, J. J., Gordon, E. K., and Durell, J., 1965, Catecholamine metabolism in affective disorders. I. Normetanephrine and VMA excretion in depressed patients treated with imipramine, *J. Psychiat. Res.* **3**:213.

Schildkraut, J. J., Green, R., Gordon, E. K., and Durell, J., 1966, Normetanephrine excretion and affective state in depressed patients treated with imipramine, *Am. J. Psychiat.* **123**:690.

Schildkraut, J. J., Draskoczy, P. R., Gershon, E. S., Reich, P., and Grab, E. L., 1971, Effects of tricyclic antidepressants on norepinephrine metabolism: basic and clinical studies, in: *Brain Chemistry and Mental Disease* (B. T. Ho and W. M. McIsaac, eds.), pp. 215–236, Plenum Press, New York.

Schou, M., 1963, Normothymotics, "mood-normalizers": are lithium and the imipramine drugs specific for affective disorders?, *Brit. J. Psychiat.* **109**:803.

Schou, M., 1968, Lithium in psychiatric therapy and prophylaxis, *J. Psychiat. Res.* **6**:67.

Seay, W., and Harlow, H., 1965, Maternal separation in the rhesus monkey, *J. Nervous Mental Disease* **140**:434.

Seay, W. Hansen, E., and Harlow, H., 1962, Mother-infant separation in monkeys, *J. Child Psychol. Psychiat.* **3**:123.

Seligman, M. E., and Maier, J. F., 1967, Failure to escape traumatic shock, *J. Exptl. Psychol.* **74**:1.

Seligman, M. E., Maier, S. F., and Geer, J. H., 1968, Alleviation of learned helplessness in the dog, *J. Abnorm. Soc. Psychol.* **73**:256.

Sheard, M. H., 1970, Effect of lithium in foot-shock aggression in rats, *Nature* **228**:284.

Sheard, M. H., 1971, Effect of lithium on human aggression, *Nature* **230**:113.

Shinfuku, N., 1965, Clinical and biochemical studies with antidepressants, *Yonago Acta Med.* **9**:100.

Shinfuku, N., Omura, M., and Kayano, M., 1961, Catecholamine excretion in manic-depressive psychosis, *Yonago Acta Med.* **5**:109.

Shopsin, B., and Gershon, S., 1973, Pharmacology—Toxicology of the lithium ion, in: *Lithium, Its Role in Psychiatric Research and Treatment* (S. Gershon and B. Shopsin, eds.), pp. 107–146, Plenum Press, New York.

Shopsin, B., Freedman, L. S., Goldstein, M., and Gershon, S., 1972, Serum dopamine-β-hydroxylase (D-β-H) activity and affective states, *Psychopharmacologia* **27**:11.

Silverman, A. J., Cohen, S. I., Shmavonian, B. M., and Kirshner, N., 1961, Catecholamines in psychophysiologic studies, in: *Recent Advances in Biological Psychiatry* Vol. 3, (J. Wortis, ed.), pp. 104–118, Grune and Stratton, New York.

Sjoerdsma, A., Vendsalu, and Engelman, K., 1963, Studies on the metabolism and mechanism of action of methyldopa, *Circulation* **28**:492.

Sloane, R. B., Hughes, W., and Haust, H. L., 1966, Catecholamine excretion in manic-depressive and schizophrenic psychosis and its relationship to symptomatology, *Can. Psychiat. Assoc. J.* **11**:6.

Smirk, H., 1963, Hypotensive action of methyl dopa, *Brit. Med. J.* **1**:146.

Smith, G. M., and Beecher, H. K., 1964, Drugs and judgement: effects of amphetamine and secobarbital on self-evaluation, *J. Psychol.* **58**:397.

Snyder, S. H., and Banerjee, S. P., 1973, Amines in schizophrenia, in: *Frontiers in Catecholamine Research* (E. Usdin and S. H. Snyder, eds.), pp. 1133–1138, Pergamon Press, New York.

Sourkes, T. L., Murphy, G. F., Chavez, B., and Zielinski, M., 1961, The action of some α-methyl and other amino acids on cerebral catecholamine, *J. Neurochem.* **8**:109.

Spector, S., Sjoerdsma, A., and Udenfriend, S., 1965, Blockade of endogenous norepinephrine synthesis of α-methyl-tyrosine, an inhibitor of tyrosine hydroxylase, *J. Pharmacol. Exptl. Therap.* **147**:86.

Sroufe, L. A., and Stewart, M. A., 1973, Treating problem children with stimulant drugs, *New Engl. J. Med.* **289**:407.

Stein, L., 1961, Effects and interactions of imipramine, chlorpromazine, reserpine and amphetamine on self-stimulation: possible neurophysiological basis of depression, in: *Recent Advances in Biological Psychiatry,* Vol. 4 (J. Wortis, ed.), p. 288, Grune and Stratton, NewYork.

Stolk, J. M., and Rech, R. H., 1970, Antagonism of *d*-amphetamine by α-methyl-L-tyrosine: behavioral evidence for the participation of catecholamine stores and synthesis in the amphetamine stimulant response, *Neuropharmacology* **9**:249.

Strom-Olsen, R., and Weil-Malherbe, H., 1958, Humoral changes in manic-depressive psychosis with particular reference to excretion of catecholamines in urine, *J. Mental Sci.* **104**:696.

Sulser, F., Bickel, M. H., and Brodie, B. B., 1964, The action of desmethylimipramine in counteracting sedation and cholinergic effects of reserpine-like drugs, *J. Pharmacol. Exptl. Therap.* **144**:321.

Takahashi, R., Nagao, Y., Tsuchiya, K., Takamizawa, M., Kobayashi, T., Toru, M., Kobayashi, K., and Kariya, T., 1968, Catecholamine metabolism of manic-depressive illness, *J. Psychiat. Res.* **6**:185.

Turner, W., and Merlis, S., 1964, A clinical trial of pargyline and dopa in psychotic subjects, *Dis. Nerv. Syst.* **24**:538.

Ungerstedt, U., 1971*a*, Adipsia and aphagia after 6-hydroxydopamine induced degeneration of the nigrostriatal dopamine system, *Acta Physiol. Scand. Suppl.* **367**:95.

Ungerstedt, U., 1971*b*, Use of intracerebral injections of 6-hydroxydopamine as a tool for morphological and functional studies on central catecholamine neurons, in: *6-Hydroxydopamine and Catecholamine Neurons* (T. Malmfors, and H. Thoenen, eds.), p. 315, North Holland, Amsterdam.

Ungerstedt, U., 1971*c*, Stereotaxic mapping of the monoamine pathways in the rat brain, *Acta Physiol. Scand. Suppl.* **367**:69.

Uretsky, N. J., and Iversen, L. L., 1970, Effects of 6-hydroxydopamine on catecholamine-containing neurons in the rat brain, *J. Neurochem.* **17**:269.

Uretsky, N. J., and Schoenfeld, R. I., 1971, *Nature (New Biol.)* **234**:157.

van Kammen, D., and Murphy, D. L., 1974, Antagonism of the euphoriant and activating effects of *d*-amphetamine by lithium carbonate treatment, *Journal de Pharmacologie, Suppl. 2,* **5**:102.

van Praag, H. M., and Korf, J., 1971, A pilot study of some kinetic aspects of the metabolism of 5-hydroxytryptamine in depressive patients, *Biol. Psychiat.* **3**:105.

Wada, J. A., Wrinch, J., Hill, D., McGeer, P. L., and McGeer, E. G., 1963, Central aromatic amine levels and behavior, *Arch. Neurol.* **9**:69.

Weil-Malherbe, H., 1960, The passage of catechol amines through the blood–brain barrier, in: *Adrenergic Mechanisms,* (J. R. Vane, G. E. W. Wolstenholme, and M. O'Connor, eds.), pp. 421–423, Ciba Foundation Symposium, Churchill, London.

Weil-Malherbe, H., 1967, Biochemistry of functional psychoses, *Advan. Enzymd.* **29**:479.

Weil-Malherbe, H., and Szara, S. I., 1971, *The Biochemistry of Functional and Experimental Psychoses,* Thomas, Springfield.

Weinshilboum, R., and Axelrod, J., 1971, Serum dopamine-β-hydroxylase activity, *Circulation Res.* **28**:307.

Weinshilboum, R. N., Raymond, F. A., Elveback, L. R., and Weidman, W. H., 1973, Serum dopamine-beta-hydroxylase activity: Sibling-sibling correlation. *Science,* **181**:943–945.

Weintraub, M. I., and van Woert, M. H., 1971, Reversal by Levodopa of cholinergic hypersensitivity in Parkinson's disease, *New Engl. J. Med.* **248**:412.

Weiss, B., and Laties, V. G., 1962, Enhancement of human performance by caffeine and the amphetamines, *Pharmacol. Rev.* **14**:1.

Weiss, J. M., Stone, E. A., and Harrell, N., 1970, Coping behavior and brain norepinephrine level in rats, *J. Comp. Physiol. Psychol.* **72**:153.

Weissman, A., and Koe, B. K., 1965, Behavioral effects of L-α-methyltyrosine, an inhibitor of tyrosine hydroxylase, *Life Sci.* **4**:1037.

Weissman, A., Koe, B. K., and Tenen, S. S., 1966, Antiamphetamine effects following inhibition of tyrosine hydroxylase, *J. Pharmacol. Exptl. Therap.* **151**:339.

Welch, A. S., and Welch, B., 1971, Isolation, reactivity and aggression: evidence for an imvolvement of brain catecholamines and serotonin in: *The Physiology of Aggression and Defeat* (B. E. Eleftheriou and J. P. Scott, eds.), pp. 97–116, Plenum Press, New York.

Wetterberg, L., Aberg, H., Ross, S. B., and Froden, O., 1972, Plasma deopamine-β-hydroxylase activity in hypertension and various neuropsychiatric disorders, *Scand. J. Clin. Lab. Invest.* **30**:283.

Wheatley, D., 1969, Comparative effects of propranolol and chlordiazepoxide in anxiety states, *Brit. J. Psychiat.* **115**:1411.

Wilk, S., Shopsin, B., Gershon, S., and Suhl, M., 1972, Cerebrospinal fluid levels of MHPG in affective disorders, *Nature* **235**:440.

Wittenborn, J. R., 1961, Efficacy of electroconvulsive therapy, iproniazid and placebo in treatment of young depressed women, *J. Nervous Mental Disease* **133**:332.

Wittenborn, J. R., 1962, Comparison of imipramine, electroconvulsive therapy and placebo in treatment of depressions, *J. Nervous Mental Disease* **135**:131.

Wooten, G. F., and Cardon, P. V., 1973, Plasma dopamine-β-hydroxylase activity, *Arch. Neurol.* **28**:103.

Wurtman, R. J., Rose, C. M., Matthysse, S., and Baldessarini, R., 1970, L-dihydroxy-phenylalanine: effect on S-adenosylmethionine in brain, *Science* **169**:395.

Wyatt, R. J., Portnoy, B., Kupfer, D. J., Snyder, F., and Engelman, K., 1971, Resting plasma catecholamine concentrations in patients with depression and anxiety, *Arch. Gen. Psychiat.* **24**:65.

Young, P. T., 1961, *Motivation and Emotion,* Wiley, New York.

Zuckerman, M., Lubin, B., and Robins, S., 1965, Validation of the multiple affect adjective checklist in clinical situations, *J. Consult. Psychol.* **29**:594.

Zung, W. W. K., 1965, A self-rating depression scale, *Arch. Gen. Psychiat.* **12**:63.

Chapter 4

Catecholamines and Depression: A Further Specification of the Catecholamine Hypothesis of the Affective Disorders

James W. Maas

Department of Psychiatry
Yale University School of Medicine
New Haven, Connecticut

1. INTRODUCTION

Several years ago three review articles appeared which summarized the then available data which suggested that some, and perhaps all, human depressive states were associated with a functional deficiency of catecholamines within the central nervous system (Schildkraut, 1965; Bunney and Davis, 1965; Schildkraut and Kety, 1967). Since that time there has been much research dealing with this suggested role between catecholamines and human depression, and while the data which have emerged are by no means conclusive, much of the more recent information is generally consistent with and supportive of the original catecholamine hypothesis of the affective disorders for some patients. In this paper some of these more recent findings will be noted and the original hypothesis further specified, in that it will be suggested that (i) there is a disorder of catecholamine metabolism or disposition in only some, and not all, depressed patients and that this group may be identified biochemically and pharmacologically, (ii) norepinephrine and *not* dopamine brain systems are principally involved in these depressive disorders, and (iii) there is another group of depressed patients in which noradrenergic systems are not altered, although serotonin systems may be. The implications of these findings for future research are noted.

2. METABOLISM OF NOREPINEPHRINE

Present knowledge as to the metabolism of norepinephrine within the central nervous system serves as a backdrop to many of the clinical studies to be described, and this information is summarized in Figure 1. The general metabolic flow as presented in this figure represents a synthesis of

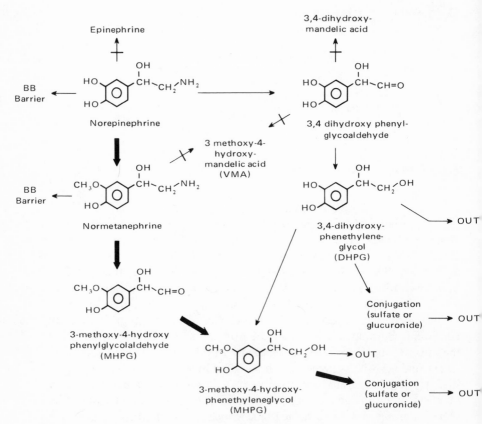

Figure 1. The metabolism of norepinephrine within the central nervous system. (See text for references and comments.)

reports from several laboratories (Mannarino *et al.*, 1963; Glowinski *et al.*, 1965; Rutledge and Jonason, 1967; Maas and Landis, 1968; Schanberg *et al.*, 1968*a,b*; Sharman, 1969). Emphasis in this figure is placed upon those ways in which the breakdown of norepinephrine centrally differs from that in peripheral organs. As is noted, there is a barrier to the movement of norepinephrine and normetanephrine out of, as well as into, brain (Glowinski *et al.*, 1965; Maas and Landis, 1966, 1968, 1971; Weil-Malherbe *et al.*, 1961). Further, the available evidence indicates that 3-methoxy-4-hydroxymandelic acid (VMA), if it is endogenously formed within the central nervous system, is present in quantities which are not detectable in brain tissue by presently available techniques. (Approximately 0.5 μg/ml of VMA is found in CSF, but the quantity was too low to allow for absolute identification [Wilk and Watson, 1974].) Similarly, it is known that very little epinephrine is present within brain (Gunne, 1962; Vogt, 1954). It therefore seems likely that assays of norepinephrine, epinephrine, normetanephrine, metanephrine, and VMA in plasma or urine will principally reflect the metabolism of norepinephrine outside the central nervous system. In contrast, the available evidence from several mammalian species indicates that norepinephrine is degraded within brain via oxidative and then reductive pathways to yield either 3-methoxy-4-hydroxyphenethyleneglycol (MHPG) or dihydroxyphenethyleneglycol (DHPG). Depending upon the species, these glycols may be further conjugated as the glucuronide or sulfate and transported out of brain and excreted into urine (Maas and Landis, 1968; Stone, 1973; Schanberg *et al.*, 1968*a*; Sharman, 1969; Sugden and Eccleston, 1971; Meek and Neff, 1972; Gordon *et al.*, 1973). It is also known that destruction of the locus coeruleus produces a decrement in cerebral MHPG, whereas stimulation leads to significant increments, and it therefore appears that not only is MHPG a major metabolic product of brain norepinephrine, but that it is formed when norepinephrine is released at nerve endings and, as such, can provide some index of functional activity of noradrenergic neurones (Korf *et al.*, 1973*a,b*; Walter and Eccleston, 1973; Arbuthnott *et al.*, 1973). For these reasons the assay of MHPG within cerebrospinal fluid and urine assumes particular significance. While assays of MHPG in these body fluids cannot yield crisp, definitive information because of questions as to the origins of CSF MHPG (Post *et al.*, 1973*a*) and to the exact fraction of urinary MHPG which is derived from central pools of norepinephrine (Maas and Landis, 1968, 1971; Maas *et al.*, 1973; Breese *et al.*, 1972; Karoum *et al.*, 1974), both approaches have been used for clinical studies of norepinephrine metabolism in patients who are either depressed or hypomanic. Results of some of these studies are presented in the following portions of this paper.

3. MHPG IN AFFECTIVE STATES

In 1968 it was reported that a heterogeneous group of depressed patients excreted significantly less MHPG into urine than did a healthy comparison group, whereas the quantities of urinary normetanephrine and metanephrine excreted by these two groups were similar (Maas *et al.,* 1968*a*). Subsequent to this, reports from three separate groups have appeared which indicate that when manic-depressive patients are followed longitudinally, they excrete less MHPG during periods of depression than they do during periods of either euthymia or hypomania, and in two of these reports it was suggested that the increments in urinary MHPG preceded the shift in the behavioral state of the patients (Greenspan *et al.,* 1970; Bond *et al.,* 1972; Jones *et al.,* 1973). Illustrative data are shown in Figure 2. It has also been noted that recovered unipolar, depressed patients excrete greater amounts of MHPG relative to the period of depression (Shaw *et al.,* 1973).

One report has appeared which indicates that decrements in urinary MHPG may be a function of activity (Ebert *et al.,* 1972), but it has also been found that strenuous exercise by healthy subjects which is sufficient to produce a three- to tenfold increase in urinary NE does not alter MHPG (Goode *et al.,* 1973). Further, no relationship between agitation or retardation in depressed patients and MHPG excretion has been found (DeLeon-Jones *et al.,* 1973*a*; Schildkraut, 1974). There are two reports, however, which indicate that stressful situations in healthy and depressed subjects may result in increases in urinary MHPG, but here there are also increases in other catecholamine metabolites (Rubin *et al.,* 1970; Maas *et al.,* 1971). This latter finding highlights the importance of assaying other metabolites of catecholamines along with MHPG, i.e., it would seem that changes in

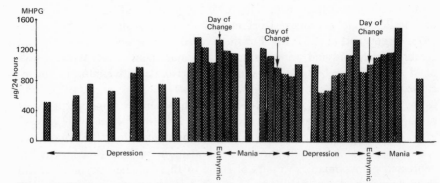

Figure 2. MHPG excretion (μg/24 hr) during manic and depressive episodes in a single patient. Note that the changes in MHPG excretion precede changes in clinical state.

Table I.   Comparison of Urinary Catecholamine Metabolite Excretion[a]

	Males			Females		
	Patients N=20	Controls N=19	p	Patients N=48	Controls N=21	p
M	114 ± 22	86 ± 9	NS	97 ± 6	83 ± 9	NS
NM	172 ± 17	196 ± 17	NS	214 ± 17	223 ± 33	NS
VMA	4601 ± 318	4165 ± 656	NS	4378 ± 257	4612 ± 408	NS
MHPG	1394 ± 89	1674 ± 117	<0.05	1155 ± 58	1348 ± 65	0.05

[a] Excretion of metanephrine (M), normetanephrine (NM), 3-methoxy-4-hydroxymandelic acid (VMA), and 3-methoxy-4-hydroxyphenethyleneglycol (MHPG) by normal subjects and diagnostically heterogeneous, hospitalized depressed patients. All values are expressed as $\mu g/24$ hr.

urinary MHPG which are not accompanied by increments or decrements in other products reflecting peripheral norepinephrine or epinephrine metabolism are of particular importance.

Studies of CSF MHPG levels in depressed versus normal subjects are contradictory in that one group of investigators find significant decrements in the patient group (Post et al., 1973b), whereas others do not (Shaw et al., 1973; Shopsin et al., 1973). These different findings may be due to the heterogeneity of the patient populations as will be detailed in other parts of this paper.

In another study in which 68 patients were compared with 40 comparison subjects, it was found that the quantities of urinary MHPG excreted by the patient groups were significantly less than that excreted by the healthy subjects, whereas the quantities of normetanephrine, metanephrine, and VMA excreted by the two groups were similar (see Table I). Furthermore, it was noted that the differences between the patient and comparison groups could not be explained in terms of age, sex, body weight, creatinine excretion, or urine volume. It should be emphasized that while the depressed patients as a group excreted significantly less MHPG than did the healthy subjects, the level of significance given the reasonably large N was modest in that the p-value was ≈ 0.05, indicating, of course, that many of the depressed patients excreted normal or even greater than normal quantities of MHPG (Dekirmenjian et al., 1973; DeLeon-Jones et al., 1973b; Maas et al., 1974). It would thus appear that, while some depressed patients excrete less than normal quantities of MHPG, this is by no means true for every patient. These findings raise the possibility that those patients who excrete less than normal amounts of MHPG may represent a particular subgroup which has special biochemical or pharmacological characteristics. (Data suggesting that the "low MHPG group" may be identified using clinical criteria have been presented by two separate groups of investigators [Maas *et al.*, 1974; Schildkraut, 1974].)

Data indicating that there is, in fact, a subgroup of depressed patients who may be identified biochemically and pharmacologically was presented in 1968 (Maas *et al.*, 1968*b*). In that report it was noted that those patients who excreted less than normal quantities of MHPG prior to treatment with imipramine or desmethylimipramine had favorable responses to treatment with these drugs, whereas those patients who excreted normal amounts of MHPG did not respond well to treatment with either desmethylimipramine or imipramine. Furthermore, it was noted that those patients who did respond to treatment had either no change or modest increments in urinary MHPG following 4 weeks of drug treatment, whereas those patients who had normal pretreatment urinary MHPG's and subsequent failure of response had decrements in the excretion of urinary MHPG. Subsequent to this original observation which was made on a series of 12 patients, a second series of 16 patients was studied in more detail. This group of patients was chosen in terms of having depression of sufficient severity to warrant hospitalization and organic treatment, and they were maintained free of all medication for 3 weeks. Nurses' depression ratings were taken daily, and any patient who showed a spontaneous change in his depression during these 3 weeks was excluded from the study. Again, in this replication study it was found that there was a direct correlation between the pretreatment MHPG level and subsequent response to imipramine, i.e., a low pretreatment MHPG predicted a favorable response to treatment with this particular antidepressant drug. Furthermore, it was found that pretreatment levels of normetanephrine, metanephrine, or VMA were not correlated with subsequent treatment response. As before, it was also found that those patients who responded to treatment with imipramine had increments in urinary normetanephrine and either no change or modest increments in urinary MHPG, whereas those patients who did not respond had rather marked decrements in both metabolites. These findings led to the suggestion that there are two populations of depressed patients who may be identified in terms of MHPG excretion (Maas *et al.*, 1972).

In support of the possibility that there are two distinct groups of patients are findings obtained with *d*-amphetamine (Fawcett *et al.*, 1972; Fawcett and Siomopoulous, 1971). In these studies patients were given, on a double-blind basis, alternately either placebo or *d*-amphetamine (15 mg b.i.d), and the effects of the *d*-amphetamine on mood elevation were noted. These studies were done originally to see if one could predict subsequent response to tricyclics by alterations in mood as induced by *d*-amphetamine. It was found that those patients who did respond with an elevation of mood to *d*-amphetamine also had favorable responses to treatment with tricyclic drugs, but interestingly, in terms of the thesis being developed in this paper, it was also found that those patients who had elevations in mood following *d*-amphetamine were those patients who excreted less than normal quantities of MHPG, whereas there was a tendency for those patients who excreted normal amounts of MHPG to have either no elevation of mood with *d*-amphetamine or a worsening. It is of interest that, as with the use of imipramine or desmethylimipramine, those patients who responded to *d*-amphetamine with a brightening of mood had increments in urinary MHPG excretion, whereas those patients who did not had decrements.

Schildkraut (1973) has reported that patients who excrete normal to higher than normal amounts of urinary MHPG have a favorable treatment response to amitriptyline, whereas those who excrete lower amounts of MHPG fail to respond to this drug. He also noted that one of the nonresponders had a history of a favorable response to imipramine treatment. More recently a study has emerged from the NIMH group which confirms and extends the above findings. Beckman *et al.* (1974) examined a group of patients who were unequivocal responders or nonresponders to either amitriptyline or imipramine in terms of their pretreatment MHPG levels. They found that those patients who had low pretreatment MHPG's responded well to imipramine, whereas those patients who had high MHPG's did not respond to treatment with this drug, and while the high pretreatment MHPG patients responded well to amitriptyline, those who excreted low quantities of this metabolite did not respond to amitriptyline. Although the number of patients per group in this study was small, it is of particular interest in that there were no cross-overs in values and all four cells were covered. These latter workers also found that those patients who responded to treatment had decrements in urinary MHPG, as did the nonresponders. In a preliminary study, however, it has been reported that, as with urinary MHPG, depressed patients who respond to treatment with tricyclic antidepressant drugs had no change in CSF MHPG levels, whereas those who do not respond have decrements in this metabolite (Post and Goodwin, 1973).

4. SUBGROUPS OF DEPRESSION

In the aggregate, these studies suggest that there are two biochemically and pharmacologically identifiable subgroups of depressed patients. The first will be called group A, and these patients are characterized by:

1. A low pretreatment MHPG.
2. A favorable response to treatment with imipramine or desmethyl-imipramine.

3. A brightening of mood following a trial of d-amphetamine.
4. Modest increments or no change in urinary MHPG following treatment with imipramine, desmethylimipramine, or a brief trial on d-amphetamine.
5. A failure to respond to amitriptyline.

The second group of patients, which is called group B, is characterized by:

1. A normal or high urinary MHPG.
2. A favorable treatment response to amitriptyline.
3. A lack of mood change during a trial of d-amphetamine.
4. Decrements in urinary MHPG following treatment with imipramine, desmethylimipramine, or a brief trial of d-amphetamine.
5. A failure to respond to imipramine.

It would thus appear that depression is a biochemically heterogeneous illness, and it is therefore likely that if depressed patients as a group are compared with normals that significant differences will be obscured. This might account for discrepant reports as to CSF MHPG levels in depressed versus normal subjects (Shaw *et al.*, 1973; Post *et al.*, 1973*b*; Shopsin *et al.*, 1973).

5. BIOCHEMICAL MECHANISMS IN AFFECTIVE DISORDERS

Given the above groups as defined, it is of use to apply the classical pharmacological strategem of examining some of the modes of action of imipramine, desmethylimipramine, d-amphetamine, and amitriptyline in order to develop hypotheses as to biological mechanisms which may be involved in these two groups of depressive disorders. To this end, a summary of some available data as to the effects of these agents on blocking amine uptake are presented in Table II (Ross and Renyi, 1967, 1969; Carlsson *et al.*, 1966, 1969*a,b*; Fuxe and Ungerstedt, 1968; Glowinski, 1960; Glowinski and Axelrod, 1964; Glowinski *et al.*, 1966; Haggendal and Hamberger, 1967; Sulser *et al.*, 1969; Alpers and Himwich, 1969; Schubert *et al.*, 1970; Coyle and Snyder, 1969; Farnebo, 1971; Schildkraut *et al.*, 1969; Iversen and Johnston, 1971; Harris *et al.*, 1973). It may be noted from Table II that in contrast to d-amphetamine, imipramine, desmethylimipramine, and amitriptyline have little or no effect on dopamine reuptake. These data, when taken in conjunction with the finding that treatment with L-dopa [which elevates brain DA and CSF hydroxyhomovanillic acid (HVA), but not CSF

Table II. A Summary of the Effects of a Variety of Antidepressant or Mood-Altering Drugs on the Blockade of Uptake of Biogenic Amines[a]

Drug	DA	NE	5-HT	GABA
d-Amphetamine	+++	+++	0	?
Imipramine	0	++	+++	0
Desipramine	0	++++	±	0
Amitriptyline	0	0	+++	0

[a] See text for references on which table is based.

MHPG (Wilk and Mones, 1971)] does not result in improvement in a significant number of depressed patients (Goodwin *et al.,* 1970), lead to the conclusion that it is unlikely that brain dopamine systems are integrally associated with depression in either subgroup A or B. [This does not exclude dopamine from having a role in the production of manic states (Murphy *et al.,* 1971).] The lack of effects of the drugs on γ-amino-butyric acid (GABA) would also seem to exclude this amine from consideration. The fact that desmethylimipramine is effective in the treatment of group A patients, that amphetamine produces a mood elevation in these subjects, and that both these agents have relatively weak effects upon blocking reuptake in serotonin (5-HT) systems suggests that 5-HT systems are not altered in the group A patients. In contrast, all agents which are effective in treating group A patients, or result in a mood elevation, block NE uptake. Further, depressed patients who respond to treatment with imipramine, desmethylimipramine, or *d*-amphetamine excrete less than normal amounts of MHPG into urine prior to treatment. It is therefore suggested that group A patients have an alteration in noradrenergic systems, probably central, which is integrally related to their depressive states. In contrast, the failure of response to imipramine, the normal to high MHPG, and the lack of a mood change with *d*-amphetamine lead to the conclusion that group B patients do not have a deficit in NE systems, although 5-HT appears to be a worthwhile candidate for investigation.

If the above conclusions are correct, one may ask why group A patients who have the postulated deficit in central NE systems do not respond to treatment with amitriptyline, i.e., amitriptyline itself is not an effective agent in blocking the reuptake of NE, but it is demethylated *in vivo* to nortriptyline which does block NE uptake (Braithwaite and Widdop, 1971; Tuck and Punell, 1973). Two explanations for this failure of type A patients to respond to amitriptyline are as follows. First, amitriptyline is demethylated *in vivo* to nortriptyline, as is imipramine to desmethylimipramine (Moody *et al.,* 1967), but the conversion of amitriptyline to the secondary amine proceeds at a slower rate than nortriptyline hydroxylation with the result that it has been found that plasma levels of amitriptyline are significantly higher than those of nortriptyline (Braithwaite and Widdop, 1971). In contrast, when imipramine is given to patients the plasma levels of desipramine are usually higher than those of imipramine (Moody *et al.,* 1967). As a consequence of the above it is possible, even likely, that when group A patients are given amitriptyline that therapeutically effective concentrations of nortriptyline are not achieved, i.e., the nortriptyline levels are not sufficient to correct the deficit in noradrenergic systems. Parenthetically, if this line of reasoning is correct it would strengthen the possibility that group B patients have a disorder in 5-HT systems (see Table II). This suggestion is testable by examining the therapeutic effects of adequate doses of nortriptyline on depressions of the A and B types as defined in this paper, i.e., group A, but not group B patients should respond to nortriptyline. Second, it is possible, even likely, that in addition to the noradrenergic, other brain amine systems than those already discussed are also involved in the genesis of depression in the type A patients. For example, the tricyclic antidepressants have been demonstrated to have significant peripheral anticholinergic properties, and while these are generally viewed as producing unwelcome side effects, it is possible that these drugs also have actions upon central cholinergic systems which when combined with their effects upon NE systems may account for their beneficial actions. This could also possibly explain why *d*-amphetamine is able to produce a mood elevation in patients but does not have a long-term therapeutic value in the treatment of depression, i.e., amphetamine has an effect on noradrenergic systems, but it does not possess significant anticholinergic properties. If this view is correct, two testable predictions emerge: (i) It would be expected that the combination of *d*-amphetamine with centrally active anticholinergic agents should be effective in the treatment of type A depression, and (ii) there should be significant differences in the effects of imipramine, desmethylimipramine, and amitriptyline upon central cholinergic mechanisms, i.e., imipramine and desmethylimipramine should be similar and both should be different from amitriptyline in their actions on cholinergic systems. In this regard it is of interest that it has recently been reported that physostigmine, which is an inhibitor of cholinesterase, is able to reverse manic states, and in patients with an affective component to their illness can produce a depressive-like syndrome (Janowsky *et al.,* 1972*a*). These data have led to the suggestion that manic-depressive illness is a function of adrenergic–cholinergic balance (Janowsky *et al.,* 1972*b*).

Inferences as to the aminergic systems involved in type B depressions are more difficult to make, but since these patients are characterized by no change in mood with d-amphetamine, have normal to high urinary MHPG values, and respond to amitriptyline (see Table II), the possibility of an alteration in 5-HT systems must be seriously considered (Van Praag and Korf, 1974).

6. SUMMARY

The generally held view that depression is a biochemically heterogeneous illness is supported by recent research findings detailed in this paper. Further, it is suggested that there is now sufficient evidence to allow for a biochemical and pharmacological identification of at least two subtypes of depressions. The implications of these data for future biochemical investigations of human depressive disorders are clear, i.e., in future studies patients should be subclassified, biochemically and pharmacologically, as much as present and future information will allow. If this is not done, new findings will be blurred and may be the cause of disparate findings between separate investigative groups.

7. REFERENCES

Alpers, H. S., and Himwich, H., 1969, An *in vitro* study of the effects of tricyclic antidepressant drugs on the accumulation of ^{14}C-5HT by rabbit brain, *Biol. Psychiat.* 1:81.

Arbuthnott, G. W., Christie, J. E., Crow, T. J., Eccleston, D., and Slater, D. S., 1973, The effects of unilateral and bilateral lesions in the locus coeruleus on the levels of 3-methoxy-4-hydroxyphenylglycol in neocortex, *Experientia* 29:52.

Beckmann, H., Jones, C. C., and Goodwin, F. K., 1974, Central norepinephrine metabolism and the prediction of antidepressant response to imipramine or amitriptyline: Studies with urinary MHPG in unipolar depressed patients. Presented at the annual meeting of the American Psychiatric Association, Detroit, Michigan.

Bond, P. A., Jenner, F. A., and Sampson, G. A., 1972, Daily variations of the urine content of MHPG in two manic-depressive patients, *Psychol. Med.* 2:81.

Braithwaite, R. A., and Widdop, B., 1971, A specific gas-chromatographic method for the measurement of "steady state" plasma levels of amitriptyline and nortriptyline in patients, *Clin. Chim. Acta* 35:461.

Breese, G. R., Prange, A. J., Howard, J. L., Lipton, M. A., McKinney, W. T., Bowman, R. E., and Bushnell, P., 1972, Noradrenaline metabolite excretion after central sympathectomy with 6-hydroxydopamine, *Nature* (*New Biol.*) 240:286.

Bunney, W. E., Jr., and Davis, J. M., 1965, Norepinephrine in depressive reactions. *Arch. Gen. Psychiat.* 13:483.

Carlsson, A., Fuxe, K., Hamberger, B., and Lindqvist, M., 1966, Biochemical and histochemical studies on the effects of imipramine-like drugs and (+)-amphetamine on central and peripheral catecholamine neurons, *Acta Physiol. Scand.* 67:481.

Carlsson, A., Corrodi, H., Fuxe, K., and Hokfelt, T., 1969a, Effect of antidepressant drugs on the depletion of intraneuronal brain 5-hydroxytryptamine stores caused by 4-methyl-α-ethyl-m-tyramine, European J. Pharmacol. 5:357.

Carlsson, A., Corrodi, H., Fuxe, K., and Hokfelt, T., 1969b, Effects of some antidepressant drugs on the depletion of intraneuronal brain catecholamine stores caused by 4,α-dimethyl-m-tyramine, European J. Pharmacol. 5:367.

Coyle, J. T., and Snyder, S. H., 1969, Catecholamine uptake by synaptosomes in homogenates of rat brain: Stereospecificity in different areas, J. Pharmacol. Exptl. Therap. 170:221.

Dekirmenjian, H., Maas, J., and Fawcett, J., 1973, Urinary excretion of norepinephrine and its metabolites in human control subjects, Presented at American Psychiatric Association annual meeting, Hawaii.

DeLeon-Jones, F., Maas, J. W., and Dekirmenjian, H., 1973a, Urinary 3-methoxy-4-hydroxyphenylethylene glycol (MHPG) excretion by female patients with agitated and retarded depressions, Presented at annual Psychosomatic Society meetings, Denver, Colorado.

DeLeon-Jones, F., Maas, J. W., Dekirmenjian, H., and Sanchez, J., 1973b, Depressive syndromes and catecholamine metabolites, Presented at American Psychiatric Association annual meeting, Hawaii.

Ebert, M. H., Post, R. M., and Goodman, F. K., 1972, Effect of physical activity on urinary MHPG excretion in depressed patients, Lancet 11:766.

Farnebo, L-O, 1971, Effect of d-amphetamine on spontaneous stimulation-induced release of catecholamines, Acta Physiol. Scand. Suppl. 371:45.

Fawcett, J., and Siomopoulous, V., 1971, Dextroamphetamine response as a possible predictor of improvement with tricyclic therapy in depression, Arch. Gen. Psychiat. 25:247.

Fawcett, J., Maas, J. W., and Dekirmenjian, H., 1972, Depression and MHPG excretion: Response to dextroamphetamine and tricyclic antidepressants, Arch. Gen. Psychiat. 26:246.

Fuxe, K., and Ungerstedt, U., 1968, Histochemical studies of the effect of (+)-amphetamine, drugs of the imipramine group, and tryptamine on central catecholamine and 5-HT neurons after intraventricular injection of catecholamines and 5-HT, European J. Pharmacol. 4:135.

Glowinski, J., 1970, Release of monoamines in central nervous system, in: New Aspects of Storage and Release Mechanisms of CA (H. J. Schumann and G. Kroneberg, eds.), p. 301, Springer-Verlag, Berlin.

Glowinski, J., and Axelrod, J., 1964, Inhibition of uptake of tritiated-noradrenaline in the intact rat brain by imipramine and structurally related compounds, Nature 204:1318.

Glowinski, J., Kopin, I. J., and Axelrod, J., 1965, Metabolism of (^{3}H) norepinephrine in rat brain, J. Neurochem. 12:25.

Glowinski, J., Axelrod, J., and Iverson, L. L., 1966, Regional studies of catecholamines in the rat brain. IV. Effects of drugs on the disposition and metabolism of ^{3}H-NE and ^{3}H-dopamine, J. Pharmacol. Exptl. Therap. 153:30.

Goode, D. J., Dekirmenjian, H., Meltzer, H. Y., and Maas, J. W., 1973, Relation of exercise to MHPG excretion in normal subjects, Arch. Gen. Psychiat. 29:391.

Goodwin, F. K., Murphy, D. L., Brodie, H. K. H., and Bunney, W. E., 1970, L-Dopa, catecholamines, and behavior: A clinical and biochemical study in depressed patients, Biol. Psychiat. 2:341.

Gordon, E. K., Oliver, J, Goodwin, F. K., Chase, T. N., and Post, R. M., 1973, Effect of probenecid on free 3-methoxy-4-hydroxyphenethyleneglycol (MHPG) and its sulfate in human cerebrospinal fluid, Neuropharmacology 12:391.

Greenspan, J., Schildkraut, J. J., Gordon, E. K., Baer, L., Aronoff, M. S., and Durell, J.,

1970, Catecholamine metabolism in affective disorders—III. 3-methoxy-4-hydroxyphenylglycol and other catecholamine metabolites in patients treated with lithium carbonate, *J. Psychiat. Res.* **7**:171.

Gunne, L. M., 1962, Relative adrenaline content in brain tissue, *Acta Physiol. Scand.* **56**:324.

Haggendal, T., and Hamberger, B., 1967, Quantitative *in vivo* studies on noradrenaline uptake and its inhibition by amphetamines, desimipramine, and chlorpromazine, *Acta Physiol. Scand.* **70**:277.

Harris, M., Hopkin, J. M., and Neal, M. J., 1973, Effect of centrally acting drugs on the uptake of ^{3}H-γ-aminobutyric acid (GABA) by slices of rat cerebral cortex, *Brit. J. Pharmacol.* **47**:229.

Iversen, L. L., and Johnston, G. A. R., 1971, GABA uptake in rat central nervous system: Comparison of uptake in slices and homogenates and the effects of some inhibitors, *J. Neurochem.* **18**:1939.

Janowsky, D. S., El-Yousef, M. K., Davis, J. M., and Hubbard, B., 1972a, Paper read at the 125th meeting of the American Psychiatric Association, Dallas, Texas.

Janowsky, D. S., El-Yousef, M. K., Davis, J. M., and Sekerke, H. J., 1972b, A cholinergic-adrenergic hypothesis of mania and depression, *Lancet* **11**:632.

Jones, F., Maas, J. W., Dekirmenjian, H., and Fawcett, J. A., 1973, Urinary catecholamine metabolites during behavioral changes in a patient with manic depressive cycles, *Science* **179**:300.

Karoum, F., Wyatt, R., and Costa, E., 1974, Estimation of the contribution of peripheral and central noradrenergic neurons to urinary 3-methoxy-4-hydroxyphenyl glycol in the rat, *Neuropsychopharmacologica* (in press).

Korf, J., Roth, R. H., and Aghajanian, G. K., 1973a, Alterations in turnover and endogenous levels of norepinephrine in the cerebral cortex following electrical stimulation and acute axotomy of cerebral noradrenergic pathways, *European J. Pharmacol.* **23**:276.

Korf, J., Aghajanian, G. K., and Roth, R. H., 1973b, Stimulation and destruction of the locus coeruleus: Opposite effects on 3-methoxy-4-hydroxyphenyl-glycol sulfate levels in the rat cerebral cortex, *European J. Pharmacol.* **21**:305.

Maas, J. W., and Landis, D. H., 1966, A technique for assaying the kinetics of norepinephrine metabolism in brain *in vivo*, *Psychosomat. Med.* **28**:247.

Maas, J. W., and Landis, D. H., 1968, *In vivo* studies of the metabolism of norepinephrine in the central nervous system, *J. Pharmacol. Exptl. Therap.* **163**:147.

Maas, J. W., and Landis, D. H., 1971, The metabolism of circulating norepinephrine by human subjects, *J. Pharmacol. Exptl. Therap.* **177**:600.

Maas, J. W., Fawcett, J. A., and Dekirmenjian, H., 1968a, 3-methoxy-4-hydroxyphenylglycol (MHPG) excretion in depressive states, *Arch. Gen. Psvchiat.* **19**:129.

Maas, J. W., Fawcett, J. A., and Dekirmenjian, H., 1968b, Catecholamine metabolism and the depressive states, Presented at American Psychiatric Association annual meeting, Boston.

Maas, J. W., Dekirmenjian, H., and Fawcett, J. A., 1971, Catecholamine metabolism and stress, *Nature* **230**:330.

Maas, J. W., Fawcett, J. A., and Dekirmenjian, H., 1972, Catecholamine metabolism, depressive illness, and drug response, *Arch. Gen. Psychiat.* **26**:252.

Maas, J. W., Dekirmenjian, H., Garver, D., Redmond, D. E., and Landis, D. H., 1973, Excretion of catecholamine metabolites following intraventricular injection of 6-hydroxydopamine in the *Macaca speciosa, European J. Pharmacol.* **23**:121.

Maas, J. W., Dekirmenjian, H., and DeLeon-Jones, F., 1974, The identification of depressed patients who have a disorder of norepinephrine metabolism and/or disposition, in: *Frontiers in Catecholamine Research,* Pergamon Press, New York.

Mannarino, E., Kirshner, N., and Nashold, B. S., 1963, The metabolism of (^{14}C) noradrenaline by cat brain *in vivo, J. Neurochem.* **10**:373.

Meek, J. L., and Neff, N. H., 1972, Acidic and neutral metabolites of norepinephrine: Their metabolism and transport from brain, *J. Pharmacol. Exptl. Therap.* **181**:457.

Moody, J. P., Tait, A. C., and Todrick, A., 1967, Plasma levels of imipramine and desmethylimipramine during therapy, *Brit. J. Psychiat.* **113**:183.

Murphy, D. L., Brodie, H. K., Goodwin, F. K., and Bunney, W., 1971, Regular induction of hypomania by L-dopa in "bipolar" manic-depressive patients, *Nature* **229**:135.

Post, R., and Goodwin, F. K., 1973, Cerebrospinal fluid MHPG in affective disorders: State dependent *vs.* state independent variables, Presented at annual meeting of the American College of Neuropsychopharmacology, Palm Springs, California.

Post, R. M., Goodwin, F. K., Gordon, E., and Watkin, D. M., 1973a, Amine metabolites in human cerebrospinal fluid: Effects of cord transsection and spiral fluid block, *Science* **179**:897.

Post, R. M., Gordon, E. K. Goodwin, F. K., and Bunney, W. E., Jr., 1973b, Central norepinephrine metabolism in affective illness: MHPG in the cerebrospinal fluid, *Science* **179**:1002.

Ross, S. B., and Renyi, A. L., 1967, Inhibition of the uptake of tritiated catecholamines by antidepressant and related agents, *European J. Pharmacol.* **2**:181.

Ross, S. B., and Renyi, A. L., 1969, Inhibition of the uptake of tritiated 5-hydroxytryptamine in brain tissue, *European J. Pharmacol.* **7**:270.

Rubin, R. T., Miller, R. G., Clark, B. R., Poland, R. E., and Arthur, R. J., 1970, The stress of aircraft carrier landings II. 3-methoxy-4-hydroxyphenyl-glycol excretion in naval aviators, *Psychosomat. Med.* **2**:589.

Rutledge, C. O., and Jonason, J., 1967, Metabolic pathways of dopamine and norepinephrine in rabbit brain *in vitro, J. Pharmacol. Exptl. Therap.* **157**:493.

Schanberg, S. M., Breese, G. R., Schildkraut, J. J., Gordon, E. K., and Kopin, I. J., 1968a, 3-methoxy-4-hydroxyphenylglycol sulfate in brain and cerebrospinal fluid, *Biochem. Pharmacol.* **17**:2006.

Schanberg, S. M., Schildkraut, J. J., Breese, G. R., and Kopin, I. J., 1968b, Metabolism of normetanephrine-^{3}H in rat brain—identification of conjugated MHPG as the major metabolite, *Biochem. Pharmacol.* **17**:247.

Schildkraut, J. J., 1965, The catecholamine hypothesis of affective disorders: A review of supporting evidence, *Am. J. Psychiat.* **122**:509.

Schildkraut, J. J., 1973, Norepinephrine metabolites as biochemical criteria for classifying depressive disorders and predicting responses to treatment: Preliminary findings, *Am. J. Psychiat.* **130**:695.

Schildkraut, J. J., 1974, Catecholamine metabolism and affective disorders, in: *Frontiers in Catecholamine Research,* Pergamon Press, New York.

Schildkraut, J. J., and Kety, S. S., 1967, Biogenic amines and emotion, *Science* **156**:21.

Schildkraut, J. J., Dodge, G. A., and Logue, M. A., 1969, Effects of tricyclic antidepressants on the uptake and metabolism of intracisternally administered norepinephrine in rat brain, *J. Psychiat. Res.* **7**:29.

Schubert, J., Nyback, H., and Sedvall, G., 1970, Effect of antidepressant drugs on accumulation and disappearance of monoamines formed *in vivo* from labelled precursors in mouse brain, *J. Pharm. Pharmacol.* **22**:136.

Sharman, D. F., 1969, Glycol metabolites of noradrenaline in brain tissue, *Brit. J. Pharmacol.* **36**:523.

Shaw, D. M., O'Keeffe, R., MacSweeney, D. A., Brooksbank, B. W. L., Noguera, R., and Coppen, A., 1973, 3-methoxy-4-hydroxyphenylglycol in depression, *Psychol. Med.* **3**:333.

Shopsin, B., Wilk, S., Gershon, S., Davis, K., and Suhl, M., 1973, Cerebrospinal fluid MHPG—an assessment of norepinephrine metabolism in affective disorders, *Arch. Gen. Psychiat.* **28**:230.

Stone, E. A., 1973, Accumulation and metabolism of norepinephrine in rat hypothalamus after exhaustive stress, *J. Neurochem.* **21**:589.

Sugden, R. F., and Eccleston, D., 1971, Glycol sulphate ester formation from (^{14}C) noradrenaline in brain and the influence of a COMT inhibitor, *J. Neurochem.* **18**:2461.

Sulser, F., Owens, M. L., Strada, S. J., and Dingell, J. V., 1969, Modification by desipramine (DMI) of the availability of norepinephrine released by reserpine in the hypothalamus of the rat *in vivo*, *J. Pharmacol. Exptl. Therap.* **168**:272.

Tuck, J. R., and Punell, G., 1973, Uptake of (^{3}H) 5-hydroxytryptamine and (^{3}H) noradrenaline by slices of rat brain incubated in plasma from patients treated with chlorimipramine, imipramine, or amitriptyline, *J. Pharm. Pharmacol.* **25**:573.

Van Praag, H. M., and Korf, T., 1974, Serotonin metabolism in depression: clinical applications of the probenecid. *Int. Pharmacopsychiatry* **9**:35:52.

Vogt, M., 1954, The concentration of sympathin in different parts of the central nervous system under normal conditions and after the administration of drugs, *J. Physiol.* **123**:451.

Walter, D. S., and Eccleston, D., 1973, Increase of noradrenaline metabolism following electrical stimulation of the locus coeruleus in the rat, *J. Neurochem.* **21**:281.

Weil-Malherbe, H., Whitby, L., and Axelrod, J., 1961, The uptake of circulating ^{3}H-norepinephrine by the pituitary gland and various areas of the brain, *J. Neurochem.* **8**:55.

Wilk, S., and Mones, R., 1971, Cerebrospinal fluid levels of 3-methoxy-4-hydroxyphenylethylene glycol in parkonsonism before and after treatment with L-dopa, *J. Neurochem.* **18**:1771.

Wilk, S., and Watson, E., 1974, VMA in spinal fluid: Evaluation of pathways of cerebral catecholamine metabolism in man, in: *Frontiers in Catecholamine Research,* Pergamon Press, New York.

Chapter 5

Catecholamines and Psychosis

John M. Davis

*Illinois State Psychiatric Institute
and
University of Chicago
Pritzker School of Medicine
Chicago, Illinois*

1. INTRODUCTION

All psychomotor stimulants which release catecholamines, such as amphetamine, methamphetamine, methylphenidate, phenmetrazine, and many others can produce a paranoid psychosis indistinguishable from paranoid schizophrenia (Kalant, 1966; Norman and Shea, 1945; Kramer et al., 1967; Kramer, 1969; Van Praag, 1968). It has been suggested that this psychosis, the amphetamine psychosis, is a useful model for schizophrenia (Kety and Matthysse, 1972; Snyder et al., 1970; Snyder, 1973a,b; Friedhoff and Schweitzer, 1971). All the drugs which benefit schizophrenia also produce extrapyramidal side effects. Lloyd and Hornkiewicz (Vol. I, Chapter 2) have discussed evidence implicating low levels of dopamine in motor function diseases. Idiopathic Parkinson's disease, drug-induced Parkinson's disease, and other motor disturbances are related to a deficit in dopaminergic function. All the agents which benefit schizophrenia block catecholamine receptors. These agents are particularly potent in blocking dopamine receptors. When psychomotor stimulants are given to a wide variety of animals, stereotyped behavior is produced. This can be blocked by all antipsychotic compounds and is useful in tests developed to screen new antipsychotic compounds (Janssen et al., 1967). The role of dopamine in the production of stereotyped behavior has been previously discussed in Volume I (Chapter 4) by Randrup et al. Thus, there is a variety of circumstantial evidence linking catecholamines, particularly dopamine to schizophrenia and noradrenaline to depression (see Chapters 3 and 4). In both cases, the theory is based primarily upon pharmacologic evidence based on the biologic actions of drugs which benefit or produce, respectively, schizophrenia, mania, or depression. The various aspects of the underlined hypothesis on an animal level has been previously discussed by Randrup *et al.,* Maas, Lloyd and Hornykiewicz, Murphy and Redmund, and others in these volumes. The purpose of this chapter is to integrate this evidence with studies of amphetamine psychosis in the schizophrenic man in order to bridge the gap between the basic knowledge, where information about pharmacologic mechanism is available, and the clinical effects of these drugs in man. For this reason, we are going to review evidence on the dopaminergic theory of schizophrenia arising from studies in man.

2. DOPAMINE THEORY OF SCHIZOPHRENIA

The dopamine theory of schizophrenia is based on two corner stones: (i) the fact that all the antipsychotic drugs cause extrapyramidal symptoms and hence, presumably block central dopamine receptors, and (ii) the fact that amphetamine can produce a paranoid psychosis. In order to examine evidence that may more specifically relate dopamine to schizophrenia, it is important to examine details of these two general classes of observation in detail. We will concern ourselves first with amphetamine psychosis.

3. AMPHETAMINE PSYCHOSIS AS A MODEL

In 1935, Prinzmental and Bloomberg (1935) found that amphetamine was useful in patients suffering from narcolepsy. A few years later, the first two cases of amphetamine psychosis were reported by Young and Scoville (1938), who reported typical paranoid schizophrenic-like episodes in narcoleptic patients receiving high doses of amphetamine, which resolved with a few days of discontinuing amphetamine. This report has been followed by numerous reports from all over the world of patients who became psychotic following the ingestion of amphetamine, methamphetamine, methylphenidate, phenmetrazine, and a variety of other psychomotor stimulants. These patients obtained the medications from physicians for narcolepsy, obesity, and so forth, on an illicit drug market or from proprietary medication, such as Benzedrene inhalers. In 1954, Herman and Nagel reported a group of eight patients who experienced the acute paranoid hallucinatory episodes which often remitted following discontinuance of drugs. This clinical study was confirmed in a much larger series in the classic monograph of Connell (1958), who collected data on 42 patients. He noted that the clinical picture is primarily a paranoid psychosis with ideas of reference, delusions of persecution, and auditory and visual hallucinations which occurred with a clear consciousness. This symptomatology is indistinguishable from acute or chronic paranoid schizophrenia. Many of these patients had their psychosis resolved over the course of several days. Other patients had some residue of psychiatric disorder, such as difficulty thinking, disturbed affect, or residual delusional ideation. Still other patients presented in the hospital with a history and with a urinary test for amphetamine but remained in a paranoid schizophrenic state for months or years. In this case, it would be reasonable to suppose that the amphetamine precipitated the psychosis, but that the psychotic episode was a schizophrenic episode, not an amphetamine psychosis *per se*. Of course, in some cases, the amphetamine ingestion could be coincidental with the development of the schizophrenic psychosis. It is, of course, quite possible that in some patients amphetamine could produce a longer-lasting and, perhaps, a permanent impairment in some central biochemical mechanism resulting in a psychosis which persisted after amphetamine had been excreted. There is ample clinical evidence from many case reports which support a wide variety of variance of amphetamine psychosis: the acute paranoid psychosis with clear consciousness which resolves in a few days, an amphetamine psychosis in a previously nonschizophrenic patient which persisted for months, episodes of schizophrenia precipitated or coincidental with ingestion of amphetamine. The following references are typical of the clinical report of amphetamine psychosis (Angrist and Gershon, 1969*a,b,* 1972*a.b*; Angrist *et al.,* 1970; Bell and Trethowan, 1961; Bell, 1965; Ellinwood, 1967, 1968; Kalant, 1966 (review); Kiloh and Brandon, 1962; Kramer *et al.,* 1967; Kramer, 1969; Monroe and Drell, 1947; Norman and Shea, 1945; Oswald and Thacore, 1963; Rylander, 1967; Smith, 1969; Young *et al.,* 1961). The most typical amphetamine psychosis is the paranoid ideation with clear consciousnesss which resolves in several days. Is this a true drug psychosis or does amphetamine precipitate a schizophrenic episode in a previously schizophrenic patient? In the clinical situation, patients are not interviewed prior to developing an amphetamine psychosis, so one does not know whether they were partially schizophrenic before they ingested the amphetamine. Empirical data to answer this question are available from experimental studies in which amphetamine was administered to volunteers. Griffith *et al.* (1968, 1970*a,b,* 1972*a,b*) administered amphetamine to nine normal volunteers in doses of 5–10 mg/hr., if the subject could tolerate the amphetamine without elevations in heart rate or blood pressure, etc. Six of these patients manifested paranoid symptoms after receiving the drug during a 1–5-day period. Two subjects had prepsychotic phases in which they experienced some paranoid ideation

with insight. The time course of the amphetamine effects were characteristic. The volunteers initially had the usual amphetamine loquacity, and
after their dose exceeded 50 mg, they appeared slightly depressed and were
hypochrondrical, irritable, faultfinding, and anorexic. Later, subjects became reserved and negativistic, giving guarded answers, although specifically denying being paranoid. After the experiment was over, the subjects
explained that they were aware of being abnormally suspicious during this
period, and tried to conceal their paranoia. Last, the onset of the frank
paranoia occurred abruptly. The subjects spoke freely about their paranoid
ideas, often feeling they suddenly gained insight into the real reason for the
project. For example, one subject thought the experiment was a way to
admit him to the hospital for his heart trouble. Another thought there was a
giant oscillator placed in the ceiling to control his thoughts. Ideas of
reference were common. One subject felt that he was being discussed on the
television. There was one case of olfactory hallucinations. There was no evidence of disorientation, clouding of consciousness, or memory disturbances.
Many of the subjects did not sleep during the first 24 hr. After this they
would take cat naps of 1–4 hr duration. That the psychosis was not due to
sleep deprivation was supported by the observation that four of the subjects
became psychotic or prepsychotic after less than two nights of sleep deprivation. The other four became psychotic or prepsychotic on the fourth or fifth
day. The total cumulative dose ingested which was necessary to produce the
psychosis varied between 100 and 800 mg of amphetamine. The subject who
did not become psychotic, received a cumulative dose of approximately 400
mg. Angrist and Gershon (1970a, 1970b) replicated and extended the work
of Griffith, giving 325–955 mg of amphetamine to volunteers, noting that
they developed a paranoid psychosis. The paranoid symptoms were quite
similar in content to those experienced in past episodes of street amphetamine psychosis. Amphetamine psychosis-produced auditory hallucinations occurred in two patients, and one subject developed signs of formal
thought disorder. The experience of Angrist on natural and experimental
psychosis confirmed the observation of Connell (1958) that amphetamine
psychosis can repeat paranoid schizophrenia in essentially all
respects—hallucinations, delusions, visual, auditory, and olfactory.

4. MECHANISM OF AMPHETAMINE PSYCHOSIS

Clinically, some patients can have as many as 15–20 paranoid
psychoses precipitated or caused by an amphetamine, which clear within a
few days of discontinuing the amphetamine. Thus, amphetamine can

produce a typical paranoid psychosis. The next question is how does amphetamine produce the psychosis. Amphetamine is a potent releaser of norepinephrine and dopamine from the neuron. It inhibits the reuptake of these amines. It is a MAO inhibitor. It has a direct receptor-stimulating effect. Its metabolites can be false transmitters (Axelrod, 1954, 1955; Davis et al., 1969; 1971a; Davis and Lemberger, 1970; Caldwell et al., 1972a–e; Dring et al., 1966, 1970; Alleva, 1963; Ellison et al., 1965). Amphetamine is metabolized by two pathways: (i) it is deaminated to benzoic acid, which is conjugated to hippuric acid and excreted; (ii) it can be very easily p-hydroxylated and then β-hydroxylated to hydroxynorephedrine (PHEP). We have found in our laboratory that amphetamine can be β-hydroxylated to norephedrine (NEF). We have two types of evidence that this can occur: (i) ^{3}H-amphetamine added to a buffer solution containing dopamine-β-oxidase was partially converted into norephedrine (Davis et al., 1971a,b); (ii) ^{3}H-norephedrine is found in the urine of patients administered ^{3}H-amphetamine. The p-hydroxynorephedrine and norephedrine are compounds structurally similar to norepinephrine and might be expected to have biologic activity. They would both be formed by the β-hydroxylation of amphetamine within the storage vesicle in the noradrenergic neuron, and it has been shown that they can fulfill the criterion for false transmitters (Davis et al., 1971a,b; Lewander, 1971; Thoenen et al., 1966). Thus, they can be released by the action potential, stimulate the receptor site, etc. Even if only relatively small amounts of these compounds were formed, they would be formed at the pharmacologically active site for storage and release. It would be reasonable to ask if amphetamine psychosis is produced by amphetamine itself or by these metabolites, namely, these false transmitters: PHEP, NEF. The false transmitter hypothesis has received extensive discussion in the animal pharmacologic literature, and there have been a multitude of investigators with an interpretation of these studies to man (Costa and Gropetti, 1970; Davis et al., 1971a, b). It is important to note that there are marked species differences in amphetamine. The rat metabolizes amphetamine to hydroxyamphetamine; in man, the important metabolic path for amphetamine is deamination to benzoic and hippuric acid. The false transmitters form a very minor route of metabolism in man, hence, one cannot generalize uncritically from the rat to the man. Both species metabolize amphetamine through quantitatively different routes. Attention is called to the elegant work of Williams and his co-workers on the metabolism of amphetamine in a wide variety of species (Caldwell et al., 1972a,b; Dring et al., 1966, 1970; Smith and Dring, 1970). There is agreement both in our previous work, in the work of Williams and his group, in the work of Anggard (1973) and of Cavanaugh et al. (1970) that the false transmitters are formed, but are a minor metabolite of amphetamine insofar as can be determined from studies in urinary metabolism of amphetamine. It is practically impossible to study how much norephedrine is formed in the human brain. The fact that norephedrine is a minor metabolite is of no "conclusive" significance. Since norephedrine and hydroxynorephedrine are formed in this storage vesicle of the noradrenergic neuron, even small amounts of it could be important physiologically.

We administered ^{3}H d-amphetamine to one amphetamine addict with an experimental amphetamine psychosis, and found amounts of norephedrine and hydroxynorephedrine in the urine similar to that found in normals. Within the limitations of the study involving one amphetamine addict, this result would suggest but not prove that addicts, during their psychotic periods, do not form larger amounts of norephedrine and hydroxynorephedrine than do controls. It is important to point out that this study was derived from urinary metabolites. One should obviously be cautious in generalization to brain.

It has been shown by Beckett and Rowland (1965) and by Asatoor *et al.* (1965) that the excretion of amphetamine is markedly dependent upon the pH of the urine. Amphetamine is readily excreted when the urine is acidic, and excreted only very slowly when the urine is alkaline. This work was extended by Davis *et al.* (1969, 1971b; Davis and Lemberger, 1970) who showed that the rate of disappearance of amphetamine from plasma, and its rate of appearance in urine is markedly influenced by the pH of the urine. When the urine is acid, the half-life of amphetamine was around 12 hr; when the urine was alkaline, the half-life was 24 to 36 hr. Davis also showed that the route of metabolism was quantitatively affected by the pH of the urine. A much greater amount of amphetamine was deaminated and p-dehydroxylated when urine was alkaline. Anggard and Gunne (1969, Anggard *et al.*, 1970; Jonsson, *et al.*, 1969a; Jonsson and Sjostrom, 1970) have confirmed this finding and have shown that patients remained psychotic for about twice as long (4 days in comparison to 2 days) when their urine was made alkaline in comparison to when it was made acid. This study does not differentiate between amphetamine psychosis being caused by amphetamine *per se* versus norephedrine, since alkaline urine would prolong the stay of both compounds in the brain. It does, however, have practical treatment implications. A more crucial piece of evidence comes from studies of d- and l-amphetamine. d-Amphetamine and its metabolite, hydroxyamphetamine, are both good substrates for dopamine-β-oxidase and, as mentioned above, are converted to norephedrine and p-hydroxynorephedrine, respectively, by dopamine-β-oxidase. l-Amphetamine is not a substrate for dopamine-β-oxidase. Therefore, L-norephedrine and L-hydroxnorephedrine are not formed from l-amphetamine (Goldstein *et al.*, 1964; Goldstein and Anagnoste, 1965). If l-amphetamine produces "an amphetamine psychosis," it cannot be caused by norephedrine or hydroxynorephedrine since these metabolites are not formed. Angrist has shown that *l*-amphetamine is quite capable of causing amphetamine psychosis, although it is about 0.8 times as potent as *d*-amphetamine. These data are consistent with the cause of amphetamine psychosis being amphetamine itself and not a metabolite such as PHEP or NEF.

4.1. Effect of Drugs on Amphetamine Psychosis

It has been clinically reported that barbiturates are not particularly effective for treating amphetamine psychosis. Barbiturates and amphetamines are in no sense opposite drugs (Bell, 1973). If amphetamine does indeed produce its psychosis by dopamine release then one should be able to block the psychosis.

Angrist *et al.,* (1974*a*) have reported that haloperidol does effectively block amphetamine psychosis and would be the drug of choice in treating amphetamine psychosis. Chlorpromazine has been found, empirically, to be a useful drug in treating amphetamine overdose in children (Espelin and Done, 1968). Presumably, in both cases, the antipsychotic agents block dopamine receptors and thus interfere with the action of catecholamines released by amphetamine. There may be a clinical pharmacologic reason for preferring haloperidol. Both drugs are potent at blocking dopamine receptors and, if the theory is correct, they would be equal in blocking amphetamine psychosis. However, chlorpromazine blocks *p*-hydroxylation of amphetamine in the rat (Lemberger *et al.,* 1970). Haloperidol does not have this property. Hence, chlorpromazine, by blocking its destruction, prolongs amphetamine's sojourn in the body, resulting in higher amphetamine levels for a longer period of time. If amphetamine produces a deleterious effect in the brain through some mechanism other than dopamine blockade, the high amphetamine levels which persist longer in the brain in the chlorpromazine-treated man may do harm. *p*-Hydroxylation is a minor route in man, so this effect will be quantitatively less important in man. Nevertheless, this clinical pharmacologic possibility would suggest that haloperidol would be the preferred drug. In trying to infer how amphetamine produces an amphetamine psychosis, it would be useful to know the drugs that would block amphetamine psychosis so that the common denominator of the pharmacologic action of these drugs could be evidence as to how amphetamine acts. Unfortunately, there have not been systematic studies of this question. There have been studies on drugs which counteract the dose-related amphetamine euphoria. Jonsson and Sjostrom, (1970; Jonnson *et al.,* 1971*b*) used amphetamine addicts in studying the effects of 200 mg iv *d*- and *l*-amphetamine. This dose produced a uniform euphoria in its quantitative intensity. These authors then explored the effects of different drugs in blocking this euphoria and showed that chlorpromazine, haloperidol, and pimoside block amphetamine euphoria.

Studies on cerebral spinal fluid HVA or 5-HIAA during amphetamine psychosis did not show any significant change with levels observed after amphetamine withdrawal. Watson *et al.* (1972) and Schildkraut *et al.* (1971) found that the clinical depression which occurs following amphetamine withdrawal was associated in a temporal manner with low levels of excretion of 3-methoxy-4-hydroxyphenylglycol (MHPG), a metabolite of norepinephrine which has been suggested as a marker for brain norepinephrine (Maas and Landis, 1968). Angrist *et al.,* (1972) found MHPG within the first 1 to 3 hr after ingestion of the last amphetamine tablet to be essentially equal to base line in three subjects. In one subject, it was slightly reduced 16 hr after the last amphetamine tablet.

To summarize thus far, we have reviewed evidence of amphetamine psychosis and found that a paranoid psychosis, indistinguishable from schizophrenia, appears following high-dose amphetamine ingestion, but clears within several days of discontinuing amphetamine. This psychosis is most likely a result of amphetamine itself and not a false transmitter, although hydroxynorephedrine or norephedrine could play a partial role. That is, in *d*-amphetamine psychosis, both the *d*-amphetamine and the false transmitters could play a role, but one can rule out the hypothesis that the psychosis is produced by the false transmitter alone.

4.2. Evidence Involving Dopamine

The next question for consideration is how does amphetamine produce the psychosis. Amphetamine-produced stereotyped behavior in a wide variety of species has been thought to be a model of amphetamine psychosis or schizophrenia (Snyder, 1972). There is a variety of pharmacologic evidence to indicate that stereotyped behavior is mediated by dopamine. This topic has been reviewed by Randrup *et al.* in Volume I, and will therefore not be repeated here.

If the stereotyped behavior model is correct, it would indicate that dopamine is the neurotransmitter involved in amphetamine psychosis. The fact that stereotyped behavior is an effective screening instrument for antipsychotic compounds is consistent with the dopamine theory of schizophrenia.

d- And *l*-amphetamine can be used safely in man (Taylor and Snyder 1970). Snyder has proposed that *d*- and *l*-amphetamine may be pharmacologic tools to differentiate between noradrenergic and dopaminergic effects. He studied stereotyped behavior in animals pretreated with a MAO inhibitor. *d*-Amphetamine is about twice as potent as *l*-amphetamine in causing stereotyped behavior in Snyder's system. Locomotor behavior is said to be under the control of norepinephrine and this, according to Snyder, may be a marker for norepinephrine. *d*-Amphetamine is ten times as potent as *l*-amphetamine in increasing locomotor behavior. This line of evidence is based upon direct measurement of stereotyped behavior and locomotor activity. Taylor and Snyder (1970; 1971) have also studied the effects of *d*- and *l*-amphetamine on the uptake of norepinephrine and dopamine in appropriate areas of the brain and have discovered similar ratios. We have been unable to replicate this in our laboratory using slightly different techniques (unpublished data). The property of blocking reuptake may not be the most important property by which *d*- and *l*-amphetamine produce its behavioral effects. These behavioral effects may be a result primarily of the releasing property. In thinking about these experiments it may be useful to keep separate three different aspects of *d*- and *l*-amphetamine comparisons: (i) the effect of *d*- and *l*-amphetamine on humans in producing amphetamine psychosis or euphoria; (ii) the effects of *d*- and *l*-amphetamine in producing stereotyped behavior or locomotor activity in rats and, (iii) the biochemical pharmacologic effects of *d*- and *l*-amphetamine in releasing norepinephrine or dopamine, blocking the reuptake of norepinephrine and dopamine, etc. The differentiation of *d*- and *l*-amphetamine in stereotyped behavior and locomotor activity may hold in the intact brain because the biochemical mechanism upon which this is based is different than that studied in synaptosomal studies of uptake of exogenous-labeled amine in an *in vivo* preparation. If the work of Snyder is valid as a behavioral model, irrespective of *in vivo* considerations, this tool can be used in man to separate noradrenergic and dopaminergic function. Namely, if in man *d*-amphetamine was also ten times as potent as *l*-amphetamine in producing behaviors mediated by norepinephrine and only two times as potent as *l*-amphetamine in producing behaviors mediated by norepinephrine and only two times as potent as *l*-amphetamine in causing dopaminergically mediated behaviors, then the relative potency of these two isomers in eliciting a given behavior may indicate whether the behavior is under dopaminergic or noradrenergic control. Angrist and Gershon (1970) and Angrist *et al.,* (1971) have produced amphetamine psychosis with both *d*- and *l*-amphetamine, and found that *d*-amphetamine is only slightly more potent (1.2) than *l*-amphetamine. This would be consistent with the dopaminergic mediation for the amphetamine psychosis. Thus far we have discussed amphetamine psychosis produced by high doses of the drugs as a model for schizophrenia. There is a second phenomenon which may relate psychomotor stimulants to schizophrenia. In our laboratory we have recently shown that one can change a moderately schizophrenic patient into a severely ill schizophrenic patient with small intravenous doses of psychomotor stimulants such as methylphenidate or *d*- and *l*-amphetamine. Normals receiving similar doses of methylphenidate (35 mg) experience a mild euphoria. Yet, schizophrenics become floridly schizophrenic, manifesting increased hallucinations, delusions, catatonic behavior, etc., when given iv 35 mg of methylphenidate or 20 mg of *d*-amphetamine. In our judgment, this worsening of psychosis provoked by psychomotor stimulants is a different phenomenon than amphetamine psychosis. Amphetamine psychosis uniformly is a paranoid schizophrenia. The worsening of psychosis produced by psychomotor stimulants in already schizophrenic patients is a worsening in the symptoms of their schizophrenia, which may or may not be paranoid symptoms. If the patient suffered from paranoid schizophrenia he would become more paranoid; however, if the patient were catatonic, he would become more catatonic. In order to discuss this second phenomenon, the psychosis-worsening phenomenon, we give below several examples of the type of experience that is seen.

Case 1. A 28-year-old schizophrenic was admitted to the hospital complaining that "spirits" were talking to him and that he "could see and sense spirits rising out of people's bodies." He showed marked loosening of associations and a flattened affect. Two weeks later, the patient showed a lessening of his loose associations and said that his talk about spirits was "crazy talk." Within 1 min of methylphenidate infusion, the patient exclaimed that the spirits had again begun to talk to him and that he could see them rising out of the interviewer's head. He also showed marked loosening of associations and increased flattening of affect.

Case 2. A 25-year-old patient was admitted to the hospital in an extremely withdrawn state, drooling, and showing near muteness. Administration of methylphenidate caused the patient to become more catatonic. Her muteness became complete, and she assumed a frozen position with catatonic posturing and waxy flexibility.

Case 3. A 26-year-old schizophrenic was admitted in a withdrawn state and exhibiting flat affect. Within 1 min of methylphenidate infusion, she became terrified, started screaming, and stated that she heard and saw her dead father. She then progressed into a state of extreme withdrawal with muteness and inactivity. She reported this phase of her interview retrospectively and stated that she had entertained paranoid thoughts and occasional hallucinations before the infusion, which she had been reluctant to discuss. These had markedly increased after administration of methylphenidate.

The worsening of psychosis produced by methylphenidate, *d*-amphetamine, or *l*-amphetamine is distinguished from amphetamine psychosis *per se* by the fact that it worsens schizophrenia with the same symptoms as the preexisting psychosis (Janowsky *et al.,* 1973*c*; Jankowsky and Davis, 1974; Davis and Janowsky, 1973). For example, catatonic patients become more catatonic. Thus, there are two psychotomimetic effects of amphetamine. We have noted above that *d*-amphetamine is slightly more potent than *l*-amphetamine in producing an amphetamine psychosis. It would be of interest to see the relative potencies of the three psychomotor stimulants, methylphenidate, *d*-amphetamine, and *l*-amphetamine in worsening schizophrenia. We have done this experiment in our laboratory (Janowsky *et al,* 1973; Jankowsky and Davis, 1974; Davis and Janowsky, 1973. It turns out that methylphenidate is clearly more potent than *d*- or *l*-amphetamine. If one rates the potency of *l*-amphetamine as 100, then *d*-amphetamine has a potency of 200, and methylphenidate has a potency of 300. These comparisons are on a molar basis. Lower doses of *d*-amphetamine, such as 10 mg and 4 mg, are less potent than equimolar doses of *l*-amphetamine (20 mg equivalent). For ethical reasons, one cannot keep acutely schizophrenic patients in a hospital for many months and administer repeated doses of psychomotor stimulants; hence, one cannot map out a dose–response curve over many doses. Within the limits of what is possible to do, we are able to bracket the relative potency of *l*-amphetamine and methylphenidate in relationship to three different doses of *d*-amphetamine. Due to the limitations inherent in doing studies on humans, one must be cautious about being overly concrete in the quantitative relationships, particularly the additive properties of our rating scale. However, these methodologic limitations notwithstanding, the descending order of potency is: methylphenidate, *d*-amphetamine, and, finally, *l*-amphetamine. This corresponds well to the study on *d*-amphetamine and *l*-amphetamine performed by Angrist and his co-workers.

5. TRANSMITTER BALANCE

In our discussions thus far, we have focused on the amphetamine psychosis or the psychosis-worsening property of psychomotor stimulants, presumably mediated by dopamine. In any consideration of a behavior, it is reasonable to ask whether that particular behavior is controlled by a balance between transmitters rather than by a single transmitter. Many peripheral autonomic functions are controlled by the balance of cholinergic and noradrenergic factors. The central autonomic nervous system, using "autonomic" in a broad sense, also has many different functions which are controlled by balances between transmitters (Janowsky *et al.,* 1972). In terms of human disease, one example of this would be motor disorder of Parkinson's disease. In a primary sense, this is due to a dopamine deficiency. However, pharmacology is under the control of both dopaminergic and cholinergic factors. Physostigmine makes Parkinson's disease worse by increasing brain acetylcholine. Anti-Parkinsonian drugs make it better by blocking central cholinergic receptors. There may be a balance between cholinergic and adrenergic factors in mania and depression. We have shown that by administering physostigmine one can reduce some manic symptoms and increase depression in patients with depressive elements in their psychiatric disorder. (Janowsky *et al.*, 1973c). In this case the balance would be high levels of norepinephrine associated with mania relative to low levels of acetylcholine; *vice versa* for depression. Could a similar dopaminergic–cholinergic balance control psychosis in the dopamine theory of schizophrenia? One associates schizophrenia with high levels of dopamine. If there is a balance controlling the schizophrenic symptoms and one were to say high dopamine–low acetylcholine produces schizophrenia, one should therefore be able to block schizophrenic symptoms with physostigmine.

Using our model of worsening psychosis with methylphenidate, we worsened the psychosis by an injection of methylphenidate and then gave physostigmine. We observed that physostigmine could terminate the methylphenidate-induced worsening of psychotic symptoms. One could also give physostigmine first, and thereby prevent methylphenidate from worsening the psychotic symptoms. Thus, in terms of the dopaminergic–cholinergic balance, one can use physostigmine to block or treat the psychosis-worsening properties of methylphenidate. This would indicate that there might be a dopamine–cholinergic balance controlling the worsening properties produced by methylphenidate. The quantitative data are summarized in Table I. Physostigmine increases acetylcholine both centrally and pe-

Table I. Effect of Physostigmine in Antagonizing or Preventing Psychosis Activation by Methylphenidate

	Base line	Physostigmine	Physostigmine–methylphenidate
Activation	5.33 ± 1.26	2.64 ± 0.74	3.71 ± 0.56
Psychosis	1.69 ± 0.55	1.61 ± 0.46	1.96 ± 0.30
		Methylphenidate	Methylphenidate–physostigmine
Activation	6.51 ± 1.13	8.37 ± 0.68	5.63 ± 1.00
Psychosis	2.21 ± 0.54	3.40 ± 0.46	2.67 ± 0.52

ripherally. Parenthetically, it might be added that in these experiments, neostigmine, a drug which does not pass the blood–brain barrier, was used as a control and did not have any mental effects. This would be evidence ruling out a peripheral effect of physostigmine as an explanation for this finding.

Insofar as stereotyped behavior may be a marker for dopamine, the relative difference in potency between *d*- and *l*-amphetamine in both (i) the amphetamine psychosis *per se,* as observed by Angrist and Gershon (1970, 1971), and (ii) the psychomotor stimulant worsening of psychosis, as observed by us, is consistent with the dopaminergic theory of schizophrenia. The latter finding seems to be under a dopamine–acetylcholine balance. Methylphenidate in the human is clearly more potent than either *d*- or *l*-amphetamine in worsening psychosis. Does this have any implications for the dopamine theory of schizophrenia? There is some equivocal evidence that methylphenidate, in a quantitative way, might be slightly more potent in effecting dopamine than norepinephrine (Ferris *et al.,* 1972). Pharmacologically, there are some important properties which differentiate two classes of psychomotor stimulants (Scheel-Kruger, 1971, 1972). Amphetamine may release norepinephrine and dopamine from storage pools. In a quantitative sense α-methyl-*p*-tyrosine (AMPT) a synthesis inhibitor, is more potent at blocking the actions of amphetamine and, indeed, in certain situations, reserpine can potentiate the effects of amphetamine. In contrast, reserpine is particularly effective in blocking methylphenidate-induced stereotyped behavior, and AMPT is relatively less effective (Scheel-Kruger, 1971, 1972). There is evidence that platelet monoamine oxidase (MAO) is reduced in schizophrenia (Murphy and Wyatt, 1972). If methylphenidate releases amines from storage, its pharmacological activities would be modulated to a greater extent by MAO. The observed data would be consistent with the known pharmacologic effect of methylphenidate in releasing amines from stores. Presumably, when amines are released from stores intracellularly, they are available for deamination with intracellular MAO. If this MAO is inhibited, more amine would therefore leak out as active dopamine. If schizophrenics have low MAO, one would expect drugs releasing amines from stores to have a greater activity. This is what we find empirically, namely, methylphenidate is the most potent of the psychomotor stimulants in worsening schizophrenic psychosis. There is evidence that AMPT alone does not benefit schizophrenia (Gershon *et al.,* 1967). This would suggest that newly synthesized dopamine is not critical to schizophrenia. However, there is evidence that AMPT reduces the dose of antipsychotic agents necessary to markedly benefit schizophrenia (Walinder and Carlsson, 1973; Carlsson *et al.,* 1973). This evidence is strongly supportive of the hypothesis that antipsychotic agents act through a catecholamine mechanism. It also suggests, since

AMPT would lower stores to some degree, that this lowering of stores may explain why AMPT markedly reduces the dose of antipsychotic drug needed to get an antipsychotic pharmacologic action. Reserpine and tetrabenazine, which decrease stores of norepinephrine and dopamine, do have a modest antipsychotic action. Thus it may be no accident that methylphenidate is more potent than the amphetamine in worsening schizophrenia.

There may be also some significance to the effects of reserpine or of AMPT in combination with an antipsychotic and the lack of the antipsychotic effect of AMPT by itself. When this evidence is coupled with the empirical data that schizophrenic patients have low MAO levels in platelets and, presumably, in the brain, the low level of brain MAO may explain the increased susceptibility of schizophrenics to agents which may act differentially through stored dopamine This line of thought is, of course, highly theoretical and is suggested only in a very tentative manner. Nevertheless, agents which directly effect stores of dopamine do have antipsychotic activity. Thus, there may be a parallel relationship with an antischizophrenic action of reserpine and AMPT to that of these drugs which antagonize methylphenidate-induced stereotyped behavior. Although we recognize that this line of thought is speculative, we would like to suggest that the dopamine involved in the undefined relationship to schizophrenia is dopamine released from the stores. Although our group feels that a dopamine theory of schizophrenia is a very promising lead, and though we are among those investigators who are investigating such a theory with active research, we would like to add a note of caution. Physostigmine does not benefit schizophrenia when given acutely, although it does antagonize the methylphenidate-induced worsening of psychosis. The phenothiazines produce their effects gradually over weeks or months.

6. TWO-FACTOR THEORY OF SCHIZOPHRENIA

One could formulate an alternative theory to the dopamine theory of schizophrenia which would be a two-factor theory of schizophrenia. It would suggest that the schizophrenic episode itself is controlled by some factor other than excess dopaminergic stimulation, such as an abnormal molecule di-O-methyldopamine (DMPEA), the first factor. This "first factor" could be related to elevation of CPK (Meltzer, 1969). Dopaminergic stimulation, however, markedly aggravates schizophrenia, the second factor. This first factor represents the "turning on" of schizophrenia, the second factor, dopaminergic stimulation, "turns up" the gain. One needs both factors in order to have an overt schizophrenic episode. Phenothiazines, in blocking dopaminergic stimulation, turn down the gains. This allows the normal reparative processes to occur so that the basic schizophrenic pathology heals after weeks or months. Conversely, methylphenidate and the amphetamines stimulate schizophrenia by turning up the gain. Physostigmine turns down the gain for a short period of time but not long enough to have the healing process take place, although it does block the psychosis-worsening property of methylphenidate. Since a single-factor theory is simpler, and perhaps the preferred theory by parsimony, one should not forget that the simplest explanation is not necessarily correct. Hence, a two-factor theory should not be prematurely excluded. Indeed, we would like to suggest an alternate interpretation to the dopamine theory, i.e., the two-factor theory of schizophrenia. Factor one is a yet unknown process (DMPEA, CPK), and factor two is a dopamine-mediated, possibly stress-related "activation of psychopathology," which acts via dopaminergic stimulation.

7. REFERENCES

Alleva, J. J., 1963, Metabolism of tranylcypromine-^{14}C and d- and l-amphetamine-^{14}C in the rat, *J. Med. Chem.* **6**:621.

Anggard, E., and Gunne, L. M., 1969, Pharmacodynamic studies on amphetamine abusers, objectives and methods, in: *Abuse of Central Stimulants* (F. Sjoqvist and M. Tottie, eds.), pp. 459–478, Almqvist and Wiksell, Stockholm.

Anggard, E., Gunne, L. M., Jonsson, L. E., and Niklasson, F., 1970, Pharmacokinetic and clinical studies on amphetamine-dependent subjects, *European J. Clin. Pharmacol.* **3**:3.

Anggard, E., Jonsson, L. E., Hogmark, A. L., and Gunne, L. M., 1973, Amphetamine metabolism in amphetamine psychoses, *European J. Clin. Pharmacol.* **14**:870.

Angrist, B. M., and Gershon, S., 1969a, Amphetamine-induced schizophreniform psychosis, in: *Schizophrenia—Current Concepts and Research* (D. V. S. Sanker, ed.), PJD Publications, Hicksville, New York.

Angrist, B. M., and Gershon, S., 1969b, Amphetamine abuse in New York City—1966–1968, *Seminars Psychiatry* **1**:195.

Angrist, B. M., and Gershon, S., 1970, The phenomenology of experimentally induced amphetamine psychosis. Preliminary observations, *Am. J. Psychiat.* **126**:95.

Angrist, B. M., and Gershon, S., 1971, A pilot study of pathogenic mechanisms in amphetamine psychosis using differential effects of d- and l-amphetamines, *Pharmacopsychiat. Neuropsychopharmakol.* **4**:64.

Angrist, B. M., and Gershon, S., 1972a, Recent studies on amphetamine psychosis. Unresolved issues, in *Current Concepts of Amphetamine Abuse*, pp., 193–204, U.S. Government Printing Office, Washington, D.C.

Angrist, B. M., and Gershon, S., 1972b, Psychiatric sequellae of amphetamine abuse, in: *Psychiatric Complications of Medical Drugs* (R. Shader, ed.), pp. 175–199, Raven Press, New York.

Angrist, B. M., Schweitzer, J., Friedhoff, A. J., Gershon, S., Hekimian, L. J., and Floyd, A., 1969, The clinical symptomatology of amphetamine psychosis and its relationship to amphetamine levels in urine, *Pharmacopsychiat. Neuropsychopharmakol.* **2**:125.

Angrist, B. M., Schweitzer, J. W., Gershon, S., and Friedhoff, A. J., 1970, Mephentermine psychosis: Misuse of the Wyamine inhaler, *Am. J. Psychiat.* **126**:1315.

Angrist, B. M., Shopsin, B., and Gershon, S., 1971, The comparative psychotomimetic effects of stereoisomers of amphetamine, *Nature* **234**:152.

Angrist, B. M., Shopsin, B., Gershon, S., and Wilk, S., 1972, Metabolites of monamines in urine and cerebrospinal fluid, after large dose amphetamine administration, *Psychopharmacologia,* **26**:1.

Angrist, B. M., Sathananthan, G., and Gershon, S., 1973, Behavioral effects of D-dopa in schizophrenic patients, *Psychopharmacologia,* 31.

Angrist, B., Lee, H. K., and Gershon, S., 1974a, The antagonism of amphetamine-induced symptomatology by a neuroleptic, *Am. J. Psychiat.* (in press).

Angrist, B. M., Sathananthan, G., Wilk, S., and Gershon, S. 1974b, Amphetamine psychosis, behavioral and biochemical aspects, *J. Psychiat. Res.* (in press).

Asatoor, A. M., Galman, B. R., Jonsson, J. R., and Milne, M. D., 1965, The excretion of dexamphetamine and its derivatives, *Brit. J. Pharmacol.* **24**:293.

Axelrod, J., 1954, Studies on sympathomimetic amines. II. The biotransformation and physiological disposition of *d*-amphetamine to *p*-hydroxyamphetamine, *J. Pharmacol. Exptl. Therap.* **110**:315.

Axelrod, J., 1955, The enzymatic deamination of amphetamine (benzedrine), *J. Biol. Chem.* **214**:753.

Beckett, A. H., and Rowland, M., 1965, Urinary excretion kinetics of amphetamine in man, *J. Pharm. Pharmacol.* **17**:628.

Bell, D. S., 1965, Comparison of amphetamine psychosis and schizophrenia, *Brit. J. Psychiat.* **113**:701.

Bell, D. S., 1973, The experimental reproduction of amphetamine psychosis, *Arch. Gen. Psychiat.* **29**:00.

Bell, D. S., and Trethowan, W. H., 1961, Amphetamine addiction and disturbed sexuality, *Arch. Gen. Psychiat.* **4**:34.

Caldwell, J., Dring, L. G., and Williams, R. T., 1972a, Norephedrines as metabolites of (^{14}C) amphetamine in urine in man, *Biochem. J.* **129**:23.

Caldwell, J., Dring, L. G., and Williams, R. T., 1972b, Biliary excretion of amphetamine and methamphetamine in the rat, *Biochem. J.* **129**:25.

Caldwell, J., Dring, L. G., and Williams, R. T., 1972c, Metabolism of (^{14}C) methamphetamine in man, the guinea pig and the rat. *Biochem. J.* **129**:11.

Carlsson, A., Persson, T., Roos, B. E., and Walinder, J., 1972, Potentiation of phenothiazines by α-methyltyrosine in treatment of chronic schizophrenia. *J. Neural Transmission* **33**:83.

Carlsson, A., Roos, B. E., Walinder, J., and Skott, A., 1973, Further studies on the mechanism of antipsychotic action: Potentiation by α-methyltyrosine of thioridazine effects in chronic schizophrenics, *J. Neural Transmission* **34**:125.

Cavanaugh, J. H., Griffith, J. D., and Oates, J. A., 1970, Effect of amphetamine on pressor response to tyramine: Formation of *p*-hydroxynorephedrine from amphetamine in man, *Clin. Pharmacol. Therap.* **11**:656.

Chen, K. K., Wu, C. K., and Henriksen, E., 1929, Relationship between the pharmacological action and the chemical constitution and figuration of the optical isomers of ephedrine and related compounds, *J. Pharmacol. Exptl. Therap.* **36**:363.

Connell, P. H., 1958, *Amphetamine Psychosis*, Maudsley Monographs, No. 5, Oxford University Press, London.

Costa, E., and Gropetti, A., 1970, Biosynthesis and storage of catecholamines in tissues of rats injected with various doses of d-amphetamine, in: *Amphetamines and Related Compounds* (E. Costa and S. Garattini, eds.), p. 231, Raven Press, New York.

Davis, J. M., and Janowsky, D. S., 1973, Amphetamine and methylphenidate psychosis, in: *Frontiers in Catecholamine Research* (E. Usdin and S. Snyder, eds.), pp. 1–10, Pergamon Press, Inc., New York.

Davis, J. M., and Lemberger, L., 1970, Pharmacologic aspects of the treatment of amphetamine abuse, *Colleg. Intern. Neuropsychopharmacol., Prague.* **1**:103.

Davis, J. M., Kopin, E. J., and Axelrod, J., 1969, Effects of urinary pH on plasma levels and metabolism of ^{3}H-amphetamine in man, *Pharmacologist* **11**:2.

Davis, J. M., Fann, E., Griffith, J., and Lemberger, L., 1971a, Pharmacological aspects of the treatment of amphetamine, in: *Advances in Neuropsychopharmacology* (O. Vinar, Z. Volava, and P. Bradley, eds.), pp. 279–282, Avicenum, Prague.

Davis, J. M., Kopin, I. J., Lemberger, L., and Axelrod, J., 1971b, Effects of urinary pH on amphetamine metabolism, *Ann. N.Y. Acad. Sci.* **179**:493.

Dring, L. G., Smith, R. L., and Williams, R. T., 1966, The fate of amphetamine in man and other animals, *J. Pharm. Pharmacol.* **18**:402.

Dring, L. G., Smith, R. L., and Williams, R. T., 1970, The metabolic fate of amphetamine in man and other species, *Biochem. J.* **116**:425.

Ellinwood, E. H., Jr., 1967, Amphetamine psychosis 1. Description of the individuals and process, *J. Nervous Mental Disease* **144**:273.

Ellinwood, E. H., Jr., 1968, Amphetamine psychosis: 11. Theoretical implications, *J. Neuropsychiat.* **4**:45.

Ellison, T. F., Gutzait, L., and Van Loon, L., 1965, The comparative metabolism of d-amphetamine-^{14}C in the rat, dog, and monkey, *J. Pharmacol. Exp. Therap.* **152**:383.

Espelin, D. E., and Done, A. K., 1968, Amphetamine poisoning effectiveness of chlorpromazine, *New Engl. J. Med.* **278**:1361.

Ferris, R. M., Tang, F., and Maxwell, R. A., 1972, A comparison of the capacities of isomers of amphetamine, deosypipradiol and methylphenidate to inhibit the uptake of tritiated catecholamines into rat cerebral cortex slices, synapsotomal preparation of rat cerebral cortex, hypothalamus and striatum and into adrenergic nerves of rabbit aorta, *J. Pharmacol. Exptl. Therap.* **181** (3):407.

Friedhoff, A. J., and Schweitzer, J. W., 1970, Amphetamine metabolism in amphetamine psychosis, 7th *Colleg. Intern. Neuropsychopharmacol., Prague.*

Gershon, S., Heikimian, L. J., Floyd, A., Jr., and Hollister, L. E., 1967. Methyl-p-tyrosine (AMT) in schizophrenia, *Psychopharmacologia* **11**:189.

Goldstein, M., and Anagnoste, M., 1965, The conversion *in vivo* of d-amphetamine to (+)-p-hydroxynorephedrine, *Biochim. Biophys. Acta* **107**:166.

Goldstein, M., McKereghan, M. R., and Lauber, E., 1964. The stereospecificity of the enzymatic amphetamine hydroxylation, *Biochim. Biophys. Acta* **89**:191.

Griffith, J. D., Oates, J., and Cavanaugh, J., 1968. Paranoid episodes induced by drugs, *J. Am. Med. Assoc.* **205**:39.

Griffith, J. D., Cavanaugh, J. H., Held, J., and Oates, J. A., 1970a. Experimental psychosis induced by the administration of d-amphetamine, in: *Amphetamines and Related Compounds* (E. Costa and S. Garattini, eds.), Raven Press, New York.

Griffith, J. D., Cavanaugh, J. H., and Oates, J. A., 1970b, Psychosis induced by the administration of amphetamine to human volunteers, in: *Psychotomimetic Drugs* D. H. Efron, (ed.), Raven Press, New York.

Griffith, J. D., Fann, W. E., and Oates, J. O., 1972a, The amphetamine psychosis, in: *Current Concepts of Amphetamine Abuse* (E. H. Ellinwood, Jr. and S. Cohen, eds.). U.S. Government Printing Office, Washington, D.C.

Griffith, J. D., et al, 1972*b*, Dextroamphetamine: evaluation of psychomimetic properties in man, *Arch. Gen. Psychiat.* **26**:97.

Herman, M., and Nagler, S. H., 1954, Psychoses due to amphetamine, *J. Nerv. Mental Disease* **120**:268.

Horn, A. S., and Snyder, S. H., 1971, Chlorpromazine and dopamine: conformational similarities that correlate with the antischizophrenic activity of phenothiazine drugs, *Proc. Natl. Acad. Sci.* (U.S.) **68**:2325.

Janowsky, D. S., and Davis, J. M., 1974, Dopamine, psychomotor stimulants and schizophrenia: effects of methylphenidate and the steroisomers of amphetamine in schizophrenics, in: *Dopamine and Behavior* (E. Usdin, ed.), Plenum Press, New York.

Janowsky, D. S., El-Yousef, M. K. Davis, J. M., *et al.*, 1972, Cholinergic antagonism of methylphenidate-induced stereotyped behavior, *Psychopharmacologia* **27**:295.

Janowsky, D. S., El-Yousef, M. K., Davis, J. M., and Sekerke, H. J., 1973a, Parasympathetic suppression of manic symptoms by physostigmine, *Arch. Gen. Psychiat.* **28**:542.

Janowsky, D. S., El-Yousef, M. K., Davis, J. M., *et al.*, 1973*b*, Provocation of schizophrenic symptoms by intravenous administration of methylphenidate, *Arch. Gen. Psychiat.* **28**:185.

Janowsky, D. S., El-Yousef, M. K., Davis, J. M., *et al.*, 1973*c*, Antagonistic effects of physostigmine and methylphenidate in man, Presented at the annual meeting of the American Psychiatric Association.

Janssen, P. A. J., Miemegeers, C. J. E., Schellekens, K. H. L., and Lenaerts, F. M., 1967, Is it possible to predict the clinical effects of neuroleptic drugs (major tranquilizers) from animal data, *Arzneimittel-Forsch.* **17**:841.

Jonsson, L. E., 1972, Pharmacological blockade of amphetamine effects in amphetamine dependent subjects, *European J. Clin. Pharmacol.* **4**:206.

Jonsson, L. E., and Sjostrom, K., 1970, A rating scale for evaluation of the clinical course and symptomatology in amphetamine psychosis, *Brit. J. Psychiat.* **177**:661.

Jonsson, L. E., Bunne, L. M., and Anggard, E., 1969a, Effects of α-methyltyrosine in amphetamine-dependent subjects, *European J. Clin. Pharmacol.* **2**:27.

Jonsson, L. E., Schuberth, J., and Sundwall, A., 1969*b*, Amphetamine effect on the choline concentration of human cerebrospinal fluid, *Life Sci.* **8**:(Part 1): 977.

Jonsson, L. E., Lewander, T., and Gunne, L. M., 1971a, Amphetamine psychosis—Urinary excretion of catecholamines and concentration of homovanillic acid (HVA) and 5-hydroxy-indoleacetic acid (5-HIAA) in the cerebrospinal fluid, *Res. Commun. Chem. Path. Pharmacol.* **2**:355.

Jonsson, L. E., Anggard, E., and Gunne, L. M., 1971*b*, Blockade of euphoria induced by intravenous amphetamine in humans, *Clin. Pharmacol. Therap.* **12**:889.

Kalant, O. J., 1966, *The Amphetamines: Toxicity and Addiction*, Alcoholism and Drug Addiction Research Foundation of Ontario, Toronto.

Kety, S., and Matthysse, S., 1972, *Neuroscis. Res. Prog. Bull.* **10**:433.

Kiloh, L. G., and Brandon, S., 1962, Habituation and addiction to amphetamines, *Brit. Med. J.* **11**:40.

Kramer, J. C., 1969, Introduction to amphetamine abuse, *J. Psychodelic Drugs* **2**:1.

Kramer, J. C., Fischman, V. S., and Littlefield, D. C., 1967, Amphetamine abuse: Pattern and effects of high doses taken intravenously, *J. Am. Med. Assoc.* **201**:305.

Lemberger, L., Witt, E. D., Davis, J. M., and Kopin, I. J., 1970, The effects of haloperidol and chlorpromazine on amphetamine metabolism and amphetamine stereotype behavior in the rat, *J. Pharmacol Exptl. Therap.* **174**:428.

Lewander, T., 1971, On the presence of *p*-hydroxynorephedrine in the rat brain and heart in relation to changes in catecholamine levels after administration of amphetamine, *Acta Pharmacol. Toxicol.* **29**:33.

Maas, J. W., and Landis, D. H., 1968, *In vivo* studies of the metabolism of norepinephrine in the central nervous system, *J. Pharmacol. Exptl. Therap.* **163**:147.

Meltzer, H. Y., 1969, Muscle enzyme release in acute psychosis, *Arch. Gen. Psychiat.* **1**:102.

Monroe, R. R., and Drell, H. J., 1947, Oral use of stimulants obtained from inhalers, *J. Am. Med. Assoc.* **135**:909.

Murphy, D. L., and Wyatt, R. J., 1972, Reduced monoamine oxidase activity in blood platelets of schizophrenic patients, *Nature* **238**:225.

Norman, J., and Shea, J., 1945, Acute hallucinosis as a complication of addiction to amphetamine sulfate, *New Engl. J. Med.* **233**:270.

Oswald, I., and Thacore, V. R., 1963, Amphetamine and phenmetrazine addiction—physiological abnormalities during the abstinence syndrome, *Brit. Med. J.* **1963**:427.

Prinzmental, M., and Bloomberg, W., 1935, Use of benzedrine for treatment of narcolepsy, *J. Am. Med. Assoc.* **105**:2051.

Rylander, G., 1967, Addiction to preludin intravenously injected, *Excerpta Med. Intern. Congr. Series* **150**:1363.

Sayers, A. C., and Handley, S. L., 1973, A study of the role of catecholamines in the response to various central stimulants, *European J. Pharmacol.* **23**:47.

Scheel-Kruger, J., 1971, Comparative studies of various amphetamine analogues demonstrating different interactions with the metabolism of the catecholamines in the brain, *European J. Pharmacol.* **14**:47.

Scheel-Kruger, J., 1972, Behavioral and biochemical comparison of amphetamine derivatives, cocaine, benztropine and tricyclic antidepressant drugs, *European J. Pharmacol.* **18**:63.

Schildkraut, J. J., Watson, R., Draskoczy, P. R. *et al.*, 1971, Amphetamine withdrawal depression and MHPG excretion, *Lancet* **2**:485.

Smith, D. E., 1969, Analysis of variables in high dose methamphetamine dependence, *J. Psychodelic Drugs* **2**:132.

Smith, R. L., and Dring, L. G., 1970, Patterns of metabolism of α-phenylisopropylamines in man and other species, in: *Amphetamines and Related compounds*, E. Costa, and S. Garattini, eds.), p. 121, Raven Press, New York.

Synder, S. H., 1972, Catecholamines in the brain as mediators of amphetamine psychosis, *Arch. Gen. Psychiat.* **27**:00

Snyder, S. H., 1973*a*, Biochemical models of drug psychosis focus on amphetamines pharmacology and the future of man, *Proc. 5th Intern. Congr. Pharmacol.* **1**:106.

Snyder, S. H., 1973*b*, Amphetamine psychosis: A "model" schizophrenia mediated by catecholamines, *Am. J. Psychiat.* **130**:61.

Snyder, S. H., 1974, Stereoselective features of catecholamine disposition and behavior implications, in: *Catecholamines and Their Enzymes in the Neuropathology of Schizophrenia* (J. Matthysse and S. S. Kety, eds.) Pergamon Press, New York (in press).

Snyder, S. H., Taylor, J. T., Coyle, J. L., and Meyerhoff, J. L., 1970, The role of brain dopamine in behavioral regulation and the action of psychotropic drugs, *Am. J. Psychiat.* **127**:199.

Taylor, K. M., and Snyder, S. H., 1970, Amphetamine: Differentiation of *d* and *l*-isomers of behavior involving brain norepinephrine or dopamine, *Science* **168**:1487.

Taylor, K. M., and Snyder, S. H., 1971, Differential effects of *d*-and *l*-amphetamine on behavior and on catecholamine disposition in dopamine and norepinephrine containing neurons of rat brain, *Brain Res.* **28**:295.

Thoenen, H., Hurlimann, Gey, K. F., and Haefely, W. E., 1966, Liberations of *p*-hydroxynorephedrine from cat spleen by sympathetic nerve stimulation after pretreatment with amphetamine, *Life Sci.* **5**:1715.

Van Praag, H. M., 1968, Abuse of, dependence on and psychosis from anorexigenic drugs, in: *Drug-Induced Diseases, Vol. 3*, pp. 281–294. Excerpta Med., Amsterdam.

Walinder, J., and Carlsson, A., 1973, Potentiation of neuroleptics by catecholamine inhibitors, *Brit. Med. J.* **1973**:551.

Watson, R., Hartmann, E., and Schildkraut, J. J., 1972, Amphetamine withdrawal: Affective state, sleep patterns, and MHPG excretion, *Am. J. Psychiat.* **129**:3.

Yara-Tobias, J. A., Diamond, B., and Merlis, S., 1970, The action of L-dopa on schizophrenic patients (preliminary report), *Current Therap. Res.* **12**:528.

Young, D., and Scoville, W. B., 1938, Paranoid psychosis in narcolepsy and the possible dangers of benzedrine treatment, *Med. Clin. N. Am.* **22**:673.

Young, G. G., Simson, C. B., and Frohman, C. E., 1961, Clinical and biochemical studies of an amphetamine withdrawal psychosis, *J. Nervous Mental Disease* **132**:234.

Chapter 6

Serum Dopamine-β-Hydroxylase in Various Pathological States*

Menek Goldstein, Richard P. Ebstein,
Lewis S. Freedman, and Dong H. Park

Department of Psychiatry
Neurochemistry Laboratories
New York University Medical Center
New York, New York

1. INTRODUCTION

Dopamine-β-hydroxylase (EC 1.14.17.1) (DβH) plays a central role in the biosynthesis of the neurotransmitter norepinephrine (NE) and the hormone of the adrenal medulla epinephrine (E). It catalyzes the hydroxylation of dopamine (DA) to NE in the only physiologically significant pathway for the formation of NE and E. The enzyme is localized to the catecholamine-containing vesicular structures in sympathetic nerve terminals (Potter and Axelrod, 1963) and in the adrenal medulla (Kirshner, 1957). The enzyme is released with catecholamines upon stimulation of sympathetic nerves and the adrenal gland by a process known as exocytosis (Viveros *et al.*, 1968; Geffen *et al.*, 1969). Although the source of circulating DβH has not been clearly defined, it is suggested that serum DβH is a reflection of peripheral sympathetic activity involving the release of catecholamines. In animals and in man stress has been shown to elevate serum DβH (Kvetnansky *et al.*, 1971; Roffman *et al.*, 1973; Wooten and Cardon, 1973; Freedman *et al.*, 1973) which suggests that the serum enzyme levels rise in a situation known to cause an increase in the release of catecholamines. Since various

* This work was supported by U.S. Public Health Service grant MH-02717.

neuropsychiatric disorders might be associated with aberrations in the disposition and metabolism of catecholamines it was of interest to investigate whether DβH measurements in the serum of such patients could be of clinical value. The purpose of this review is to summarize and to evaluate some studies on serum DβH levels in various neuropsychiatric disorders.

2. DETERMINATION OF DβH ACTIVITY IN HUMAN SERUM

A sensitive and specific enzymatic assay for determination of DβH activity in sympathetic innervated tissues and in serum was described (Goldstein *et al.*, 1971; Molinoff *et al.*, 1971). The principle of the assay is outlined in the following reaction scheme:

$$\text{Tyramine} \xrightarrow{\text{D}\beta\text{H}} \text{Octopamine} \xrightarrow[\text{}^{14}\text{C-SAM}]{\text{PNMT}} N\text{-methyl-}^{14}\text{C-octopamine}$$

When tyramine is used as a substrate, in the first of coupled enzymatic reactions tyramine is converted by DβH to octopamine; in the second reaction the octopamine is further converted by added phenylethanolamine-N-methyltransferase (EC 2.1.1.28) (PNMT) to radioactively labeled N-methyl octopamine. In presence of S-adenosyl-L-methionine-methyl-^{14}C (^{14}C-SAM) the final reaction product N-methyl-^{14}C-octopamine (synephrine) is separated from the radioactive S-adenosyl-L-methionine by solvent extraction and its radioactivity is determined. In this procedure endogenous inhibitors of DβH must be inactivated by addition of N-ethyl maleimide (Goldstein *et al.*, 1971) or by cupric ions (Molinoff *et al.*, 1971) at the beginning of the incubation.

3. DETERMINATION OF IMMUNOREACTIVE (IR) DβH LEVELS IN HUMAN SERUM

The technique of radioimmunoassay is now a well established laboratory procedure which has been applied to the estimation of various hormones and enzymes in human serum. The principle of this procedure is outlined in the following scheme:

$$\begin{array}{ll} \text{Ag*} + \text{Ab} \rightleftarrows \text{Ag*} \cdot \text{Ab} & \text{Ag: unlabeled antigen} \\ \qquad + & \text{Ag*: labeled antigen} \\ \qquad \text{Ag} & \text{Ab: specific antibody} \\ \qquad \updownarrow & \\ \text{Ag} \cdot \text{Ab} & \end{array}$$

Labeled antigen (Ag*) binds to specific antibody (Ab) to form a labeled antigen–antibody (Ag · Ab) complex. The unlabeled antigen in serum competes with labeled antigen for antibody and thereby inhibits the binding of labeled antigen. As a result of competitive inhibition the binding of labeled antigen to antibody is diminished. The concentration of the antigen in the serum is obtained by comparing the inhibition of the serum sample with that of a standard solution containing known amounts of the antigen.

Recently a solid-phase radioimmunoassay utilizing antibodies to sheep adrenal DβH and I^{125}-labeled sheep adrenal DβH was described (Rush and Geffen, 1972). Since there is a considerable cross-species loss in immunoreactivity (Ohuchi et al., 1972), we have modified the radioimmunoassay for determination of human DβH by using I^{125}-labeled human DβH to inhibit competitively the binding of human DβH to antibody directed toward human enzyme (Ebstein et al., 1973). The results of our study have shown that the radioimmunoassay of human serum DβH could be used in monitoring changes of sympathetic activity in various physiological and pathological states (Ebstein et al., 1973; Freedman et al., 1973).

4. SERUM DβH LEVELS: ENZYMATIC ASSAY VERSUS RADIOIMMUNOASSAY

The DβH activity in the serum represents only a small fraction of the total enzyme protein (Goldstein, Freedman, Ebstein, and Park, unpublished data). The enzyme activity in the serum may not reflect the amount of the enzyme released from synaptic vesicles following sympathetic stimulation, since the enzyme might be inactivated to some extent prior to its removal from the circulation. It is noteworthy that DβH is a copper enzyme (Goldstein et al., 1965; Blumberg et al., 1965; Friedman and Kaufman, 1965) and that the valence of the copper undergoes cyclic changes during the enzymatic hydroxylation reaction. The Cu^{2+} of the enzyme can be reduced by ascorbate or by other reducing agents, and the reduced enzyme intermediate loses its activity more readily than the native cupric form of the enzyme (Goldstein and Freedman, unpublished data). Thus, the enzyme activity might be affected by the concentration of reducing agents in the serum. We are therefore investigating the effects of oral administration of ascorbate on DβH activity in the serum.

On the other hand, the radioimmunoassay is not dependent on the labile enzyme activity and, therefore, this procedure could be more advantageous. Although we have shown a significant correlation between IR-enzyme protein levels and enzyme activity levels in sera obtained from the normal population (Ebstein et al., 1973), it is conceivable that in some pathological states the IR-protein levels may not correlate with DβH activity levels. A correlation or lack of correlation between these two assays will indicate whether the alteration in circulatory enzyme levels are due to changes in the rate of enzyme release or to changes in the rate of enzyme inactivation prior to its elimination from the circulation.

5. SERUM DβH ACTIVITY IN NEUROBLASTOMA

Neuroblastoma and its variant, ganglioneuroma, are the second most common solid malignant tumors of infants and children (Lingley *et al.,* 1967). In view of the common histogenetic origin of the chromaffin cells and of the sympathetic nerve cells it was reasonable to assume that pheochromocytoma and neuroblastoma tumors are metabolically active in a similar manner. Indeed, both tumors were shown to be associated with an increase in the urinary excretion of catecholamines. However, the urinary excretion pattern of catecholamines and their metabolites in patients with neuroblastoma is variable. Some patients excrete large quantities of dopamine and its major metabolite homovanillic acid (HVA), others excrete both dopamine and norepinephrine and their respective major metabolites, HVA and vanilmandelic acid (VMA) (Bell, 1963).

Serum DβH activity and urinary catecholamine levels were monitored in 20 children with active neuroblastoma and 11 patients with inactive or "cured" disease (Goldstein *et al.,* 1972*a,b*; Freedman *et al.,* 1973). Serum DβH activity was elevated (activity greater than two standard deviations above control mean value) in 9 of 20 active cases. In these patients urinary catecholamine excretion was characterized by abnormal levels of NE and VMA. No correlation of serum DβH and dopamine or HVA was apparent. Thus, serum DβH levels paralleled the catecholamine secretory processes of the active tumor. However, high serum DβH activity was also observed in six of ten "cured" patients (Freedman *et al.,* 1973). Long-term studies are underway to ascertain whether serum DβH activity may be predictive of tumor reoccurence in these patients. Thus, the monitoring of serum DβH in conjunction with other diagnostic tests might be of significant usefulness in the diagnosis and prognosis of neuroblastoma.

6. SERUM DβH ACTIVITY IN FAMILIAL DYSAUTONOMIA

Familial dysautonomia (F.D.) is an inherited autosomal recessive disease with protean neurological manifestations, dysfunctions of the autonomic nervous system as indicated by vasomotor instability with hypertensive episodes, postural hypotension, and exaggerated responses to norepinephrine (NE). Histological studies of sural nerve biopsies have revealed neuronal degeneration in patients with F.D. (Aguayo *et al.,* 1971). We and others (Freedman *et al.,* 1972; Weinshilboum and Axelrod, 1971) have investigated serum DβH activities in patients with this disorder. We have extended our studies to a larger population and the results are summarized in Figure 1.

Patients with F.D. show a similar variability in serum enzyme activity levels as the control population. There is no significant difference in serum DβH activity levels as compared to the control subjects in the age group 1–5 years. In the six and older age group the mean level in F.D. is slightly but significantly lower. Some F.D. patients have serum DβH activity levels one or more standard deviations below the mean of the control subjects, but some have enzyme activity levels higher than one standard deviation above the mean. The parents of the dysautonomia patients had a mean value similar to the age-matched control population. Enzyme activity levels in patients with F.D. correlate significantly with the levels of their mothers (correlation coefficient = 0.45; $p < 0.05$). A very good correlation exists in patients with F.D. between enzyme activity levels and IR-DβH levels (correlation coefficient = 0.80; $p < 0.01$).

The low values in serum DβH of some patients with F.D. might result from the diminution in the number of neurons in the sympathetic and sensory ganglia. However, over half of the analyzed patients with F.D. failed to have a low level of serum DβH. It seems therefore, that the disease may have some effect on the circulating levels of DβH but not a decisive one. This point is perhaps best illustrated with the results obtained with one family. Three sons are affected with the disease; two have low levels and one has a normal serum DβH level. The healthy parents have normal serum DβH levels. F.D. is an autosomal recessive disease affecting one ethnic group, the Ashkenazi Jew, suggesting that the disease is genetically homogeneous. Thus, the findings that two affected siblings have low enzyme levels while the third has normal levels do not support the previously presented idea that a subgroup of "DβH negative" patients have a genetic defect involving DβH as the cause of this disease (Weinshilboum and Axelrod, 1971).

7. SERUM DβH LEVELS IN DOWN'S SYNDROME

Patients who suffer from Down's syndrome (a constellation of clinical symptoms with aberrations of the chromosome designated as the 21st) have

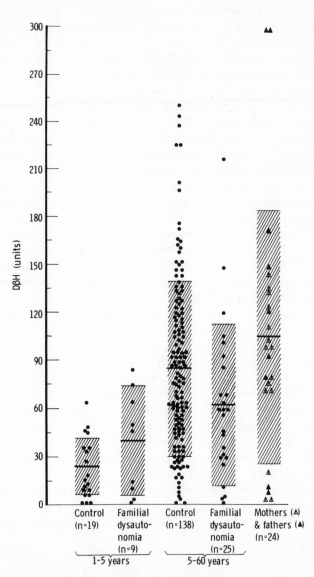

Figure 1. The distribution of DβH activity in patients with familial dysautonomia and in their parents as well as in age-matched controls. The horizontal lines represent the means and the bars represent ± S.D. The mean values ± S.D. are: controls (age group 1–5) 24.0 ± 21.06; patients with familial dysautonomia (age group 1–5) 34.0 ± 33.12; controls (over 6 yr of age) 86.1 ± 54.31; patients with familial dysautonomia (age group over 6 yr of age) 62.7 ± 49.61; parents of patients with familial dysautonomia, 105.5 ± 29.68.

been reported to have idiosyncratic responses to drugs affecting the parasympathetic and sympathetic system (O'Brien *et al.*, 1960). In the past decade, several studies have shown that platelet serotonin levels are low in patients with Down's syndrome (Boullin *et al.*, 1969), but no comparable studies were made on blood norepinephrine levels.

More recently it was reported that patients with Down's syndrome have low serum DβH activity (Wetterberg *et al.*, 1972*b*; Coleman *et al.*, 1973). We have now extended these studies on a large population of patients. The results presented in Figure 2 show that there is a preponderance of sera with low serum DβH activity among patients with Down's syndrome. The mean serum DβH activity value was significantly lower in patients with Down's syndrome than in either the age-matched normal controls or the age-matched nonmongoloid mentally disturbed children. It is of interest to note that the mean serum DβH activity of the nonmongoloid mentally disturbed children is higher than that of the normal children. However, it is necessary to corroborate this finding in a study of a larger population.

The mean value of serum IR-DβH levels in patients with Down's syndrome is also significantly lower than that of age-matched normal controls. This finding indicates that the diminished serum DβH activity levels in the mongoloid patients cannot be attributed to an increased rate of enzyme inactivation prior to its removal from the circulation. To determine whether the diminished serum DβH levels in patients with Down's syndrome reflect hereditary patterns or are related to trisomy 21, we are now investigating the correlation between serum DβH levels of parents and their children. The low serum DβH values in mongoloids may not be attributed to heredity but rather may reflect the chromosomal aberrations characteristic for this disorder. However, if the low serum DβH levels of patients with Down's syndrome are due to familial factors, then the serum enzyme levels of prospective parents might be of prognostic value.

8. SERUM DβH ACTIVITY IN AFFECTIVE STATES

Sympathetic nervous discharge has been associated with affective states of fear and anxiety in humans. The norepinephrine hypothesis of affective disorders has been useful for further studies on the etiopathogenesis underlying this group of endogenous illnesses. In our previous studies we found no differences in serum DβH levels between patients with affective states and the age-matched control population (Shopsin *et al.*, 1972). The results presented in Figure 3 show that serum DβH activity in the psy-

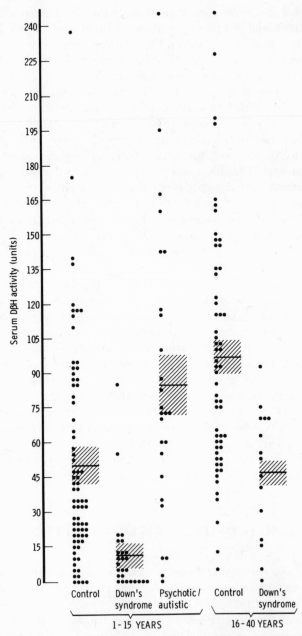

Figure 2. The distribution of DβH activity in Down's syndrome patients, in normal controls and in nonmongoloid mentally disturbed patients. The horizontal lines represent the mean and the bars represent ± S.E.M.

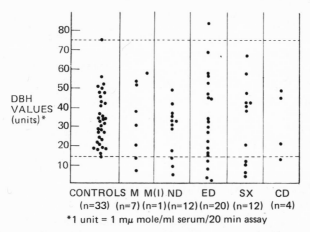

Figure 3. Serum DβH activity in psychiatric patients. M is the cyclic (bipolar) manic depressive in manic phase. M(I) is the manic in interphase which is asymptotic. ND is neurotic depressives. ED is unipolar (endogenous) depressives. SX is schizophrenics. CD is character disorders.

chiatric populations explored failed to differentiate between different diagnostic entities and were compatible with values obtained from normal age-matched control subjects (Shopsin *et al.*, 1972). In two separate studies it was confirmed that patients with schizophrenia and manic-depressive disorders had a mean and variation of serum DβH activity similar to that of normal age-matched controls (Wetterberg *et al.*, 1972*a,b*; Dunner *et al.*, 1973).

Since hereditary factors are important in the etiology of schizophrenia (Kety *et al.*, 1968) and also influence serum dβH levels (Ross *et al.*, 1973; Weinshilboum *et al.*, 1973) it is now of interest to investigate whether there is any correlation between the inheritance patterns of schizophrenics and serum DβH levels. It is possible that variation in serum DβH levels caused by hereditary differences may mask changes caused by the disease.

Recently it was reported that DβH is decreased in postmortem brain obtained from schizophrenic patients (Wise and Stein, 1973), and these results were interpreted as consistent with the hypothesis that noradrenergic "reward pathways" are damaged in schizophrenia. Further studies are now required to corroborate or deny this challenging hypothesis.

Inherent in the biochemical study of the human brain is the inability to obtain fresh material such as that used with laboratory animals. The measurement of DβH activity in postmortem brains could yield erroneous results since enzymatic activity of DβH is labile and could vary with storage time. Furthermore, the enzymatic activity could be influenced by a variety of clinical and postmortem conditions (i.e., drug treatment, interfering disease processes, time interval between death and freezing of the brain). Since radioimmunoassay measures the total DβH protein which might not be as sensitive to postmortem conditions as the labile enzyme activity, we have modified the radioimmunoassay for measurements of DβH in human postmortem brain and in other tissues. The radioimmunoassay for measuring DβH in postmortem brain could represent a new approach for investigating the role of the noradrenergic system in schizophrenia.

9. DISCUSSION AND CONCLUSIONS

DβH is released with NE into the circulation, and the levels measured in the serum do not necessarily reflect tissue enzyme levels. The determination of serum DβH by either enzymatic assay or by radioimmunoassay measures only the balance between rate of the release of the enzyme and its clearance from the blood. The steady state level of circulatory DβH may be pictured as follows (Goldstein *et al.*, 1972*a,b*):

Release
from sympathetic $\longrightarrow$ Circulatory DβH $\longrightarrow$ Clearance
nerve terminals   from the circulation

Recent evidence suggests that the mechanisms controlling the basal levels of human serum DβH involves not only sympathetic activity but also genetic factors (Ross *et al.*, 1973; Weinshilboum *et al.*, 1973; Goldstein *et al.*, 1973). The great variation between individuals in serum DβH levels indicates that other factors besides sympathetic activity are involved in determining the DβH levels in serum. It is not yet known whether the sympathetic nerve activity or the turnover rate of the enzyme in the serum is genetically influenced. The findings that familial factors significantly influence the basal levels of circulating DβH are of importance in the interpretation of clinical studies.

The variations in serum DβH levels caused by hereditary differences could mask changes caused by the disease. Thus, the comparison of serum DβH levels of patients with a specific disease with the serum DβH levels of the patients family might be useful in the interpretation of the data.

ACKNOWLEDGMENT

The clinical studies were carried out in collaboration with Dr. Felicia Axelrod and Dr. Joseph Dancis of the Department of Pediatrics, New York

University Medical Center, Dr. Magda Campbell and Dr. Baron Shopsin of the Department of Psychiatry, New York University Medical Center, Dr. Larry Helson of Sloan-Kettering Institute for Cancer Research, New York City, and Dr. Mary Coleman of Children's Brain Research Clinic, Washington, D.C.

10. REFERENCES

Aguayo, A. J., Nair, C. P. V., and Brag, G. M., 1971, Peripheral nerve abnormalities in the Riley-Day Syndrome, *Arch. Neurol.* **24**:106.

Bell, M., 1963, The clinical chemistry of neuroblastomas, in: *The Clinical Chemistry of Monoamines* (H. Varley and A. H. Gowenlock, eds.), pp. 82–91, Elsevier Publishing Co., New York.

Blumberg, W. E., Goldstein, M., Lauber, E., and Peisach, J., 1965, Magnetic resonance studies on the mechanism of the enzymic β-hydroxylation, *Biochim. Biophys. Acta* **99**:188.

Boullin, D. J., Coleman, M., and O'Brien, R. A., 1969, Defective binding of 5-hydroxytryptamine by blood platelets from children with the trisomy 21 form of Down's syndrome, *J. Physiol. (London)* **204**:104.

Coleman, M., Lodge, A., Barnett, A., and Cytryn, L., 1973, *Serotonin in Down's Syndrome*, North Holland Publishing Co., Amsterdam.

Dunner, D. L., Cohn, C. K., Weinshilboum, R. M., and Wyatt, R. J., 1973, The activity of dopamine-β-hydroxylase and methionine-activating enzyme in blood of schizophrenic patients, *Biol. Psychiat.* **6**(3):215.

Ebstein, R. P., Park, D. H., Freedman, L. S., Levitz, S. M., Ohuchi, T., and Goldstein, M., 1973, A radioimmunoassay of human circulatory dopamine-β-hydroxylase, *Life Sci.* **13**:769.

Freedman, L. S., Ohuchi, T., Goldstein, M., Axelrod, F., Fish, I., and Dancis, J., 1972, Changes in human serum dopamine-β-hydroxylase with age, *Nature* **236**:310.

Freedman, L. S., Roffman, M., and Goldstein, M., 1973, Changes in human serum dopamine-β-hydroxylase in various physiological and pathological states, in: *Frontiers in Catecholamine Research,* Pergamon Press, New York pp. 1109–1114.

Freedman, L. S., Ebstein, R. P., Park, D. H., Levitz, S. M., and Goldstein, M., 1973, The effect of cold pressor test in man on serum immunoreactive dopamine-β-hydroxylase and on dopamine-β-hydroxylase activity, *Res. Commun. Chem. Path. Pharmacol.* **6**:873.

Friedman, S., and Kaufman, S., 1965, 3,4-Dihydroxyphenylethylamine β-hydroxylase: a copper enzyme, *J. Biol. Chem.* **240**:552.

Geffen, L. B., Livett, B. G., and Rush, R. A., 1969, Immunohistochemical localization of protein components of catecholamine storage vesicles, *J. Physiol. (London)* **204**:593.

Goldstein, M., Lauber, E., and McKereghan, M. R., 1965, Studies on the purification and characterization of 3,4-dihydroxyphenylethylamine-β-hydroxylase, *J. Biol. Chem.* **240**:2066.

Goldstein, M., Freedman, L. S., and Bonnay, M., 1971, An assay for dopamine-β-hydroxylase activity in tissues and in serum, *Experientia* **27**:632.

Goldstein, M., Freedman, L. S., Bohuon, A. C., and Guerinot, F., 1972a, Serum dopamine-β-hydroxylase activity in neuroblastoma, *New Engl. J. Med.* **286**:1123.

Goldstein, M., Fuxe, K., and Hökfelt, T., 1972b, Characterization and tissue localization of catecholamine-synthesizing enzymes, *Pharmacol. Rev.* **24**:293.

Goldstein, M., Freedman, L. S., Ebstein, R. P., Park, D. H., and Kashimoto, T., 1974, Human serum dopamine-β-hydroxylase: Relationship to sympathetic activity in physiological and pathological states. in: *Neuropsychopharmacology of Monoamines and Their Regulatory Enzymes* (E. Usdin, ed.), Raven Press, New York, pp. 105–119.

Kety, S. S., Rosenthal, D., Wender, P. H., and Schulsinger, F., 1968, The types and prevalence of mental illness in the biological and adoptive families of adopted schizophrenics. in: *The Transmission of Schizophrenia* (D. Rosenthal and S. S. Kety, eds.), p. 345, Pergamon Press, New York.

Kirshner, N., 1957, Pathway of noradrenaline formation from dopa, *J. Biol. Chem.* **226**:821.

Kvetnansky, R., Gewirtz, G. P., Weise, V. K., and Kopin, I. J., 1971, Enhanced synthesis of adrenal DβH induced by repeated immobilization in rats, *Mol. Pharmacol.* **7**:81.

Lingley, J. F., Sagerman, R. H., and Santulli, T. V., 1967, Neuroblastoma: management and survival, *New Engl. J. Med.* **277**:1227.

Molinoff, P. B., Brimijoin, S., and Weinshilboum, R. M., 1970, Neurally mediated increase in dopamine-β-hydroxylase activity, *Proc. Natl. Acad. Sci. (U.S.)* **66**:453.

Molinoff, P. B., Weinshilboum, R., and Axelrod, J., 1971, A sensitive enzymatic assay for dopamine-β-hydroxylase, *J. Pharmacol. Exptl. Therap.* **178**:425.

O'Brien, D., Haake, M. W., and Brand, B., 1960, Atropine sensitivity and serotonin in mongolism, *Am. J. Diseases Children* **100**:873.

Ohuchi, T., Joh, T. H., Freedman, L. S., and Goldstein, M., 1972, *Fifth Intern. Cong. Pharmacol.* (abstr. 1022), p. 171.

Potter, L., and Axelrod, J., 1963, Properties of norepinephrine storage particles of the rat heart, *J. Pharmacol. Exptl. Therap.* **142**:299.

Roffman, M., Freedman, L. S., and Goldstein, M., 1973, The effect of acute and chronic swim stress on dopamine-β-hydroxylase activity, *Life Sci.* **12**:369.

Ross, S. B., Wetterberg, L., and Myrhed, M., 1973, Genetic control of plasma dopamine-β-hydroxylase, *Life Sci.* **12**(12):529.

Rush, R. A., and Geffen, L. B., 1972, Radioimmunoassay and clearance of circulating dopamine-β-hydroxylase, *Circulation Res.* **31**:444.

Shopsin, B., Freedman, L. S., Goldstein, M., and Gershon, S., 1972, Serum dopamine-β-hydroxylase (DβH) activity and affective states, *Psychopharmacologia* **27**:11.

Viveros, O. H., Arqueros, L., and Kirshner, N., 1968, Release of catecholamines and dopamine-β-oxidase from the adrenal medulla, *Life Sci.* **7**:609.

Weinshilboum, R. M., and Axelrod, J., 1971, Reduced plasma dopamine-β-hydroxylase activity in familial dysautonomia, *New Engl. J. Med.* **285**:938.

Weinshilboum, R. M., Raymond, F. A., Elveback, L. R., and Weidman, W. H., 1973, Serum dopamine-β-hydroxylase activity: Sibling–Sibling correlation, *Science* **181**:943.

Wetterberg, L., Aberg, H., Ross, S. B., and Froden, O., 1972*a*, Plasma dopamine-β-hydroxylase activity in hypertension and various neuropsychiatric disorders, *Scand. J. Clin. Lab. Invest.* **30**(3):283.

Wetterberg, L., Gustavson, K.-H., Backstrom, M., Ross, S. B., and Froden, O., 1972*b*, Low dopamine-β-hydroxylase activity in Down's syndrome, *Clin. Genet.* **3**:152.

Wise, C. D., and Stein, L., 1973, Dopamine-β-hydroxylase deficits in the brains of schizophrenic patients, *Science* **181**:344.

Wooten, G. F., and Cardon, P. V., 1973, Plasma dopamine-β-hydroxylase: Elevation in man during cold pressor tests and exercise, *Arch. Neurol.* **28**:103.

Chapter 7

Possible Roles of Catecholamines in the Action of Narcotic Drugs

Doris H. Clouet

Testing and Research Laboratory
New York State Drug Abuse Control Commission
Brooklyn, New York

1. INTRODUCTION

The relation between brain catecholamines and the pharmacological responses induced by morphine and other narcotic analgesic drugs has been investigated extensively in order to determine whether the brain amines play a role in the responses to acute drug treatment, and to examine the possibility that catecholaminergic mechanisms in the central nervous system are involved in the development of tolerance to chronic drug treatment. It is important to distinguish between the effects produced by a single exposure of animal or man to morphine or other narcotic analgesic drugs, and the effects produced by chronic drug exposure, because these effects, both pharmacological and biochemical, are modulated by the intensity and duration of drug exposure (Eddy *et al.*, 1965). At moderate doses, the acute administration of a narcotic drug produces mainly depressant effects: e.g., respiratory depression, narcosis, sedation, analgesia, hypotension, hypothermia, inhibition of REM sleep, decreased performance in behavioral tests, and alterations in EEG patterns. Other central responses presumably nondepressant, produced by moderate doses include euphoria (in man), increased locomotor activity (in mice), and manic activity (in cats). At very high doses, the acute administration of an opiate produces convulsions and death. The predominant responses are dose- and species-dependent, as are the potency and duration of activity of each drug (Hug, 1972). The active

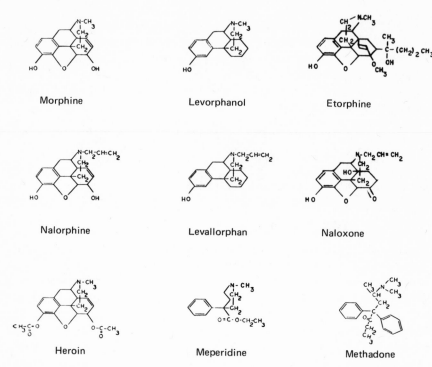

Figure 1. Structures of opiate agonists and antagonists. Nalorphine, levallorphan, and naloxone are mainly antagonists. All of the other compounds are narcotic agonists.

agonists differ structurally from morphine, the prototype agonist, both toward simpler structures, such as meperidine, and toward more complex structures, such as etorphine (Figure 1). Studies of structure–activity relationships have demonstrated that the drugs have stereospecificity in potency (Beckett and Casy, 1965), and that there are a number of determinant sites for activity on the drug molecule (Lewis *et al.*, 1971; Bentley and Lewis, 1973). The acute effects of narcotic agonists are blocked by narcotic antagonists. The antagonists, which are closely related chemically to the narcotic agonists (Figure 1), differ from agonists in the substituents on the tertiary nitrogen atom (Lewis *et al.*, 1971). Many antagonists, such as nalorphine and diprenorphine, also have agonistic activity, and are termed partial agonist-antagonists, while others such as naloxone, are considered pure antagonists (Harris, 1971).

Upon chronic exposure of subjects to opiates, tolerance develops in most of the depressant effects produced by acute administration, and in other effects which cannot be classified as depressant, such as increased locomotor activity in mice (Hug, 1972). Tolerance develops at a rate which is dose-dependent and dependent on the interval between doses and on the mode of drug administration. In order to maintain a constant level of response, it is necessary to increase the dose of drug at intervals during chronic treatment. In tolerant individuals, antagonist administration produces a set of symptoms termed the withdrawal reaction. In addition to the phenomena of tolerance and physical dependence (manifested by withdrawal symptoms), a third phenomenon, psychic dependence, is required in order to characterize chronic drug use as drug dependence (Schuster, 1970). Psychic dependence is demonstrated in its simplest form by showing drug-seeking behavior in man or animals. Drug-seeking behavior has been demonstrated in animals in choice situations in which the animal (mouse, rat, monkey) specifies the amount of drug to be administered (Weeks, 1962; Thompson and Schuster, 1964; Wikler and Pescor, 1967). The quantitation of drug-seeking behavior in animals has become precise with the introduction of self-administration techniques (Yanagita et al., 1965; Weeks and Collins, 1964; Brady, 1973), and the reinforcing effect of opiates and its antecedent variables have been established (Woods and Schuster, 1970; Goldberg et al., 1972).

The sites of action in the CNS of narcotic analgesic drugs administered acutely has been defined operationally in the terms of several disciplines: Anatomically, opiates act throughout the CNS with a polysynaptic circuit as a minimal requirement (Borison, 1971); physiologically, opiates impair sensory input, association, and integration of input, and seem to have some effects on central efferent motor activity (Domino, 1968); subcellularly, opiates interfere in impulse transmission at the level of the neuronal membrane and alter neurotransmitter function (Clouet, 1972); molecularly, opiates, bind in homogenates and synaptic membranes of brain (Terenius, 1973; Pert and Snyder, 1973; Simon et al., 1973). With this emphasis on central neuronal function as the focus of drug action, it would be most surprising if catecholamines and other neurotransmitters were not involved in the mechanisms of action. However, whether narcotic drugs act directly on some aspect of the synthesis, storage, release, catabolism, or receptor activity of norepinephrine and/or dopamine in the CNS, or whether some initial drug–tissue interaction triggers responses in neurotransmitter systems, remains an open question, as is whether the catecholamine system is important in physiological adaptation, or tolerance, to chronic drug use. In succeeding sections of this chapter, I shall review evidence bearing on the role of catecholamines in the action of narcotic analgesic drugs, garnered mainly from pharmacological and biochemical studies, and then attempt to make an orderly interpretation of these data in the light of present knowledge.

2. EFFECTS OF OTHER DRUGS ON OPIATE ACTIVITY

2.1. Monoamine Oxidase Inhibitors

MAO inhibitors increase the levels of brain catecholamines by inhibiting their catabolism. Pretreatment of experimental animals with MAO inhibitors, such as pargyline, tranylcypromine, or iproniazid, increases the acute pharmacological effects produced by morphine and other narcotic analgesic drugs: in mice, pargyline potentiated the locomotor hyperactivity induced by morphine (Carroll and Sharp, 1972; Villarreal *et al.*, 1973) and by levorphanol (Hollinger, 1969); in rabbits, pargyline decreased the toxicity of meperidine (Fahim *et al.*, 1972); in rats, the analgetic response to morphine was potentiated by iproniazid and nialamide (Gupta and Kulkarni, 1966); in mice, the acute toxicity of morphine, meperidine, and phenazocine was potentiated by iproniazid or tranylcypromine (Rogers and Thornton, 1969), and in decerebrate cats, morphine-induced respiratory depression was enhanced by pretreatment with pargyline or tranylcypromine (Florez *et al.*, 1972). MAO inhibitors also enhance the pharmacological responses to opiates in opiate-dependent animals by reducing the degree of tolerance: both the analgetic responses in morphine-dependent rats (Vedernikov, 1970) and the locomotor hyperactivity in morphine-dependent mice (Iwamoto *et al.*, 1971) were increased by pargyline treatment in response to a test dose of morphine. In abstinence, MAO inhibitors alter the intensity of the withdrawal symptoms: in morphine-dependent mice, naloxone-induced stereotypic jumping was exacerbated by pargyline (Maruyama *et al.*, 1971; Iwamoto *et al.*, 1971), and iproniazid lengthened the time period during which nalorphine induced withdrawal symptoms (Maggiolo and Huidobro, 1965).

2.2. Tricyclic Antidepressants

The tricyclic antidepressants increase catecholamine levels at the synapse by blocking reuptake into the nerve ending. There are few studies on the interaction of these drugs with opiates: the pretreatment of mice with imipramine, desimipramine, or nortriptyline potentiated the locomotor hyperactivity induced by morphine (Carroll and Sharp, 1972) and, in abstinence, the administration of imipramine enhanced the intensity of withdrawal signs in morphine-dependent mice (Chiosa *et al.*, 1968).

2.3. Adrenergic Blocking Agents

In most studies on the influence of α-adrenergic or β-adrenergic blockers on the acute actions of morphine, no alterations of responses have been found: propranolol (β-blocker) and azapetine (α-blocker) had no effect on morphine ED_{50}s in the tail-flick test (Dewey *et al.,* 1970); phenoxybenzamine (α-blocker) had no effect on morphine analgesia in mice (Vanderwende and Spoerlein, 1973); propranolol had no effect on responses to morphine in the mouse (Fennessey and Lee, 1970); and neither phenoxybenzamine nor propranolol blocked morphine-induced mania in cats (Dhasmana *et al.,* 1972). However, slight decreases in pharmacological responses to the acute administration of morphine have been described: in mice, locomotor hyperactivity was decreased by pretreatment with phentolamine (α-blocker) or phenoxybenzamine, but not with propranolol (Carroll and Sharp, 1972); and, in rats, the analgesic response to morphine was decreased by propranolol (Heller *et al.,* 1968). In the abstinent spinalectomized dog, the signs of withdrawal were not affected by phenoxybenzamine (Martin and Eades, 1967).

2.4. Amine Depletors

Reserpine, tetrabenazine, and oxypertine differ in their activity in depleting brain monoamines: reserpine causes the depletion of serotonin as well as dopamine and norepinephrine, tetrabenazine depletes only catecholamines, and oxypertine has a short duration of activity in depleting catecholamines in the CNS. When oxypertine was administered 30 min prior to morphine, the morphine ED_{50} in the tail-flick test in mice was elevated, indicating an antagonism to the opiate. The antagonism was not found when oxpertine was administered 1 hr prior to morphine, or if the two drugs were administered simultaneously (Dewey *et al.,* 1970). Tetrabenazine causes depletion over a longer time period: pretreatment of animals with tetrabenazine 1–18 hr prior to the administration of morphine blocked or diminished the effects of morphine in the tail-flick test in mice and the manic response in cats (Dewey *et al.,* 1970; Dhasmana *et al.,* 1972). The time-dependent effect of tetrabenazine on catecholamine levels in brain and on acute morphine analgesia were shown by Takagi and his colleagues (1964; Takagi and Nakama, 1968). The daily administration of tetrabenazine 2 hr prior to morphine for 10 days partially blocked the development of tolerance to morphine (Takagi and Kuriki, 1969).

Reserpine has been shown to antagonize various acute agonist effects of narcotic analgesics in various animal species: analgesia in rats (Sigg *et al.*, 1958); respiratory depression in cats (Florez *et al.*, 1972); levorphanol- or morphine-induced locomotor hyperactivity in mice (Hollinger, 1969; Carroll and Sharp, 1972; Villarreal *et al.*, 1973); mania in cats (Dhasmana *et al.*, 1972), analgesia in rabbits (Verri *et al.*, 1968), and meperidine toxicity in mice (Sethy *et al.*, 1970). Just as there are temporal dimensions to the central amine depletion induced by reserpine, there are temporal dimensions to its antagonistic activity to morphine: when reserpine was administered simultaneously with morphine, there was no antagonism of the acute effects, but when given 16 hr prior to morphine, the ED_{50} of morphine was increased sixfold (Dewey *et al.*, 1970). In mice implanted with morphine pellets, reserpine produced sedation. However, if withdrawal was then induced by the administration of nalorphine, severe symptoms were evoked of convulsions and death (Maggiolo and Huidobro, 1965).

2.5. Inhibitors of Catecholamine Synthesis

The usual effect of prior inhibition of the biosynthesis of brain catecholamines is blockage of the acute effects of narcotic analgesics at the time when brain catecholamine levels are depressed. Pretreatment of animals with an inhibitor of tyrosine hydroxylase, α-methyl-p-tyrosine (AMPT): prevented the hyperactivity response in mice induced by morphine (Hollinger, 1969; Carroll and Sharp, 1972); blocked morphine-induced analgesia (Eidelberg and Schwartz, 1970; Verri *et al.*, 1968), and meperidine-induced analgesia (Sethy *et al.*, 1970). However, single or multiple doses of AMPT were not found to block the alerting effect of morphine, or its effect on REM sleep in cats (Echols and Jewett, 1969). The development of tolerance in mice was blocked by the simultaneous administration of AMPT with morphine (Marshall and Smith, 1973). Prior treatment with AMPT decreased abstinence symptoms in morphine-treated animals (Maggiolo and Huidobro, 1965; Maruyama and Takemori, 1973; Marshall and Smith, 1973). AMPT also blocked withdrawal aggression in rats (Puri and Lal, 1973) and blocked the self-administration of morphine in addicted monkeys (Pozuelo and Kerr, 1972). AMPT decreased the acquisition of morphine self-administration in rats (Davis and Smith, 1972).

The administration of α-methyldopa, an inhibitor of dopa decarboxylase, had little effect on responses to morphine administered either acutely (Rudzik and Mennear, 1965; Vanderwende and Spoerlein, 1972) or chronically (Maggiolo and Huidobro, 1965; Ross and Ashford, 1967).

Inhibitors of dopamine-β-hydroxylase also seem to have little effect on acute responses to morphine, although pretreatment with diethyldithiocarbamate (disulfiram) prior to morphine enhanced the analgesic response in rats (Watanabe *et al.,* 1969). Alterations in the intensity of withdrawal symptoms have been found after the administration of disulfiram: naloxone-induced "wet dog" shakes in tolerant rats were decreased by disulfiram, but the hyperthermic responses were increased (Schwartz and Eidelberg, 1970); disulfiram inhibited the naloxone-induced stereotypic jumping in tolerant mice (Maruyama and Takemori, 1973). Another inhibitor of dopamine-β-hydroxylase, 1-phenyl 3-(2-thiazolyl)-2 thiourea, also decreased the signs of precipitated abstinence in mice (Bhargava *et al.,* 1972).

2.6. Catecholamines and Precursors

The administration of large doses of dopa peripherally and smaller doses of dopamine or norepinephrine centrally has been shown to increase the level of brain catecholamines. In mice, the administration of dopa produces effects similar to those induced by narcotic analgesics. Large doses of dopa decreased the reaction time to the hot-plate analgesia test to lower than that of controls (Major and Pleuvry, 1971) and also altered the locomotor activity in mice in a biphasic pattern similar to that induced by opiates (Stromberg, 1970). Dopamine and norepinephrine also produced sedative and hyperactive motor effects in rodents when introduced into the CNS (Calcutt *et al.,* 1973).

The injection of dopa with morphine produced various effects related both to the pharmacological response measured, and to the time interval between dopa administration and drug administration: when administered intraperitoneally 15 or 30 min prior to morphine, dopa blocked the analgesic response to morphine, but had no effect when injected after morphine (VanderWende and Spoerlein, 1972). Similar antagonism to acute morphine effects have been described by Major and Pleuvry (1971), and Sparkes and Spencer (1971). However, a potentiation of morphine-induced locomotor activity was seen in mice injected with dopa 30 min prior or together with morphine (Carroll and Sharp, 1972). Dopa administration also increased the nociceptive threshold and enhanced the analgetic effects of meperidine and methodone (Radouco-Thomas *et al.,* 1967). Dopa reversed the effects of tetrabenazine (Takagi and Kuriki, 1969), AMPT (Eidelberg and Schwartz, 1970), and reserpine (Saarnivarra, 1969). In tolerant animals, dopa enhanced the withdrawal aggression seen 72 hr after the last injection of morphine (Puri and Lal, 1973).

The injection of dopamine either blocked (Contreras and Tamayo, 1966) or potentiated (Calcutt *et al.,* 1971) the analgesic response to morphine. When administered intracisternally, dopamine decreased the severity of abstinence symptoms in rats (Sharkawi, 1973).

Seemingly contradictory effects are also induced by norepinephrine administration. In rats, the intraventricular injection of norepinephrine depressed the analgesic effect of morphine (Sparkes and Spencer, 1971). However, norepinephrine potentiation of acute morphine effects has been reported more often (Sigg et al., 1958; Nott, 1968; Verri et al., 1968; Saarnivaara, 1969). In these experiments the biogenic amine was administered centrally. The intraventricular injection of norepinephrine produced an immediate attenuation of the nociceptive response to morphine in rats and mice, the completeness and duration of the potentiation being determined by the dose of norepinephrine (Calcutt et al., 1973).

2.7. Amphetamines and Cocaine

Both amphetamines and cocaine increase extrasynaptic levels of catecholamines in the CNS. Amphetamine, metamphetamine, ephedrine, and metaraminol have analgesic activity per se of brief duration (Colville and Chaplin, 1964). Pretreatment with amphetamine increased the analgesic response to acute morphine in mice, as measured by the hot-plate test (Major and Pleuvry, 1972) and in the tail-flick test (Dewey et al., 1970), and in rats, amphetamine potentiated the analgesic response to acute morphine (Vedernikov, 1970).

Cocaine increases synaptic levels of catecholamines by inhibiting the uptake of the biogenic amines into nerve endings (Herrting et al., 1961). Treatment of morphine-tolerant rats with cocaine restored the analgesic response to a dose of morphine to which the animals were tolerant (Vedernikow, 1970). Cocaine has also been shown to serve as a reinforcer in the maintenance of opiate self-administration in monkeys (Hofmeister and Schlichting, 1972).

2.8. Neuroleptic Drugs

Catecholamine receptors are blocked specifically by butyrophenones, such as haloperidol, and by phenothiazines, such as chlorpromazine, fluphenazine, and perphenazine (Andén, 1970; 1972). Pretreatment of cats with chlorpromazine or haloperidol blocked the characteristic manic response induced by morphine in this species (Quinn and Brodie, 1961; Dhasmana et al., 1972). Pretreatment of mice with either chlorpromazine or haloperidol blocked the morphine-induced locomotor hyperactivity (Carroll and

Sharp, 1972). In tolerant and abstinent animals neuroleptic drugs also alter responses to opiates: in rats and monkeys made tolerant to morphine by self-administration, haloperidol blocked bar-pressing for morphine (Hanson and Cimini-Venema, 1972; Pozuelo and Kerr, 1972), and in abstinent mice withdrawal aggression was blocked by haloperidol in a dose-dependent way (Puri and Lal, 1973). The hypothermic effect induced in morphine-dependent mice by abstinence has been reversed by morphine, and also by a conditioned stimulus. Haloperidol was able to block the reversal of this hypothermic effect by the conditioned stimulus (Drawbaugh and Lal, 1973).

2.9. Apomorphine and Amantadine

Apomorphine and amantadine have a direct stimulatory effect on dopaminergic structures (Andén et al., 1967; Stromberg, 1970). A secondary effect of both drugs on norepinephrine neurons is attributed to the primary effect of these drugs on dopamine neurons (Persson and Waldeck, 1970; Major and Pleuvry, 1972). Both apomorphine and amantadine have been shown to antagonize some responses to acute morphine administration in mice and rats (VanderWende and Spoerlein, 1973; Kuschinsky and Hornykiewicz, 1972), while in other experiments, apomorphine enhanced the analgesic effects of morphine (Vedernikov and Afrikanov, 1969) or had no effect (Florez et al., 1972). Since the aggressive response to withdrawal from morphine by tolerant rats was enhanced by apomorphine and reversed by morphine and methodone (Lal and Puri, 1972), the effect of apomorphine may also be classified as antagonistic to morphine. It is possible that the contradictory results of apomorphine on morphine-induced pharmacological responses are dose-related, since the effect of apomorphine on dopamine-sensitive adenyl cyclase in the caudate nucleus is dose-dependent, being stimulatory at 3 to 10 μM and inhibitory above 100 μM (Kebabian et al., 1972).

2.10. 6-Hydroxydopamine

6-Hydroxydopamine (6-OHDA) has a long-lasting effect in depleting brain catecholamines brought about by a selective degeneration of adrenergic nerve terminals when the drug is introduced into the CNS (Uretsky and Iversen, 1970). In general, the administration of 6-OHDA to animals antagonizes many of the pharmacological responses to opiates; the analgesis response in naive rats was decreased (Ayhan, 1972; Friedler et al., 1972), the stimulation threshold for morphine was decreased in rats (Bläsig et al.,

1973), and the latency of the tail-flick response was restored in tolerant mice (Nakamura *et al.,* 1973). Since 6-OHDA must be introduced into the CNS, it has been possible to eliminate possible sites of action by microinjection of the drug into discrete sites in brain. Microinjection into the ventricular system produced antagonism to morphine. However, injection into hypothalamic nuclei had no effect on morphine responses (Nakamura *et al.,* 1973).

When rats were injected with 6-OHDA at two weeks of age, less than half of the normal component of brain catecholamines were present six weeks later. In these animals, the analgesic responses to morphine were also completely abolished (Elchisak and Rosencrans, 1973).

3. OPIATE-INDUCED ALTERATIONS IN THE LEVELS OF BRAIN CATECHOLAMINES

The acute administration of morphine and other opioids to laboratory animals induces alterations in the content of catecholamines in the CNS. A depletion of catecholamines in the hypothalamus and midbrain of the cat by acute morphine administration was described by Vogt in 1954. This observation has been amply confirmed (Moore *et al.,* 1965; Laverty and Sharman, 1965; Reis *et al.,* 1969). The levels of biogenic amines fall in whole brain also after a single injection of morphine in cats or dogs (Schneider, 1954; Quinn and Brodie, 1961; Gunne, 1963; Maynert and Klingman, 1962, Maynert and Levi, 1964) and rodents (Maynert and Klingman, 1962; Gunne, 1963). In studies in which dopamine was separated from norepinephrine, both amines have been shown to be affected by narcotic analgesics. In mouse brain, the fall in dopamine levels was found to precede the fall in norepinephrine levels (Takagi and Nakama, 1966). The magnitude of the effect was shown to be dose-dependent with maximal depletion at intermediate doses of morphine (Fukui and Takagi, 1972; Fennessey and Lee, 1972). Not only morphine but also codeine, methadone, etorphine, levorphanol, meperidine, ketobemidone, and pentazocine produced falls in catecholamine levels in brain (Rethy *et al.,* 1971; Ahtee, 1973), and the antagonists nalorphine and naloxone were able to block the depleting action of morphine (Fukui and Takagi, 1972; Rethy *et al.,* 1971). These antagonists and inactive related compounds such as dextrorphan, thebaine, and *d*-methadone were not able to cause amine depletion (Rethy *et al.,* 1971). The dynamic state of the biogenic amines in the CNS is emphasized by the many reports of time-dependent and multiphasic responses in monoamine levels after morphine administration. The pattern of change in the levels of dopamine catabolites in brain after a single injection of morphine illustrates the state of brain amine flux: both homovanillic acid and dihydroxyphenyla-cetic acid levels in brain change in a manner related both to dose of morphine and to the time after morphine administration (Fukui and Takagi, 1972). In our experiments, we found that the content of dopamine in rat striatum was altered biphasically by morphine at doses of 5, 20, or 60 mg/kg (Clouet et al., 1973) and that the content of norepinephrine varied similarly in most areas of brain. With the use of histofluorometric techniques, increases in dopamine in dopaminergic cell bodies in the substantia nigra and ventromedial tegmental areas, and norepinephrine in noradrenergic cell bodies in the midbrain reticular formation were seen before increases in catecholamine levels in nerve terminals after morphine administration (Heinrich et al., 1971).

In tolerant animals, brain catecholamine levels are either normal or slightly above normal, depending on the species examined and the dose of opiate attained. The depleting effect of the initial dose of morphine was not found after chronic treatment in dogs, cats and rats (Maynert and Klingman, 1972; Gunne, 1963). Tolerance in catecholamine depletion was also found in methadone- or leveorphanol-tolerant animals (Akera and Brody, 1968). In tolerant rabbits and rats, brain catecholamines levels were above normal, especially when the dose of morphine was increased during chronic treatment (Maynert and Klingman, 1962; Sloan et al., 1963). It took 38 days for tolerance to the catecholamine-depleting effect of metha-done to be established when tolerance was produced slowly by supplying methadone in drinking water (Ahtee, 1973). However, shorter exposure to higher doses of morphine resulted in tolerance to catecholamine depletion at earlier times (Rethy et al., 1971; Fukui and Takagi, 1972). Cross-tolerance was exhibited between morphine, levorphanol, methadone, and meperidine (Rethy et al., 1971). The increased fluorescense in dopaminergic cell bodies invoked by a single injection of morphine was not seen after chronic mor-phine treatment (Leinhart et al., 1973).

The most common effect of withdrawal from chronic opiate use is de-pletion of dopamine and norepinephrine in brain after either antagonist-in-duced withdrawal or discontinuance of drug use (Maynert and Klingman, 1962; Gunne, 1963). In some studies this depleting effect was not demonstrated (Sloan et al., 1963; Gunne et al., 1969). An attempt has been made to correlate the variation in responses during opiate withdrawal to the predominance of excitatory or depressant states in the animals during withdrawal (Gunne, 1963; Martin, 1967).

4. OPIATE-INDUCED ALTERATIONS IN THE TURNOVER OF BRAIN CATECHOLAMINES

The multiphasic nature of the responses in brain catecholamine levels after opioid administration suggests that the drugs may induce alterations in the turnover of the amines as well as in the amine content. Using α-methyltyrosine to block tyrosine hydroxylase activity, Gunne and colleagues (1969) found that brain dopamine levels fell after acute morphine, indicating an increased turnover, with little change in norepinephrine levels. The rate of dopamine synthesis from ^{14}C-tyrosine in rat brain was increased by a single injection of morphine with most of the increase due to biosynthesis in the striatum and hypothalamus (Clouet and Ratner, 1970). In mice, the same stimulatory effect of morphine on the rate of brain dopamine synthesis was found, and a smaller increase in the rate of biosynthesis of norepinephrine was detected (Smith et al., 1972). The effect was dose-dependent in both mice (Smith et al., 1972) and rats (Johnson et al., 1974; Clouet et al., 1973), and was induced by levorphanol (Smith et al., 1972), methadone (Perez-Cruet et al., 1972; Gessa, 1973), viminol (Costa et al., 1973), and pentazocine (Sugrue, 1974), but not by d-methadone or propoxyphene (Gessa, 1973).

The major increase in dopamine biosynthesis after opiates occurs in the striatum (Clouet and Ratner, 1970; Perez-Cruet et al., 1972; Sugrue, 1974; Gauchy et al., 1973; Costa et al., 1973). The increased rate of dopamine biosynthesis is also seen in vitro in striatal slices prepared from morphine-treated rats (Gauchy et al., 1973). Seemingly contradictory results have been reported concerning the doses of narcotic analgesic drug necessary to stimulate dopamine turnover. In mice, the dose dependency has been well-established for morphine and levorphanol (Rosenman and Smith, 1972; Loh et al., 1973). In rats, stimulation of striatal dopamine biosynthesis has been found after morphine doses of 60 mg/kg (Gauchy et al., 1973), 20 mg/kg (Fukui et al., 1972), 16 mg/kg (Berney and Buxbaum, 1973), and 60, 20, and 5 mg/kg (Clouet et al., 1973), while doses less than 20 mg/kg have been reported to be without effect (Costa et al., 1973). Strain differences in rats to the effects of opiates have been described, which may affect the doses of narcotic analgesic drugs which are equipotent in various strains.

Morphine has a greater effect on the turnover of dopamine than on its content in the same tissue. The relative stability of the brain levels of this monamine is maintained by an increased rate of catabolism of dopamine after morphine treatment. Homovanillic acid and dihydroxyphenylacetic acid levels were increased to 155% and 140% of control levels 30 min after an injection of 20 mg/kg morphine, with smaller increases after 5 or 10 mg/kg (Fukui *et al.*, 1972). In these studies, partial tolerance to the increased catabolism of dopamine was found after 9 days of morphine treatment. In other studies, an increase was found in ^{14}C-methoxylated catabolites derived from precursor ^{14}C-tyrosine, suggesting that extraneuronal catabolism of the catecholamines was accelerated (Hitzemann and Loh, 1971).

Tolerance develops to the stimulatory effect of narcotic analgesic drugs on catecholamine turnover during chronic drug adminstration. In several studies, however, an acceleration of dopamine biosynthesis above that after the first injection was seen after the next few injections. In mice injected every 6 hr at a very high dose of morphine (100 mg/kg), the second, third, and fourth injection of morphine evoked increases in the rates of synthesis above that evoked by the first injection (Rosenman and Smith, 1972). In mice tolerant to one dose of morphine in this biochemical parameter, an increased dose was able to recall the stimulatory effect. In rats injected with morphine once a day for 10 days, or implanted with morphine pellets, the stimulation of dopamine and norepinephrine synthesis in the CNS was greater than after the first injection (Clouet and Ratner, 1970; Clouet *et al.*, 1973). As in mice, an increase in the dose produced a new increase in dopamine turnover in the striatum of rats tolerant to a lower dose of drug (Costa *et al.*, 1973). Tolerance in the brain amine turnover parameter coincided with tolerance in several other pharmacological parameters (Smith *et al.*, 1972). Since the term "tolerance" includes a wide variety of conditions arrived at in a wide variety of treatment schedules, it is not surprising that some differences have been found in the ability of morphine to induce increases in catecholamine biosynthetic rates in the brains of "tolerant" animals.

In tolerant animals, abstinence induces a depletion of brain catecholamines similar to that induced by the initial injection of drug (Gunne *et al.*, 1969), which is mirrored by an increased rate of biosynthesis of the biogenic amines in abstinent animals (Rosenman and Smith, 1972).

5. EFFECTS OF OPIATES ON THE TRANSPORT OF CATECHOLAMINES

The rates of uptake and release of biogenic monamines in brain tissue are altered by many drugs. The possibility that narcotic analgesics may influence the rate of transport of the catecholamines in brain slices or in isolated nerve ending preparations has been explored in several laboratories. Pretreatment of rats with morphine enhanced the synthesis of dopamine in striatal slices prepared from the animals, and also influenced the rate at which dopamine was released from the slices (Gauchy et al., 1973). The addition of morphine to slices prepared from untreated mice inhibited both the high affinity and the low affinity uptake of dopamine into cortex or diencephalon (Hitzemann and Loh, 1973). Kinetic analysis of this inhibition by morphine indicated a "mixed" inhibition. The addition of naloxone partially reversed the inhibition of dopamine uptake with a K_1 value suggesting that only low affinity uptake was sensitive to the antagonist.

In isolated nerve ending preparations, the synaptosomes, the uptake of dopamine into the predominantly dopaminergic striatal synaptosomes, and the uptake of norepinephrine into hypothalamic synaptosomes, was inhibited by morphine in concentrations higher than 5×10^{-6} M (Clouet and Williams, 1974). As in slices, kinetic analysis indicated that the inhibitory effect was nonspecific since only low affinity uptake of catecholamines was affected. A lack of specificity was also found in earlier experiments in which morphine, methadone, thebaine, and naloxine all inhibited the uptake of norepinephrine into nerve endings from whole brain with similar I_{50}s in the vicinity of 10^{-4}M (Ciofalo, 1973). Pretreatment of rats with heroin or morphine has been reported to result in less amine uptake by synaptosomal preparations from the animals (Boykin and Martin, 1973). There was no direct effect of morphine on the release of labeled dopamine or norepinephrine from preloaded synaptosomes (Clouet and Williams, 1974).

6. EFFECTS OF OPIATES ON THE ADENYL CYCLASE SYSTEM IN BRAIN

The transient effects of opiates on the levels and the rates of synthesis of biogenic amines in brain suggest that function at the synaptic junction might be altered by the drugs. A postjunctional element shown to be sensitive to neurohormones is the cAMP-adenyl cyclase system. This sensitivity has been demonstrated in vitro in studies in which the addition of dopamine (Kebabian et al., 1972) or norepinephrine (VanHungen and Robertis, 1973) increased the activity of adenyl cyclase in appropriate areas of brain in a dose-dependent stimulation of enzyme activity. The effects of the administration of neurotransmitters on the levels or rates of biosynthesis of cAMP seem to be temporally disparate: the intraventricular administration of norepinephrine to rats caused an increase in cAMP levels in whole brain 2 min after the injection with a return to normal levels by 15 min (Burkard, 1972), while the administration of the same amount of the neuroamine by the same route caused an increase in cerebral adenyl cyclase activity which was maximal 24 hr after the administration of the neuroamine (Chou *et al.*, 1971). In these studies, the levels of norepinephrine in the cerebral cortex were increased by exogenous amine for only a few hours.

In isolated nerve–muscle preparations, methadone potentiated the contractile effect of epinephrine, and also potentiated the effect of aminophylline, which acts to increase cAMP levels by inhibiting phosphodiesterase, and reversed the effect of imidazole, which activates phosphodiesterase (Huidoboro *et al.*, 1972). Opposite effects were obtained in *in vivo* studies: the systemic administration of imidazole to mice enhanced morphine-induced analgesia (Contreras *et al.*, 1972), and the systemic administration of theophylline or dibutyryl-cAMP antagonized morphine effects (Ho *et al.*, 1972). Morphine antagonism, as demonstrated by an increase in the ED_{50}, was also found 1 hr after systemic or intracerebral injection of cAMP. The maximal effect was found 1 hr after intracerebral injection of cAMP and 6 hr after systemic injection of a larger amount of the cyclic nucleotide. Since it is unlikely that cAMP crosses cell membranes (Robison *et al.*, 1965), the possibility that a part of the cAMP molecule was responsible for the antagonism was examined. Adenine, adenosine, AMP, and ATP each increased the ED_{50} for morphine in mice in two tests of analgesia: hot-plate and stretch response to phenylbenzoquinone (Gourley and Beckner, 1973). Hypoxanthine, uridine, and 2-deoxyadenosine were without activity. These results suggest that adenine is the active component, but do not, however, exclude the possibility that an increased rate of synthesis of cAMP in the CNS is the mechanism of antagonism.

The activity of adenyl cyclase in synaptic membrane preparations was inhibited by the addition of morphine *in vitro* at 0.1 mM concentration (Iwatsubo and Clouet, 1973). However, the inhibition was not related to drug concentration, and was not limited to active opiate agonists, since thebaine and dextrorphan had inhibitory activity. When homogenates of various brain regions (cerebral cortex, cerebellum, or thalamus–hypothalamus) were examined for cyclase activity 1 hr after a single injection of morphine, or in tolerant rats, there was no alteration in enzyme activity (Singhal *et al.*, 1973). However, a more detailed time-curve of adenyl cyclase activity in synaptic membrane preparations from six areas of rat brain after acute morphine or levorphanol injection showed biphasic alteration in cyclase activity; an increase 30 min after the injection, followed by a fall well below control levels after 2 hr (Iwatsubo, Gold, and Clouet, unpublished results). Larger increases in cyclase activity in all brain regions were measured in tolerant rats. Similarly, long-term morphine treatment produced increases in adenyl cyclase activity in mouse brain (Naito and Kuriyama, 1973). Since only half of the cyclase activity of a brain homogenate is in the synaptic membrane fraction (DeRobertis *et al.*, 1967), it is possible that the changes which we have detected in membrane preparations after acute morphine treatment would have not been seen in whole tissue homogenates. The time required for the preparation of synaptic membranes seems to eliminate the possibility that endogenous neurotransmitters produced the variations in enzyme activity after a single injection of an opiate. Enzyme induction (or translocation) is not ruled out in tolerant animals.

The levels of cAMP in homogenates of brain regions also followed a biphasic pattern after acute morphine: increases in cAMP levels in cerebral cortex, midbrain, striatum, and cerebellum, peaking 15 min after the injection, and, then significant decreases in most areas 2 hr after the opiate was given. In most brain areas in tolerant rats, the levels of cAMP were not altered following morphine (Iwatsubo, Gold, and Clouet, unpublished results).

The hydrolysis of cAMP was not found to be affected by opiate treatment in two studies: neither acute nor chronic morphine treatment had any effect of brain phosphodiesterase activity (Chou et al., 1971; Naito and Kuriyama, 1973). Another enzyme involved in cAMP action, protein kinase, was influenced by the pharmacological states induced by narcotic analgesics. Brain preparations from rats made tolerant to morphine by daily infusions of morphine for 8 hr contained significantly less protein kinase activity when assayed in the presence or absence of cAMP, and significantly higher activity when nalorphine was used to induce withdrawal in the animals (Clark et al., 1972).

7. DOPAMINE RECEPTOR HYPOTHESIS

Dopaminergic pathways in the corpus striatum have been implicated in the mechanism of opiate action by the results of numerous studies, some of which have been described in the preceding sections of this review. Manifestations of opiate-induced activity (catalepsy, muscle rigidity, analgesia, mania, stereotypy, locomotor activity, abstinence aggression, self-administration of opiates, crowding aggression, and drug hunger in man) have been associated with striatal dopamine metabolism. That many of these responses to opiates can also be induced by other drugs, or drug combinations; i.e., manic response by apomorphine (Dhasmana et al., 1972), catalepsy by chlorpromazine or haloperidol (Kuschinsky and Hornykiewicz, 1972; Lal and Puri, 1972), crowding hyperactivity, stereotypy, and aggression by apomorphine or dopa plus amphetamine (Andén et al., 1970; Puri and Lal, 1973), sedation by the central administration of norepinephrine or dopamine (Calcutt et al., 1973) and algesia by dopa (Major and Pleuvry, 1971) is an indication that common mechanisms and sites of action are involved. Histofluorescent studies have shown that the most potent antipsychotic neuroleptics selectively blocked dopamine receptors in brain, both in the neostriatum and in the mesolimbic neurons (Andén *et al.*, 1970), while other studies localize the effects in the nigrostriatal pathways.

Drugs which affect dopamine metabolism in such a way that dopamine levels at the putative dopamine receptor are altered, or might be presumed to be altered, either antagonize or potentiate the pharmacological responses to the acute administration of morphine or other opiates according to the direction of the change in the levels of the biogenic amine (Figure 2). Thus, the administration of tyrosine, dopa, dopamine, apomorphine, iproniazid, disulfiram, or cocaine potentiated opiate responses, while the administration of α-methyltyrosine, haloperidol, or pretreatment with reserpine antagonized the responses. Naturally, the effects of such other drugs are time- and dose-dependent so that experimental evidence indicating opposite or no modulation of opiate responses have also been obtained. The influence of

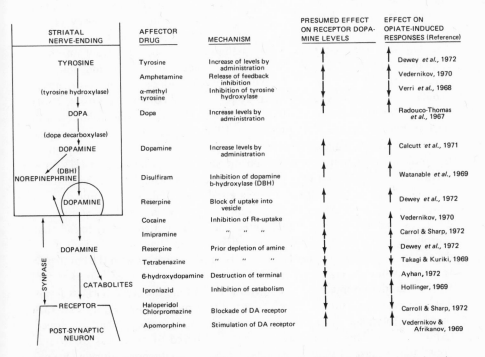

Figure 2. Relationship of dopamine to opiate activity. On the left is depicted a dopaminergic nerve terminal. The sites at which affector drugs act, by the specified mechanisms, to alter dopamine levels at the receptor are indicated, as are the effects of the affector drugs on the pharmacological responses to the acute administration of narcotic analgesics.

reserpine on acute morphine effects is an example in which seemingly contradictory evidence has been accumulated over the years, but in which a careful study has shown that when brain amines were depleted by prior administration of an adequate dose of reserpine, the morphine effect was blocked, while the simultaneous administration of reserpine and morphine produced a slight enhancement of morphine action (Dewey *et al.*, 1970). Similarly, contradictory effects of dopamine introduced centrally were resolved by a study showing that small doses of dopamine potentiated morphine-induced analgesia, while larger doses of dopamine antagonized the analgesic response (Calcutt *et al.*, 1971).

Because many of the other drugs also produce effects on norepinephrine levels as well as on dopamine levels, efforts have been made to differentiate between the two catecholamines. Haloperidol blocks dopamine receptors while chlorpromazine blocks both amines (Andén *et al.*, 1970) so that when chlorpromazine effects coincide with haloperidol effects these effects can be ascribed to dopaminergic pathways. The lack of effect of the administration of specific α- and β-blockers of norepinephrine activity, phenoxybenazmine, and propranolol on analgesia in mice (Dewey *et al.*, 1970; Fennessey and Lee, 1970) or mania in cats (Dhasmana *et al.*, 1972) also suggests that norepinephrine pathways are not important in these responses. However, antagonistic effects of these blockers on morphine-induced behavior have been observed in other studies: morphine-disrupted avoidance in mice was antagonized by propranolol (Black and Grosz, 1974) and morphine-induced activation in mice was blocked by phentolamine and phenoxybenzamine (Carroll and Sharp, 1972). An examination of the metabolic products of catecholamines in the CNS also differentiates dopamine metabolism from that of norepinephrine since homovanillic acid (HVA) is exclusively derived from dopamine. In studies of HVA levels in the rat caudate nucleus and their relation to opiate-induced catalepsy, Sasame and his colleagues (1972) observed a parallelism between methadone-induced catalepsy and HVA levels, and Ahtee and Kaarianinen (1973) found that morphine, codeine, etorphine, meperidine, and methadone produced dose-dependent increases in HVA levels which again coincided with the cataleptic response, while cyclazocine and thebaine were inactive in each parameter. During the development of tolerance to methadone the striatal HVA levels were increased maximally after 32 days of treatment. However, in these rats there was tolerance in the cataleptic response and stereotypy had developed (Ahtee, 1973). This latter response was attributed to an excess of striatal dopamine because of induced increases in dopamine turnover during chronic opiate treatment.

The formal dopamine receptor hypothesis for the mechanism of action of opiates is confined to the striatum, and to catalepsy as a measure of opiate activity. Since methadone produced both an increased dopamine turnover and increased HVA levels in the striatum, Sasame and his colleagues (1972) have suggested that methadone and other opiates block the striatal postsynaptic dopamine receptor, and stimulate dopamine synthesis by a compensatory feedback mechanism. Following Sharman's suggestion for etorphine action (1966), Kuschinsky and his colleagues have modified the hypothesis to include both blockade of the postsynaptic receptor and a presynaptic diversion of dopamine to sites of catabolic degradation (Kuschinsky and Hornykiewicz, 1972, Kuschinsky, 1973). Since naloxone antagonized the effect of morphine on HVA levels and catalepsy but did not antagonize the effects of chlorpromazine on the same parameters, it is possible that while chlorpromazine and other neuroleptics have a direct effect on the dopamine receptor, opiates act at a step other than receptor blockade (Kuschinsky and Hornykiewicz, 1972). However, both classes of drugs might block the receptor, but by different chemical reactions, so that naloxone would only displace the opiate-type interaction, as pointed out by VanderWende and Spoerlein (1973). Haloperidol and chlorpromazine have been shown to have a direct effect on dopamine-induced adenyl cyclase activity, an enzyme activity which has been suggested as the dopamine receptor (Kebabian et al., 1972). Opiates do not have a similar effect on dopamine-induced adenyl cyclase activity in striatal synaptic membrane preparations (Iwatsubo and Clouet, 1975), except a nonspecific inhibitory action at high drug concentrations, thus indicating a difference between neuroleptics and opiates. It is not even necessary to implicate the dopaminergic nigrostriatal pathways as the initial site of opiate action, since transsynaptic activation of these neurons by other neurotransmitters has been observed (Cheramy et al., 1970). Because the complex brain neuronal pathways are interrelated, and because the neurotransmittory systems are interrelated, disturbances on one pathway reverberate throughout the brain. It has been suggested many times that the activity in any pathway relative to other pathways depends more on the ratios of activity than on the levels of a single neurotransmitter.

8. DISCUSSION AND CONCLUSIONS

8.1. A Unique Role for a Single Neurotransmitter

As the subject of this paper is catecholamines, the relationship between the metabolism and function of these neurotransmitters and opiate activity have been reviewed. However, equally important roles have been suggested for acetylcholine and serotonin on the basis of studies of the relationship of opiates and these neurotransmitters. Early experiments by Paton (1957) and Schaumann (1957) demonstrated that morphine inhibited the release of acetylcholine in isolated nerve–muscle preparations from guinea pig ileum. Increases in brain levels of acetylcholine, presumably derived from inhibited release, were described (Herken et al., 1957; Hano et al., 1964), as was the reversal of the morphine effect by nalorphine (Howes et al., 1970). The depletion of brain acetylcholine by hemicholinium was blocked by morphine, and tolerance developed during chronic morphine treatment (Wilson and Domino, 1970). An interaction between acetylcholine and dopamine in the striatum was demonstrated in experiments in which haloperidol-induced increases in HVA levels were blocked by anticholinergic drugs (Andén and Bedard, 1971), and in which an increase in acetylcholine output followed the blockade of the dopamine receptor by haloperidol (Stadler et al., 1973).

An antagonism of morphine-induced responses by p-chlorophenyl-alanine, an inhibitor of serotonin biosynthesis, has been shown in several laboratories (Tenen, 1968; Way et al., 1968; Berney and Buxbaum, 1973). The importance of the serotonin-to-catecholamine ratios has been indicated in morphine-induced analgesia (Sparkes and Spencer, 1971), temperature regulation (Feldberg and Sherwood, 1954) and oxytremorine analgesia (Calcutt et al., 1973). In these studies, norepinephrine antagonized morphine effects and serotonin potentiated them.

No role has been ascribed to GABA in opiate action. However, GABA neurons in the substantia nigra modulate the nigrostriatal dopamine pathway (Andén and Stock, 1973). It is interesting that while GABA increased the turnover of striatal dopamine by blocking the nigrostriatal pathways, stimulation of these pathways also increased dopamine turnover (Roth et al., 1973). Thus, a lack of impulse flow increased dopamine turnover by feedback from the receptor while an increase in impulse flow increased dopamine turnover by a release of end product inhibition of tyrosine hydroxylase activity.

The preceding discussion forces the conclusion that there is no neurotransmitter which is uniquely involved in the mechanism of action of narcotic analgesic drugs. Even though a good case has been made for the importance of striatal dopamine nerve terminals, the modulation of these pathways by inhibitory GABA neurons in the substantia nigra, and the increase in acetylcholine release consequent to dopamine receptor blockade, are evidence that no neurotransmitter stands (or falls) alone in the CNS. However, that brain catecholamines are involved in the mechanism of opiate action is amply documented.

8.2. Role of Catecholamines in Dependence

The development of tolerance to chronic opiate treatment is blocked by a number of drugs that alter catecholamine levels in brain. Abstinence signs after opiate withdrawal are also enhanced or diminished by drugs that alter the levels of biogenic amines in the CNS. There is a *caveat* for the interpretation of some of the results of studies in which several classes of drugs are used. The measured pharmacological responses are complex and may involve pathways sensitive to the modulator drugs, but not near the initial site of opiate action; i.e., the *expression* of the response may be inhibited by the action of the modifying drug. However, direct evidence that neurochemical tolerance develops to chronic opiate treatment is found in experiments in which the increase in turnover of brain catecholamines that is elicited by the initial opiate exposure is no longer found in tolerant animals (Fukui and Takagi, 1972; Smith *et al.*, 1972). Although the first few doses of morphine or other narcotic analgesic drugs seem to increase further the rates of dopamine turnover in striatum and norepinephrine in other brain areas (Clouet and Ratner, 1970; Rosenman and Smith, 1972), subsequent opiate treatment no longer results in increased rates of catecholamine turnover, unless the dose of opiate is raised to a level which also produces pharmacological responses (Costa *et al.*, 1973). Regulatory influences on the rates of catecholamine biosynthesis occur at the first biosynthetic step, the hydroxylation of tyrosine to dopa, catalyzed by tyrosine hydroxylase. The activity of this enzyme is controlled by endproduct inhibition by dopamine and norepinephrine for short-term control (Fukui *et al.*, 1972). A prolonged increase in tyrosine hydroxylase activity occurs through transsynaptic induction in which new enzyme protein is synthesized (Mueller *et al.*, 1969). The induction of tyrosine hydroxylase in the caudate nucleus of rats treated for 15 days with morphine was shown by Reis *et al.* (1970). In our experiments, in which tyrosine hydroxylase was partially purified from brain samples before assay, enzyme induction was found in the striatum and hypothalamus only after long-term treatment (Clouet *et al.*, 1973). It is possible that tyrosine hydroxylase is induced after a single injection but requires time for the amount of additional enzyme to be measurable. In the peripheral sympathetic nervous system, the induction of tyrosine hydroxylase is mediated by an increased liberation of acetylcholine from preganglionic nerve terminals (Thoenen *et al.*, 1969) and is accompanied by an induction of preganglionic choline acetyltransferase (Oesch, 1974). If this is a general phenomenon and not confined to the peripheral nervous system it is possible that the induction of biosynthetic enzyme systems may be a homeostatic response to chronic opiate treatment. Indeed, the activity of adenyl cyclase in striatal synaptic membranes is also induced in morphine-tolerant rats (Iwatsubo and Clouet, 1975).

8.3. Site of Opiate Action

Since a cursory review of the many studies on the anatomical sites of opiate action could not do justice to these studies, I shall confine my discussion of this topic to those physiological sites that are related to catecholamine metabolism or function. A concentration of radioactively labeled opiate in nerve ending fractions was found after the incubation of drug and brain tissue *in vitro* (Terenius, 1973; Pert and Snyder, 1973b), and after the injection of the labeled drug in pharmacologically effective doses to rats (Clouet and Williams, 1974). A plausible site for opiate binding is membranes, especially synaptic membranes. In preliminary experiments, we have shown that naloxone pretreatment reduced the amount of tritiated etorphine bound in synaptic membrane fractions after injection of both drugs to rats in dose ratios effective in blocking pharmacological responses (Mule', Casella, and Clouet, 1974). In addition, a stereospecific binding of labeled levorphanol to a lipoprotein fraction of brain membranes has been recently reported (Goldstein et al., 1974). Such binding of narcotic analgesics and antagonists to synaptic membranes would be expected to alter neuronal function. Although the effect of opiates on the uptake and release of catecholamines in isolated nerve endings seems to be nonspecific and, therefore, unimportant mechanistically, an enhanced synthesis of dopamine and an increased release in striatal slices from morphine-treated rats (Gauchy et al., 1973) argues for an effect of opiates on dopamine transport *in vivo*. The inhibition by narcotic analgesics of the release of acetylcholine from perfused brain (Beleslin and Polak, 1965), from brain slices (Richter and Marchbanks, 1971) and from isolated nerve ending particles (Clouet and Williams, 1974) appears to be a general phenomenon, perhaps related more closely to the site of the initial drug: tissue interaction. If so, presynaptic membranes would be implicated. It is, of course, possible that membranes throughout the nervous system accumulate opiates through specific binding reactions, with an apparent disturbance in function occurring only when a critical disruption of membrane activity obtains. It is possible, but less likely, that the involvement of specific neurotransmitter systems is related to their accessibility to the opiates, and to the size of the disruption required to affect function.

9. REFERENCES

Ahtee, L., 1973, Catalepsy and stereotyped behavior in rats treated chronically with methadone: relation to brain homovanillic acid levels, *J. Pharm. Pharmacol.* **25**:649.
Ahtee, L., and Kaarianinen, I., 1973, The effect of narcotic analgesics on the homovanillic acid
content of rat caudate nucleus, *J. Neurochem.* **20**:206.
Akera, T., and Brody, M., 1968, The addiction cycle to narcotics in the rat and its relation to
catecholamines, *Biochem. Pharmacol.* **17**:675.
Andén, N. E., 1970, Effects of amphetamine and some other drugs on central catecholamine
mechanisms, in: *Amphetamines* (E. Costa and S. Garattini, eds.), pp. 447–462, Raven
Press, New York.
Andén, N. E., 1972, Dopamine turnover in the corpus striatum and the limbic system after
treatment with neuroleptic and anticholinergic drugs, *J. Pharm. Pharmacol.* **24**:905.
Andén, N. E., and Bedard, P., 1971, Influences of cholinergic mechanisms on the formation
and turnover of brain dopamine, *J. Pharm. Pharmacol.* **23**:460.
Andén, N. E., and Stock, G., 1973, Inhibitory effect of γ-hydroxybutyric acid and γ-
aminobutyric acid on dopamine cells in the substantia nigra, *Naunyn-Schmiedebergs
Arch. Pharmakol.* **279**:89.
Andén, N. E., Rubenson, A., Fuxe, K., and Hökfelt, T., 1967, Evidence for dopaminergic
receptor stimulation by apomorphine, *J. Pharm. Pharmacol.* **19**:627.
Andén, N. E., Butcher, S. G., Corradi, H., Fuxe, K., and Ungerstedt, U., 1970, Receptor
activity and turnover of dopamine and noradrenalin after neuroleptics, *European J.
Pharmacol.* **11**:303.
Ayhan, J. H., 1972, Effect of 6-hydroxydopamine on morphine analgesia, *Psychopharmaco-
logia* **25**:183.
Beckett, A. H., and Casey, A. F., 1965, Analgesics and their antagonists: biochemical aspects
and structure-activity relationships, in: *Progress in Medicinal Chemistry, Vol. 4* (G. P.
Ellis and G. B. West, eds.), pp. 171–218, Butterworths, London.
Beleslin, D., and Polak, R. L., 1965, Depression by morphine and chloralose of acetylcholine
release from cat's brain, *J. Physiol.* **177**:411.
Bentley, K. W., and Lewis, J. W., 1973, The relationship between structure and activity in the
6,14-endoethenotetrahydro-thebaine series of analgesics, in: *Agonist and Antagonist Actions of Narcotic Analgesic Drugs*, (H. W. Kosterlitz, H. O. J. Collier, and J. E. Villar-
real, eds.), pp. 6–16, University Park Press, London.
Berney, S. A., and Buxbaum, D. M., 1973, The effect of morphine on catecholamine turnover
and its relationship to morphine-induced motor activity, *Pharmacologist* **15**:202.
Bhargava, H. N., Ho, I. K., and Way, E. L., 1972, Effect of dopamine-β-hydroxylase inhibi-
tion on morphine analgesia, tolerance and physical dependence, *Fifth Intern. Cong.
Pharmacol.* p. 21 (abtr).
Black, W. C., and Grosz, H. J., 1974, Propranolol antagonism of morphine-influenced be-
havior, *Brain. Res.* **65**:362.
Bläsig, J., Reinhold, K., and Herz, A., 1973, Effect of 6-hydroxydopamine, 5,6-
dihydroxytryptamine and raphe lesions on the antinociceptive actions of morphine in rats,
Psychopharmacologia **31**:111.
Borison, H., 1971, Sites of action of narcotic analgesic drugs in the nervous system, in: *Nar-
cotic Drugs: Biochemical Pharmacology* (D. H. Clouet, ed.), pp. 342–365, Plenum Press,
New York.
Boykin, M. E., and Martin, R. H., 1973, Preliminary observations on the uptake of cate-
cholamines in synaptosomes of opiate-treated animals, *J. Pharm. Pharmacol.* **25**:484.

Brady, J., 1973, Standardization of self-administration techniques, Presented at NAS-NRC meeting of the Committee on Problems of Drug Dependence, Chapel Hill, North Carolina.

Burkard, W. P., 1972, Catecholamine induced increase of cyclic AMP in rat brain *in vivo, J. Neurochem.* **19**:2615.

Calcutt, C. R., Dogett, N. S., and Spencer, P. S. J., 1971, Modification of the antinociceptive activity of morphine by centrally administered ouabain and dopamine, *Psychopharmacologia* **21**:111.

Calcutt, C. R., Handley, S. L., Sparkes, C. G., and Spencer, P. S. J., 1973, Roles of noradrenaline and 5-hydroxytryptamine in the antinociceptive effects of morphine, in: *Agonist and Antagonist Actions of Narcotic Analgesic Drugs* (H. W. Kosterlitz, H. O. J. Collier, and J. E. Villarreal, eds.), University Park Press, London.

Carroll, B. J., and Sharp, P. T., 1972, Monoamine mediation of the morphine-induced activation of mice, *Brit. J. Pharmacol.* **46**:124.

Cheramy, A., Besson, M. J., and Glowinski, J., 1970, Increased release of dopamine from striatal dopaminergic terminals in the rat after treatment with a neuroleptic, thioproperazine, *European J. Pharmacol.* **10**:206.

Chiosa, L., Dumitrescu, S., and Banaru, A., 1968, The influence of imprapine on the "abstinence syndrome" to morphine in mice, *Intern. J. Neuropharmacol.* **7**:161.

Chou, W. S., Ho, A. K. S., and Loh, H. H., 1971, Neurohormones on brain adrenyl cyclase activity *in vivo, Nature* (New Biol.) **233**:280.

Ciofalo, F. R., 1973, Effects of some narcotics and antagonists on synaptosomal H-norepinephrine uptake, *Life Sci.* **11**:573.

Clark, A. G., Jovic, R., Ornellas, M. R., and Weller, M., 1972, Brain microsomal protein kinase in the chronically morphinized rats, *Biochem. Pharmacol.* **21**:1989.

Clouet, D. H., 1972, Theoretical biochemical mechanisms for drug dependence in: *Chemical and Biochemical Aspects of Drug Dependence* (S. J. Mule' and H. Brill, eds.), pp. 545–561, CRC Press, Cleveland, Ohio.

Clouet, D. H., and Ratner, M., 1970, Catecholamine biosynthesis in brains of rats treated with morphine, *Science,* **168**:854.

Clouet, D. H., and Williams, N., 1974, The effect of narcotic analgesic drugs on the upake and release of neurotransmitters in isolated synaptosomes, *J. Pharmacol. Exptl. Therap.* **188**:419.

Clouet, D. H., Johnson, J. C., Ratner, M., Williams, N. and Gold, G. J., 1973, The effect of morphine on rat brain catecholamines, turnover *in vivo* and uptake in isolated synaptosomes, in: *Frontiers in Catecholamine Research* (E. Costa and E. Usdin, eds.), pp. 1039–1042, Pergamon Press, N.Y.

Colville, K. I., and Chaplin, E., 1964, Sympathomimetics as analgetics, *Life Sci.* **3**:315.

Contreras, E., and Tamayo, L., 1966, Effect of drugs acting in relation to sympathetic functions on the analgesic action of morphine. *Arch. Intern. Pharmacodyn.* **160**:312.

Contreras, E., Castillo, S., and Quijada, L., 1972, Effect of drugs that modify 3′ 5′ cAMP concentration on morphine analgesia, *J. Pharm. Pharmacol.* **24**:65.

Costa, E., Carenzi, A., Guidotti, A. and Reuvelta, A., 1973, Narcotic analgesics and the regulation of neuronal catecholamine stores, in: *Frontiers in Catecholamine Research* (E. Costa and E. Usdin, eds.), pp. 1003–1010, Pergamon Press, New York.

Davis, W., and Smith, S. G., 1972, Alpha-methyl tyrosine to prevent self-administration of morphine and amphetamine, *Current Therap. Res.* **14**:814.

De Robertis, E., De Lores Arnaiz, G. R., Alberici, M., Butcher, R. W., and Sutherland, E. W., 1967, Subcellular distribution of adenyl cyclase and cyclic phosphodiesterase in rat brain cortex, *J. Biol. Chem.* **242**:3487.

Dewey, W. L., Harris, L. S., Howes, J. F., and Nuite, J. A., 1970, The effect of various neurohumoral modulators on the activity of morphine and the narcotic antagonists in the tailflick phenylquinone tests, *J. Pharmacol. Exptl. Therap.* **175**:435.

Dhasmana, K. M., Dixit, K. S., Jaju, B. P., and Gupta, M. L., 1972, Role of central dopaminergic receptors in manic response of cats to morphine, *Psychopharmacologia* **24**:380.

Domino, E. F., 1968, Effects of narcotic analgesics on sensory input, activating system and motor output, in: *The Addictive States* (A. Wikler, ed.), pp. 117–149, Williams and Wilkins Co., Baltimore.

Drawbaugh, R., and Lal, H., 1974, Reversal by narcotic antagonist of a narcotic action elicited by a conditional stimulus, *Nature* **247**:65.

Echols, S. D., and Jewett, R. E., 1969, The effect of morphine on the sleep of cats, *Pharmacologist* **11**:254.

Eddy, N. B., Halbach, H., Isbell, H., and Seevers, M. H., 1965, Drug dependence—its significance and characteristics, *Bull. World Health Organ.* **32**:721.

Eidelberg, E., and Schwartz, A. S., 1970, Possible mechanisms of action of morphine on brain, *Nature* **225**:1152.

Elchisak, M. A., and Rosecrans, J. A., 1973, Effect of central catecholamine depletions by 6-OH dopamine on morphine antinociceptive rats: Involvement of brain dopamine, *Pharmacologist* **15**:(66):167.

Fahim, I., Ismail, M., and Osman, O. H., 1972, The role of 5-hydroxytryptamine and noradrenaline in the hyperthermic reaction induced by pethidine in rabbits pretreated with pargyline, *Brit. J. Pharmacol.* **46**:416.

Feldberg, W., and Sherwood, S. L., 1954, Injection of drugs into the lateral ventricles of the cat, *J. Physiol.* **107**:372.

Fennessey, M. R., and Lee, J. R., 1970, Modification of morphine analgesia by drugs affecting adrenergic and tryptaminergic mechanisms, *J. Pharm. Pharmacol.* **22**:930.

Fennessey, M. R., and Lee, J. R., 1972, Comparison of the dose-response effects of morphine on brain amines, analgesia and activity in mice, *Brit. J. Pharmacol.* **45**:240.

Florez, J., Delgado, G., and Armijo, J. A., 1972, Adrenergic and serotonergic mechanisms in morphine-induced respiratory depression, *Psychopharmacologia* **24**:258.

Friedler, G., Bhargava, H. N., Quock, R., and Way, E. L., 1972, The effect of 6-hydroxydopamine on morphine tolerance and physial dependence, *J. Pharmacol. Exptl. Therap.* **183**:49.

Fukui, K., and Takagi, H., 1972, Effect of morphine on cerebral contents of metabolites of dopamine in normal and tolerant mice: its possible relation to analgesic action, *Brit. J. Pharmacol.* **44**:45.

Fukui, K., Shiomi, H., and Takagi, H., 1972, Effect of morphine on tyrosine hydroxylase activity in mouse brain, *European J. Pharmacol.* **19**:123.

Gauchy, C., Agid, Y., Glowinski, J., and Cheramy, A., 1973, Acute effects of morphine on dopamine synthesis and release and tyrosine metabolism in the rat striatum, *European J. Pharmacol.* **22**:311.

Gessa, G. L., Vargiu, L., Biggio, G., and Tagliamonte, A., 1973, Effect of methadone and other narcotic analgesics on brain dopamine metabolites, in: *Frontiers of Catecholamine Research*, (E. Costa and E. Usdin, eds.), pp. 1011–1014, Pergamon Press, New York.

Goldberg, S. R., Hoffmeister, F., and Schlichting, U. U., 1972, Morphine antagonists: Modification of behavioral effects by morphine dependence, in: *Drug Addiction, Vol. I* (J. M. Singh, L. H. Miller, and H. Lal, eds.), pp. 31–48, Futura Publishing Co., Mount Kisco, New York.

Goldstein, A., Lowney, L. I., Schultz, K., and Lowery, P. J., 1974, Partial purification of an opiate receptor from mouse brain, *Science* **183**:749.

Gourley, D. R. H., and Beckner, S. K., 1973, Antagonism to morphine analgesia by adenine, adenosine and adenine nucleotides, *Proc. Soc. Exptl. Biol. Med.* **144**:774.

Gunne, L. M., 1963, Catecholamines and 5-hydroxytryptamine in morphine-tolerance and withdrawal, *Acta Physiol. Scand. Suppl. 204,* **58**:1.

Gunne, L. M., Jonsson, J., and Fuxe, K., 1969, Effects of morphine intoxication on brain catecholamine neurons, *European J. Pharmacol.* **5**:338.

Gupta, S. K., and Kulkarni, H. J., 1966, Modification of morphine analgesia in rats by MAO inhibitors, *J. Indian Med. Assoc.* **46**:197.

Hano, K., Kaneto, H., Kakunaga, T., and Moribayashi, N., 1964, The administration of morphine and changes in acetylcholine metabolism by mouse brain, *Biochem. Pharmacol.* **13**:441.

Hanson, H. M., and Cimini-Venema, C. A., 1972, Effects of haloperidol on self-administration of morphine in rats, *Federation Proc.* **31**:503.

Harris, L. S., 1971, Structure : activity relationships, in: *Narcotic Drugs: Biochemical Pharmacology* (D. H. Clouet, ed.), pp. 89–98, Plenum Press, New York.

Heinrich, U., Lichtensteiger, W., and Langemann, H., 1971, Effect of morphine on the catecholamine content of midbrain nerve cell groups in rat and mouse, *J. Pharmacol. Exptl. Therap.* **179**:259.

Heller, B., Saavedra, J. M., and Fischer, E., 1968, Influence of adrenergic blocking agents upon morphine and catecholamine analgesic effect, *Experientia* **24**:804.

Herken, H., Maibauer, D., and Müller, S., 1957, Acetylcholingehalt des Gehirns und Analgesie nach Einwickung von Morphin und einigen 3-oxymorphinanen, *Arch. Exptl. Pathol. Pharmakol.* **230**:313.

Herrting, G., Axelrod, J., and Whitby, L. G., 1961, Effect of drugs on the uptake and metabolism of H^3-norepinephrine, *J. Pharmacol. Exptl. Therap.* **134**:146.

Hitzemann, R. J., and Loh, H. H., 1973, Effect of morphine on the transport of dopamine into mouse brain slices, *European J. Pharmacol.* **21**:121.

Ho, I. K., Loh, H. H., and Way, E. L., 1972, Effect of cyclic AMP on morphine analgesia, tolerance and physical dependence, *Nature* **238**:397.

Hofmeister, F., and Schlichtung, U. U., 1972, Reinforcing properties of some opiates and opioids in rhesus monkeys with histories of cocaine and codeine self-administration, *Psychopharmacologia* **23**:55.

Hollinger, M., 1969, Effect of reserpine, α-methyl-p-tyrosine, p-chlorophenylalanine and pargyline on levorphanol-induced running activity in mice, *Arch. Intern. Pharmacodyn.* **179**:419.

Howes, J. F., Harris, L. D., and Dewey, W. L., 1970, The effect of morphine, nalorphine, naloxone, pentazocine, cyclazocine, and oxotremorine on the synthesis and release of acetylcholine by mouse cerebral cortex slices *in vitro, Arch. Intern. Pharmacodyn.* **184**:267.

Hug, C. c., 1972, Characteristics and theories related to acute and chronic tolerance development, in: *Chemical and Biological Aspects of Drug Dependence* (S. J. Mule´ and H. Brill, eds.), pp. 307–358, CRC Press, Cleveland.

Huidobro, F., Contreras, E., and Tamayo, L., 1972, The influence of drugs affecting cyclic AMP levels on methadone induced potentiation of adrenalin effects, *Arch. Intern. Pharmacodyn.* **198**:29.

Iwamoto, E. T., Shen, F., Loh, H. H., and Way, E. L., 1971, The effects of pargyline on morphine tolerant-dependent mice, *Federation Proc.* **30**:278.

Iwatsubo, K., and Clouet, D. H., 1973, The effects of narcotic analgesic drugs on the levels and the rates of synthesis of cAMP in six areas of rat brain, *Federation Proc.* **32**:536.

Iwatsubo, K. and Clouet, D. H., 1975, Dopamine-sensitive adenylate cyclase of the caudate nucleus of rats treated with morphine or haloperidol, *Biochem. Pharmacol.* (in press).

Johnson, J. C., Ratner, M., Gold, G. J., and Clouet, D. H., 1974, Morphine effects on levels and turnover of rat brain catecholamines, *Res. Comm. Chem. Path. Pharmacol.* **9**:41.

Kebabian, J. W., Petzold, G. L., and Greengard, P., 1972, Dopamine-sensitive adenylate cyclase in caudate nucleus of rat brain and its similarity to the "dopamine receptor," *Proc. Natl. Acad. Sci. (U.S.)* **8**:2145.

Kuschinsky, K., 1973, Evidence that morphine increases dopamine utilization in corpora striata of rats, *Experientia* **29**:1365.

Kuschinsky, K., and Hornykiewicz, O., 1972, Morphine catalepsy in the rat: relation to striatal dopamine metabolism, *European J. Pharmacol.* **19**:119.

Lal, H., and Puri, S. K., 1972, Morphine withdrawal aggression: role of dopaminergic stimulation, in: *Drug Addiction, Vol. I,* (J. M. Singh, L. Miller, and H. Lal, eds.), pp. 301–310, Futura Publishing Co., Mt. Kisco, New York.

Laverty, R., and Sharman, D. F., 1965, Modification by drugs of the metabolism of 3,4 dihydroxy phenylethylanine in tissues, *Brit. J. Pharmacol.* **24**:759.

Leinhart, R., Lichtensteiger, W., and Langemann, E. H., 1973, Studies on midbrain dopamine neurons in morphine-tolerant mice, *Experientia* **29**:764.

Lewis, J. W., Bentley, K. W., and Cowan, A., 1971, Narcotic analgesics and antagonists, *Ann. Rev. Pharmacol.* **11**:241.

Loh, H. H., Hitzemann, R. J., and Way, E. L., 1973, Effect of acute morphine administration on the metabolism of brain catecholamines, *Life Sci.* **12**:33.

Maggiolo, C., and Huidobro, F., 1965, Actions of drugs that mobilize aromatic alkylamines on the intensity of the abstinence syndrome to morphine in white mice, *Acta Physiol. Latinoam.* **15**:292.

Major, C. T., and Pleuvry, B. J., 1971, Effects of α-methyl-*p*-tyrosine, *p*-chlorophenylalanine, *l*-β-(3,4-dihydroxyphenyl)alanine, 5-hydroxytryptophan and diethyldithiocarbamate on the analgesic activity of morphine and methylamphetamine in the mouse, *Brit. J. Pharmacol.* **45**:512.

Marshall, I., and Smith, C. B., 1973, Blockade of the development of physical dependence on morphine by chronic inhibition of tyrosine hydroxylase, *Pharmacologist* **15**:243.

Martin, W. R., 1967, Opioid antagonists, *Pharmacol. Rev.* **19**:463.

Martin, W. R., and Eades, C. G., 1967, Pharmacological studies of spinal cord, adrenergic and cholinergic mechanisms and their relation to physical dependence on morphine, *Psychopharmacologia* **11**:195.

Maruyama, Y., and Takemori, A. E., 1973, The role of dopamine and norepinephrine in the naloxone-induced abstinence of morphine-dependent mice, *J. Pharmacol. Exptl. Therap.* **185**:602.

Maruyama, Y., Hayashi, G., Smits, S. E., and Takemori, A. E., 1971, Studies on the relationship between 5-hydroxytryptamine turnover in brain and tolerance and physical dependence in mice, *J. Pharmacol. Exptl. Therap.* **178**:20.

Maynert, E. W., and Klingman, G., 1962, Tolerance to morphine. I. Effects on catecholamines in the brain and adrenal glands. *J. Pharmacol. Exptl. Therap.* **135**:285.

Maynert, E. W., and Levi, R., 1964, Stress-induced release of brain noradrenalin and its inhibition by drugs, *J. Pharmacol. Exptl. Therap.* **143**:90.

Moore, K. E., McCarthy, L. E., and Borison, H. L., 1965, Blood glucose and brain catecholamine levels in the cat following the injection of morphine into the CSF, *J. Pharmacol. Exptl. Therap.* **148**:169.

Mueller, R. A., Thoenen, H., and Axelrod, J., 1969, Inhibition of transsynaptically increased tyrosine hydroxylase activity by cycloheximide and actinomycin D, *Mol. Pharmacol.* **5**:463.

Mule', S. J., Casella, G., and Clouet, D. H., 1974, Localization *in vivo* of naracotic analgesics in synaptic membranes of rat brain, *Res. Comm. Chem. Path. Pharmacol.* **9**:55.

Naito, K., and Kuriyama, K., 1973, Effect of morphine administration on adenyl cyclase and 3'5 cyclic nucleotide phosphodiesterase activities in the brain, *Japan J. Pharmacol.* **23**:274.

Nakamura, K., Kuntzman, R., Maggio, A., and Conney, A. H., 1973, Restoration of morphine analgesia in morphine-tolerant rats after the intraventricular administration of 6-hydroxydopine, *J. Pharm. Pharmacol.* **25**:584.

Nott, M. W., 1968, Potentiation of morphine analgesia by cocaine in mice, *European J. Pharmacol.* **5**:93.

Oesch, F., 1974, Transsynaptic induction of choline acetyltransferase in the preganglionic neuron of the peripheral sympathetic neurons system, *J. Pharmacol. Exptl. Therap.* **188**:439.

Paton, W. D. M., 1957, The action of morphine and related substances on contraction and on acetylcholine output of co-axially stimulated guinea pig ileum, *Brit. J. Pharmacol.* **12**:119.

Perez-Cruet, J., Chiara, G., Di, and Gessa, G. L., 1972, Accelerated synthesis of dopamine in the rat brain after methadone, *Experientia* **28**:926.

Persson, T., and Waldeck, B., 1970, Is there an interaction between dopamine and noradrenaline containing neurons in the brain?, *ActaPhysiol. Scand.* **78**:142.

Pert, C. B., and Snyder, S. H., 1973a, Properties of opiate receptor binding in rat brain, *Proc. Natl. Acad. Sci. (U.S.)* **70**:2243.

Pert, C. B., and Snyder, S. H., 1973b, Opiate receptor: demonstration in nervous tissue, *Science* **179**:1011.

Pozuelo, J., and Kerr, W. L., 1972, Suppression of craving and other signs of dependence in morphine-addicted monkeys by administration of α-methyl-p-tyrosine, *Mayo Clin. Proc.* **47**:621.

Puri, S. K., and Lal, H., 1973, Effect of dopaminergic stimulation or blockade on morphine-withdrawal aggression, *Psychopharmacologia* **32**:113.

Quinn, G. P., and Brodie, B. B., 1961, Effect of chlorpromazine and reserpine on the central actions of morphine in the cat, *Med. Exp.* **4**:349.

Radouco-Thomas, S., Singh, P., Garcia, F., and Radouco-Thomas, C., 1967, Relationship between experimental analgesia and brain monoamines, catecholamines and 5-hydroxytryptamine, *Arch. Biol. Med. Exp.* **4**:42.

Reis, D. J., Rifkin, M., and Corvelli, A., 1969, Effects of morphine on cat brain norepinephrine in regions with daily monoamines rhythms, *European J. Pharmacol.* **8**:149.

Reis, D. J., Hess, P., Azmitia, E. C., 1970, Changes in enzymes subserving catecholamine metabolism in morphine tolerance and withdrawal in the rat, *Brain Res.* **20**:309.

Rethy, C. R., Smith, C. B., and Villarreal, J., 1971, Effects of narcotic analgesics upon locomotor activity and brain catecholamine content of the mouse, *J. Pharmacol. Exptl. Therap.* **176**:472.

Richter, J. A., and Marchbanks, R. M., 1971, Synthesis of radioactive acetylcholine from H³-choline and its release from cerebral cortex slices *in vitro, J. Neurochem.* **18**:691.

Robison, G. A., Butcher, R. W., Oye, I., Morgan, H. E., and Sutherland, E. W., 1965, The effect of epinephrine on cAMP levels in isolated perfused rat heart, *Mol. Pharmacol.* **1**:168.

Rogers, K. J., and Thornton, J. A., 1969, The interaction between monoamine-oxidase inhibitors and narcotic analgesics, *Brit. J. Pharmacol.* **36**:470.

Rosenman, S. J., and Smith, C. B., 1972, ¹⁴C-Catecholamine synthesis in mouse brain during morphine withdrawal, *Nature* **240**:153.

Ross, J. W., and Ashford, A., 1967, The effect of reserpine and α-methyl-dopa on the analgesic action of morphine in the mouse, *J. Pharmacol. Exptl. Therap.* **19**:709.

Roth, R. H., Walters, J. R., and Aghajanian, G. K., 1973, Effect of impulse flow on the release and synthesis of dopamine in the striatum, *Life Sci.* **13**:139.

Rudzik, A. D., and Mennear, J. H., 1965, Antagonism of analgesics by amine-depleting agents, *J. Pharm. Pharmacol.* **17**:326.

Saarnavaara, L., 1969, Analgesic activity of some sympathetic drugs and their effect on morphine analgesics in rabbits, *Ann. Med. Exptl. Biol. Fenniae (Helsinki)* **47**:180.

Sasame, H. A., Perez-Cruet, J., DiChiara, G., Tagliamonte, G., Tagliamonte, P., and Gessa, G. L., 1972, Evidence that methadone blocks dopamine receptors in the brain. *J. Neurochem.* **19**:1953.

Schaumann, W., 1957, Inhibition by morphine of the release of acetylcholine from the intestine of the guinea pig, *Brit. J. Pharmacol.* **12**:115.

Schneider, J. A., 1954, Reserpine antagonism of morphine analgesia, *Proc. Soc. Exptl. Biol. Med.* **87**:614.

Schuster, C. R., 1970, Psychological approaches to opiate dependence and self-administration in laboratory animals, *Federation Proc.* **29**:205.

Schwartz, A., and Eidelberg, E., 1970, Role of biogenic amines in morphine dependence in the rat, *Life Sci.* **9**:613.

Sethy, V. H., Pradhan, R. J., Mandrekar, S. S., and Sheth, U. K., 1970, Role of brain amines in the analgesic action of meperidine hydrochloride, *Psychopharmacologia* **17**:320.

Sharkawi, M., 1973, Possible involvement of central dopaminergic and cholinergic mechanisms in morphine tolerance and withdrawal, *The Pharmacologist* **15**:168.

Sharman, D. F., 1966, Changes in the metabolism of 3,4-dihydroxyphenylethylamine (dopamine) in the striatum of the mouse induced by drugs, *Brit. J. Pharmacol.* **28**:153.

Sigg, E. B., Caprio, G., and Schneider, J. A., 1958, Synergism of amines and antagonism of reserpine to morphine analgesia, *Proc. Soc. Exptl. Biol. Med.* **97**:97.

Simon, E. J., Hiller, J. M., and Edelman, I., 1973, Stereospecific binding of the potent narcotic analgesic H³-etorphine to rat-brain homogenate, *Proc. Natl. Acad. Sci. (U.S.)* **70**:1947.

Singhal, R. L., Kacew, S., and Lafreniere, R., 1973, Brain adenyl cyclase in methadone treatment of morphine dependency, *J. Pharm. Pharmacol.* **25**:1022.

Sloan, J. W., Brooks, J. W., Eisenmann, A. J., and Martin, W. R., 1963, The effect of addiction to and abstinence from morphine on rat tissue catecholamine and serotonin levels, *Psychopharmacologia* **4**:261.

Smith, C. B., Sheldon, M. I., Bednarczyk, H. J., and Villarreal, J. E., 1972, Morphine-induced increases in the incorporation of ¹⁴C-tyrosine into ¹⁴C-dopamine and ¹⁴C-norepinephrine in the mouse brain: Antagonism by naloxone and tolerance, *J. Pharmacol. Exptl. Therap.* **180**:547.

Sparkes, C. G., and Spencer, P. S. J., 1971, Antinociceptive activity of morphine after injection of biogenic amines in the cerebral ventrides of the conscious rat, *Brit. J. Pharmacol.* **42**:230.

Stadler, H., Lloyd, K. G., Gadea-Ciria, M., and Bartholini, G., 1973, Enhanced striatal acetylcholine release by chlorpromazine and its reversal by apomorphine, *Brain Res.* **55**:476.

Stromberg, U., 1970, Dopa effects on motility in mice, potentiation by MK-485 and hexachlorpheniramine, *Psychopharmacologia* **18**:58.

Sugrue, M. F., 1974, Effects of morphine and pentazocine on the turnover of noradrenaline and dopamine in various regions of the rat brain, *Brit. J. Pharmacol.* **52**:159.

Takagi, H., and Kuriki, H., 1969, Suppressive effect of tetrabenazine on the development of tolerance to morphine and its reversal by dopa, *Intern. J. Neuropharmacol.* **8**:195.

Takagi, H., and Nakama, M., 1966, Effect of morphine and nalorphine on the content of dopamine in mouse brain, *Japan. J. Pharmacol.* **16**:483.

Takagi, H., and Nakama, M., 1968, Studies on the mechanism of action of tetrabenazine as a morphine antagonist, *Japan. J. Pharmacol.* **18**:54.

Takagi, H., Takashima, T., and Kimura, K., 1964, Antagonism of the analgesic effect of morphine in mice by tetrabenazine and reserpine, *Arch. Intern. Pharmacodyn.* **149**:484.

Tenen, S. S., 1968, Antagonism of the analgesic effect of morphine and other drugs by *p*-chlorophenylalanine, a serotonin depletor, *Psychopharmacologia* **12**:278.

Terenius, L., 1973, Stereospecific interaction between narcotic analgesics and a synaptic plasma membrane fraction of rat cerebral cortex, *Acta Pharmacol. Toxicol.* **32**:317.

Thoenen, H., Mueller, R. A., and Axelrod, J., 1969, Increased tyrosine hydroxylase activity after drug-induced alteration of sympathetic transmission, *Nature* **221**:1264.

Thompson, T., and Schuster, C. R., 1964, Morphine self-administration, food reinforced and avoidance behaviors in Rhesus monkeys, *Psychopharmacologia* **587**:94.

Uretsky, N.Y., and Iversen, L. L., 1970, Effects of 6-hydroxydopamine on catecholamine containing neurons in the rat brain, *J. Neurochem.* **17**:269.

VanderWende, C., and Spoerlin, M. T., 1972, Antagonism by dopa of morphine analgesia. A hypothesis for morphine tolerance, *Res. Commun. Chem. Path. Pharmacol.* **3**:37.

VanderWende, C., and Spoerlin, M. T., 1973, Role of dopaminergic receptors in morphine analgesia and tolerance, *Res. Commun. Chem. Path. Pharmacol.* **5**:35.

VanHungen, K., and Robertis, S., 1973, Adenylate-cyclase receptors for adrenergic neurotransmitters in rat cerebral cortex, *European J. Biochem.* **36**:391.

Vedernikov, Y. P., 1970, The role of brain catecholamines in morphine analgesic action in morphine-tolerant rats, *J. Pharm. Pharmacol.* **22**:238.

Vedernikov, Y. P., and Afrikanov, I. I., 1969, On the role of a central adrenergic mechanism in morphine analgesic action, *J. Pharm. Pharmacol.* **21**:845.

Verri, R. A., Graeff, F. B., and Corrado, A. P., 1968, Effect of reserpine and α-methyltyrosine on morphine analgesia, *Intern. J. Neuropharmacol.* **7**:283.

Villarreal, J. E., Guzman, M., and Smith, C. B., 1973, A comparison of the effects of *d*-amphetamine and morphine upon the locomotor activity of mice treated with drugs which alter brain catecholamine content, *J. Pharmacol. Exptl. Therap.* **187**:1.

Vogt, M., 1954, The concentration of sympathin in different parts of the CNS under normal conditions and after the administration of drugs, *J. Physiol. (London)* **123**:451.

Watanabe, K., Matsui, Y., and Iwata, H., 1969, Enhancement of the analgesic effect of morphine by sodium diethyldithio carbamate in rats, *Experientia* **25**:950.

Way, E. L., Loh, H., and Shen, F. H., 1968, Morphine tolerance, physical dependence and the synthesis of brain serotonin, *Science* **162**:1290.

Weeks, J. R., 1962, Experimental morphine addiction: Method for autonomic intravenous injections in unrestrained rats, *Science* **138**:143.

Weeks, J. R. and Collins, R. J., 1964, Factors affecting voluntary morphine intake in self-maintained addicted rats, *Psychopharmacologia* **6**:267.

Wikler, A., and Pescor, F. T., 1967, Classical conditioning of a morphine abstinence phenomenon, reinforcement of opioid drinking behavior and "relapse," *Psychopharmacologia* **10**:255.

Wilson, A. E., and Domino, E. F., 1970, Inhibitory effects of morphine on brain acetylcholine depletion following intraventricular hemicholinium, *Pharmacologist* **12**:294.

Woods, J. H., and Schuster, C. R., Jr., 1970, Regulation of self-administration, in: *Drug Dependence, Advances in Mental Science, II* (R. T. Harris, W. M. McIsaac, and C. R. Schuster, eds.), pp. 158–169, University of Texas Press, Austin, Texas.

Yanagita, T., Deneau, G. A. and Seevers, M. H., 1965, Evaluation of pharmacologic agents in the monkey by long-term intravenous self or programmed administration, *Excerpta Med. Intern. Congr. Ser.* **87**:453.

Chapter 8

Metabolic Adaptation to Antidepressant Drugs: Implications for Pathophysiology and Treatment in Psychiatry*

Arnold J. Mandell, David S. Segal,
and Ronald Kuczenski

Department of Psychiatry, School of Medicine
University of California, San Diego
La Jolla, California

1. BIOCHEMICAL INDICES OF PSYCHOTROPIC DRUG ACTION

In late 1969 and early 1970 our group first presented a model of adaptive regulation as a potentially significant mechanism underlying the action of many psychotropic drugs (Segal *et al.,* 1971). Shifting our attention from levels of biogenic amines and indices of amine turnover in brain, we began to see that chronic administration of psychotropic drugs led to alterations in biosynthetic capacity and receptor sensitivity that appeared to counteract the acute drug effect. For example, when given chronically, drugs that release or block reuptake of biogenic amines at central synapses resulted in a decrease in such biosynthetic enzymes as tyrosine hydroxylase and tryptophan hydroxylase. On the other hand, agents that impair synaptic transmission, e.g., reserpine or receptor blockers like the phenothiazines or propanalol, led to the inverse effect, an increase in those brain enzymes as well as to a kind of functional supersensitivity of the receptors. The latencies and durations of these changes in presynaptic enzymes and recep-

* This work is supported by NIMH Grants DA-00265-03 and DA-00046-04 and Friends of Psychiatric Research of San Diego, Inc. Dr. Segal is the recipient of NIMH Research Scientist Award MH-70183-02.

tor function ranged from hours to weeks, and helped us explain one of the striking paradoxes of clinical psychopharmacology, the time-to-action of many agents (lithium, the phenothiazines, the tricyclics). The latencies began to represent to us the time necessary for compensatory macromolecular changes to occur in the brain, and we felt they had functional import in the mechanism of action of psychotropic drugs. We were suggesting that the compensatory changes, rather than the acute alterations in synaptic neurotransmitter mobility, were responsible for the behavioral effects of such drugs. The first integrated presentation of this theoretical model was made at a meeting in San Francisco, and was included in a book of those proceedings edited by James McGaugh (Mandell *et al.,* 1972). At that time several discussants, including Morris Lipton and Seymour Kety, suggested that those interesting shifts in indices of brain capacity to synthesize amines probably represented compensatory changes that were the mirror images of, and therefore only confirmed, the original conceptions of acute drug mechanisms. We answered with speculation that since the latency to action of the drugs administered approximated the time to the changes in biosynthetic enzymatic capacity, perhaps the enzymic and receptor changes were, indeed, most significant. We speculated that depression might be viewed as a reflection of a state of pathological activation of central biogenic amine neurons that could be tuned down by antidepressants and would be tuned up by the rauwolfia alkaloids and the phenothiazines.

We continued to focus on neurobiological mechanisms of adaptation in central biogenic amine synapses. By careful regional dissection of rat brain we have specified and isolated regions in which the cell bodies and nerve endings of various biogenic amine systems predominate, and we studied the chemical alterations that occur in these subcellular areas with carefully controlled parameters of psychotropic drug dose and time. And we have been able to elucidate further those mechanisms that we speculated were directed toward adaptive regulation of synaptic function, as well as additional mechanisms.

We shall review briefly the five adaptive mechanisms that we have been studying in central synaptic systems, and then focus on the long-term changes in tyrosine hydroxylase, the apparent rate-limiting enzyme in the biosynthesis of catecholamines (CA), following the chronic administration of drugs. These changes will be related to chronic unit discharge activity in biogenic amine neurons and discussed in relation to a biochemical model of depression as pathological activation (Segal *et al.,* 1974*a*).

2. ADAPTIVE MECHANISMS IN CENTRAL SYNAPSES

Figure 1 is a diagram summarizing some of the mechanisms with which our group has been working. Number (1) was deduced from a series of ex-

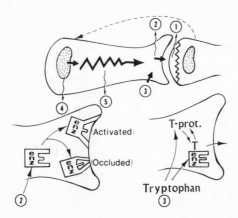

Figure 1. Macromolecular mechanisms involved in the regulation of neurotransmitter synthesis and efficacy. (1) The receptor function is thought to increase or decrease in sensitivity to infused neurotransmitter. (2) Enzymes in the nerve ending may be inhibited by occlusion or activated by alterations in physical conformation resulting in decreased K_m for cofactor or substrate or increased V_{max}. (3) Uptake is thought to involve a drug-sensitive mechanism, a storage pool, and a direct conversion pathway. (4) Nuclear enzyme synthesis or degradation is probably affected by intra- or interneuronal feedback communication. (5) Axoplasmic flow is thought to affect the latency of increases or decreases in amounts of enzyme acting in the nerve ending.

periments that suggest that impairment of synaptic transmission in the rat brain by such agents as α-methyltyrosine or 6-hydroxydopamine (6-OHDA) leads to supersensitivity of central CA receptors as reflected by behavioral responses to chronic intraventricular infusion of low doses of norepinephrine (NE). Part of this behavioral supersensitivity, particularly that appearing after 6-OHDA, has been attributed to the loss of the presynaptic uptake mechanism, at least early on. Later changes, however, appear to involve the receptor. We blocked reuptake with acute high doses of a tricyclic antidepressant in rats that served as controls for the 6-OHDA experiment. Behavioral sensitivity to NE and dopamine (DA) infusions was much greater in experimental animals that had received 2–3 weeks of 6-OHDA treatment than shortly after the initial administration of 6-OHDA or than in rats that had received the tricyclic agent (Segal *et al.,* 1974*b*).

The second mechanism noted in Figure 1 has to do with alterations in the physical state of critical biosynthetic enzymes in biogenic amine systems, specifically tyrosine hydroxylase in the nerve ending. We have been able to demonstrate *in vitro* at least two, and perhaps three, models for the physical state of tyrosine hydroxylase in nerve endings from rat striatum: (i) occluded, (ii) membrane-bound, allosterically activated, and (iii) unbound, soluble (Kuczenski and Mandell, 1972*a,b;* Kuczenski, 1973*a,b*). There is evidence that certain drug effects with short latency may alter the physical state and therefore the activity of this rate-limiting enzyme. Certain aspects of activation by membrane binding can be mimicked by the specific mucopolysaccharide heparin. Recent work in our laboratory and by Fisher and Kaufman (1972) has suggested the possibility that tryptophan hydroxylase may also be regulated by membrane binding. The physical state of the presynaptic enzyme is one among several complex factors for intrasynaptosomal regulation of enzyme activity, including product-feedback inhibition, cofactor supply, and substrate supply.

The third regulatory mechanism involves the uptake of the amino acid precursors of biogenic amine neurotransmitters. We have yet to find significant or systematic alterations in tyrosine uptake associated with the administration of various drugs or environmental manipulations. We therefore doubt that alterations in the active uptake of tyrosine normally play a significant role in the regulation of CA biosynthesis. However, in the serotonergic system the uptake of radioactive tryptophan is influenced by various agents (e.g., inhibited by cocaine and stimulated by acute administration of lithium or tryptophan loads) and, in turn, alters the capacity of synaptosomes to convert tryptophan to serotonin (Knapp and Mandell, 1972*a,b*; 1973*a,b*). The specific function of the high affinity, drug-sensitive tryptophan uptake systems remains to be elucidated.

The fourth and fifth mechanisms in Figure 1 have to do with alterations in the synthesis of biosynthetic enzymes in the cell body, which we deduce are probably regulated by either feedback information from the postsynaptic cell or by the electrical firing rate of the cell itself for specifiable periods of time. In our experiments the time constants for these alterations in enzyme levels have generally been days to weeks; for example, drugs that impair transmission (e.g., reserpine) take 1–3 weeks to result in an increase in tyrosine hydroxylase in the nerve ending (Segal *et al.,* 1971), whereas tricyclics take a like amount of time to do the reverse.

For the most part these adaptive mechanisms begin to operate hours to weeks after the initiation of chronic administration of psychotropic drugs and appear to have as the major facet of their organization the development of the capacity to compensate for the acute effects of the drugs.

3. ENZYMATIC ADAPTATION TO CHRONIC DRUG ADMINISTRATION

We should like to focus attention now on the long-latency adaptive changes in tyrosine hydroxylase in various regions of rat brain after chronic administration of reserpine, a drug that impairs central biogenic amine transmission, and after chronic administration of desmethylimipramine (DMI), an agent that (at least acutely) potentiates biogenic amine transmission in the brain by blocking reuptake in the nerve ending. We are particularly interested in the changes that occur one or two weeks after initiation of the latter drug—a ramification of our mystification as to why tricyclics block reuptake of biogenic amines almost immediately but have their therapeutic effect weeks later.

As can be seen in Figure 2, chronic treatment with reserpine (0.5 mg/kg q.d. for 8 days) produced increases in tyrosine hydroxylase activity in all the regions of rat brain studied, including locus coeruleus (a noradrenergic cell body region), hippocampus (a noradrenergic nerve ending region), caudate (a dopaminergic nerve ending region), and (not shown) substantia nigra (a dopaminergic cell body region) and hypothalamus. Such elevations had not been present 24 hr after a single administration of reserpine. The largest increase, in the locus coeruleus, reached 250% of control.

In contrast to the effects of reserpine, repeated administration of DMI (10 mg/kg b.i.d. for 8 days) produced a significant decline in enzyme activity, with the most pronounced reduction in the hippocampal cortex (a

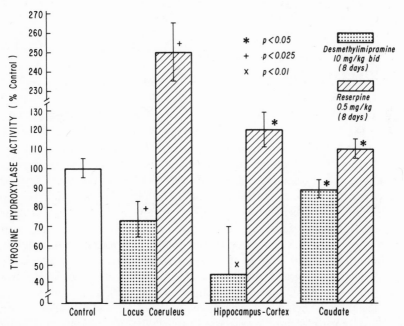

Figure 2. A comparison of the effects of chronic administration of reserpine and chronic administration of desmethylimipramine on tyrosine hydroxylase activity in various regions of rat brain.

noradrenergic nerve ending region). This was about 50% of corresponding controls. No significant change in enzyme activity was observed 24 hr after a single administration of a large dose of DMI (25 mg/kg).

The data presented here are consistent with those from many of our previous studies in which the independent variable was genetic strain, sensory isolation, one of various drugs, or hormonal manipulation (Emlen *et al.*, 1972; Segal *et al.*, 1972, 1973). The greater the amount or effect of central biogenic amine neurotransmission, the less presynaptic biosynthetic activity and/or receptor responsiveness we found, and the converse. In some instances the presynaptic alterations appeared to be due to change in the amount of rate-limiting enzyme; in other instances they appeared to result from rapid change in enzyme in the nerve ending due to factors like physical state or substrate supply. The question, "Do enzymes responsible for the biosynthesis of the biogenic amines function inversely to drugs that affect biogenic amine synaptic function?" now becomes, "What is the functional significance of the biosynthetic enzymes?" In other words, are these enzyme changes merely inverse images of synaptic alterations and therefore consistent with current theories of psychotropic drug action, or do they introduce another factor to consider in attempts to understand the mechanism of action of some of these drugs?

4. A MODEL FOR NEUROCHEMICAL ADAPTATION TO TRICYCLIC DRUGS

Our own model for these adaptations has two phases (Figure 3). We envision the initial effect of tricyclic antidepressant drugs as facilitation of transmission with a compensatory decrease in the firing rate of neurons. Table I shows the effects of three psychoactive drugs on reticular multiple unit activity in cat brain (Wallach *et al.*, 1969). A reduction in reticular unit activity occurred in the ventromedial midbrain about 30 min after tricyclic injection and lasted between 24 and 36 hr. In a tricyclic-treated system we think the (probably feedback regulated) decrease in unit discharge rate promptly balances the facilitated transmission. This might account for the fact that there is very little in the way of acute effects from tricyclics. In general, pharmaceutical houses are unable to use acute behavioral effects of tricyclics alone as a screening technique for the drugs. Except for some early sleepiness (which could even be the result of an acute shutdown in the arousal system firing rate [Segal and Mandell, 1970]), patients may notice only the side effects of these drugs during the initial days of treatment.

The second phase of adaptation we envision as occurring within the

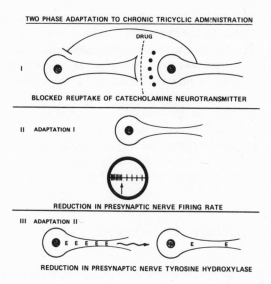

Figure 3. We postulate that Adaptation I, the reduction in presynaptic nerve firing rate, results from feedback following the facilitation of transmission when reuptake of amine is blocked by a drug. Adaptation II, the decrease in the synthesis and flow of tyrosine hydroxylase to the nerve ending, we think results from the decreased firing rate.

presynaptic neuron. Here our premise is that the synthesis of biosynthetic enzyme is a function of the discharge rate of the cell, particularly over some critical time period (e.g., the change in firing rate must be maintained to produce macromolecular changes, much as the presence of an addicting drug must be maintained to produce tolerance). This has been the implication of studies in the periphery by Thoenen, Mueller, and Axelrod (Axelrod, 1971), who used denervation, receptor blockade, and other means to show that postural feedback and cardiovascular feedback (expressed through reflexes in the spinal cord) resulted in increases in tyrosine hydroxylase in the adrenal and sympathetic nerves. These data from peripheral systems suggest

Table I. Psychotropic Drug Effects on Neuronal Discharge in the Midbrain of the Cat[a]

Drug	Reticular unit activity as % of that during REM Sleep
Chlorpromazine (15 mg/kg)	95.0 ± 2.2 (s.d.)
Imipramine (10 mg/kg)	56.0 ± 6.6
Desmethylimipramine (10 mg/kg)	67.3 ± 4.9

[a] After Wallach *et al.* (1969).

that the amount of tyrosine hydroxylase is some function of the firing rate, particularly over time. In the peripheral studies, time constants varied upward from two days. In some instances slow axoplasmic flow was suggested. In other instances it may have taken time for the biosynthetic apparatus to "decide" to make such a major alteration. In our experiments with rat brain, the gradual decrease in tyrosine hydroxylase activity in the presence of daily doses of tricyclic medication is, we think, consequent to the maintenance of a decreased discharge rate. In the presence of reserpine, in contrast, there probably is a marked increase in the presynaptic unit firing rate to compensate for the impaired transmission, and that increased firing rate leads to an increase in tyrosine hydroxylase.

5. A REVISED THEORY OF DEPRESSIVE ILLNESS

Only recently has the evaluation of the predominant effects of drug treatments on biogenic amine systems in the brain been possible, by stop-flow analyses of metabolites in the CSF of depressive patients and normal subjects after the administration of probenecid. Inhibiting the egress of biogenic amine acid metabolites from the CSF, Frederick Goodwin and his associates (1973) have measured the rate of metabolite accumulation and provided an opportunity for deductions about the net effects of the mechanisms involved in the synthesis, storage, and release of central biogenic amines. Their findings appear directly relevant to the question of the functional significance of the drug-induced adaptive mechanisms that we are studying.

Studies of endogenously depressed patients show that they have low levels of biogenic amine acids in their CSF (Coppen, 1970; Sjostrom and Roos, 1972; Goodwin *et al.*, 1973). However, recently Goodwin *et al.* (personal communication) found that treating depressed patients with tricyclic drugs chronically did not reverse the abnormally low levels of biogenic amine metabolites in their CSF, rather it reduced still further the apparent rate of the overall synthesis, release, and metabolism of 5-hydroxyindoleacetic acid, 4-hydroxy-3-methoxy-phenylacetic acid (homovanillic acid), and 3-methoxy-4-hydroxy-phenylglycol (MHPG) in particular. After probenecid, the clinical response to tricyclic medication corresponded in time to a drug-induced decrease in the synthesis of biogenic amines in the brain as reflected in the rate of accrual of acid metabolites after the blockade. Thus decreased brain capacity for amine synthesis because of decreased enzymatic activity appears, at least in depressed patients, to be reflected by a decrease in the synthesis and accumulation of acid metabolites in the CSF.

We think Goodwin's work and the work in our laboratory are indications for revising the neurochemical theories of depressive illness. We have developed a proposition incorporating many recent findings from the NIH Laboratory of Clinical Science and from our own work (Figure 4). In the studies done in Bethesda, low measures of catechol-*O*-methyltransferase (COMT) in red blood cells and clinical responsiveness to tricyclic antidepressant medication clustered in a population of patients suffering from unipolar endogenous depression (Bunney *et al.*, 1970; Dunner *et al.*, 1971; Goodwin *et al.*, 1970). This suggests the possibility that depression, particu-

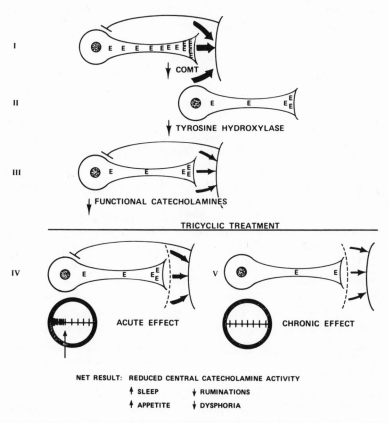

Figure 4. A model for the pathophysiology of depression and its treatment with tricyclic antidepressant drug (I) A congenitally low level of COMT allows overstimulation of catecholamine receptors. (II) Partial compensation is achieved by the decreased firing rate of the presynaptic catecholamine neuron that is accompanied by a decrease in neural tyrosine hydroxylase (reflected by low catechol acids in CSF and a decrease in functional catecholamines) (III). (IV) Treatment with tricyclic antidepressants temporarily facilitates transmission, leading to further compensatory decreases in firing rate and (V) in neuronal tyrosine hydroxylase (reflected in a further drop in CSF catechol acids).

larly unipolar depression, could be a manifestation of a congenital deficiency in COMT, which might produce functionally supersensitive receptors if the capacity to remove CA were lost with "lost" COMT. With an initial endogenous compensatory decrease in spontaneous firing rate there would ensue a decrease in tyrosine hydroxylase activity, resulting in low base line measures of catechol acids in the CSF. Tricyclics given to people with endogenous unipolar depression would initially potentiate transmission, which would decrease the firing rate and tyrosine hydroxylase still further, and certainly not reverse the low catechol acids in the CSF. That is, unsuccessful endogenous attempts to dampen apparently supersensitive receptors would be made more vigorous by tricyclic potentiation of synaptic transmission and reflexive decreases in neuronal discharge rate and enzyme synthesis.

This concept of a functionally hyperactive central system in depression provokes speculation about the clinical phenomena of depression. Classical theories of the role of central biogenic amines do allow that one manifestation of an "overfunctioning" system might be a pathological state of activation. This would include, for example, loss of sleep, loss of weight, and persistent rumination—a hyperactivity of the internal arousal system that the patient could not "turn off." The valence of that internal discomfort usually has had something to do with whether it has been called "depression" or not. Regardless, such clinical phenomena are consonant with our proposition. Certainly the reserpine-induced depression has biochemical similarities to this model. That is, impairment in transmission leads to an increase in presynaptic nerve firing, thence to an increase in tyrosine hydroxylase that would tend, if the functional correlation holds, to increase the CA in the brain. Another comparable syndrome in which we have seen an increase in brain tyrosine hydroxylase is hypothyroidism in the rat (Emlen *et al.*, 1972). In man also, hypothyroidism, like the effect of chronic reserpine administration, mimics endogenous depression.

Thus, although functional deductions from basic biochemical changes are fraught with risks involving differences in strain, in the complexity of animal brains, in the dynamics of pharmacology, and in the relationships between dose and efficacy, we think the work at NIH with catechol and indole acids in the CSF can be linked to our findings in the chemistry of the rat brain. Is it possible that depression is due to increased activity in biogenic amine systems, and that tricyclics initially make the matter a bit worse but then achieve therapeutic efficacy by means of the adaptive mechanisms we have described? It is interesting in this regard that Oswald *et al.* (1972), who gave tricyclics to normal subjects in whom they were studying sleep, report that the first several days of tricyclic administration led to transient depression, after which the patients returned to their previous normal mood. Although some might attribute this to the nonspecific side effects, or the sleepiness, it may represent a fundamental aspect of tricyclic action.

In summary, we are suggesting that, rather than being mirror images or epiphenomenal changes, compensatory changes in biosynthetic enzymes may be intrinsically related to the therapeutic efficacy of psychotropic drugs. The efficacy of tricyclics in a group of unipolar depressive patients, who reveal in their red blood cells primary or secondary deficiency of COMT, suggests a syndrome of hyperactive central biogenic amine systems and that the tricyclics quiet the agitation by prompting the lagging compensatory mechanisms to further decrease the neuronal firing rate and, consequently, the enzymatic capacity to synthesize neurotransmitter, thereby protecting the receptors.

6. REFERENCES

Axelrod, J., 1971, Noradrenaline: fate and control of its synthesis, *Science* **173**:598.

Bunney, W. E., Jr., Brodie, H. K. H., Murphy, D. L., and Goodwin, F. K., 1970, Psychopharmacological differentiation between two subgroups of depressed patients, *Proc. Am. Psychol. Assoc.* **5**:829.

Coppen, A. J., 1970, The chemical pathology of the affective disorders, *Sci. Basis Med.,* p. 179.

Dunner, E. L., Cohn, C. K., Gershon, E. S., and Goodwin, F. K., 1971, Differential catechol O-methyltransferase activity in unipolar and bipolar affective illness, *Arch. Gen. Psychiat.* **25**:348.

Emlen, W., Segal, D. S., and Mandell, A. J., 1972, Effects of thyroid state on pre- and postsynaptic central noradrenergic mechanisms, *Science* **175**:79.

Fisher, D. B., and Kaufman, S., 1972, The stimulation of rat liver phenylalanine hydroxylase by phospholipids, *J. Biol. Chem.* **247**:2250.

Goodwin, F. K., Murphy, D. L., Brodie, H. K. H., and Bunney, W. E., 1970, L-dopa, catecholamines, and behavior: a clinical and biochemical study in depressed patients, *Biol. Psychiat.* **2**:341.

Goodwin, F. K., Post, R. M., Dunner, E. L., and Gordon, E. K., 1973, Cerebrospinal fluid amine metabolites in affective illness: the probenecid technique, *Am. J. Psychiat.* **130**:73.

Knapp, S., and Mandell, A. J., 1972a, Narcotic drugs: effects on serotonin biosynthetic systems of the brain, *Science* **177**:1209.

Knapp, S., and Mandell, A. J., 1972b, Parachlorophenylalanine: its three phase sequence of interactions with the two forms of brain tryptophan hydroxylase, *Life Sci.* **2**:761.

Knapp, S., and Mandell, A. J., 1973a, Some drug effects on the functions of the two physical forms of tryptophan-5-hydroxylase: influence on hydroxylation and uptake of substrate, in: *Serotonin and Behavior* (J. Barchas and E. Usdin, eds.), pp. 61–71, Academic Press, New York.

Knapp, S., and Mandell, A. J., 1973b, Short- and long-term lithium administration: effects on the brain's serotonergic systems, *Science* **180**:645.

Kuczenski, R., 1973*a*, Soluble, membrane-bound, and detergent-solubulized rat striatal tyrosine hydroxylase: *p*H-dependent cofactor binding, *J. Biol. Chem.* **248**:5074.

Kuczenski, R., 1973*b*, Striatal tyrosine hydroxylases with high and low affinity for tyrosine: implications for the multiple-pool concept of catecholamines, *Life Sci.* **13**:247.

Kuczenski, R., and Mandell, A. J., 1972*a*, Allosteric activation of hypothalamic tyrosine hydroxylase by ions and sulfated mucopolysaccharides, *J. Neurochem.* **19**:131.

Kuczenski, R., and Mandell, A. J., 1972*b*, Regulatory properties of soluble and particulate rat brain tyrosine hydroxylase, *J. Biol. Chem.* **247**:3114.

Mandell, A. J., Segal, D. S., Kuczenski, R., and Knapp, S., 1972, Some macromolecular mechanisms in CNS neurotransmitter pharmacology and their psychobiological organization, in: *The Chemistry of Mood, Motivation, and Memory* (J. McGaugh, ed.), pp. 105–147, Plenum Press, New York.

Oswald, I., Brezinova, V., and Dunleavy, D. L. F., 1972, On the slowness of action of tricyclic antidepressant drugs, *Brit. J. Psychiat.* **120**:673.

Segal, D. S., and Mandell, A. J., 1970, Behavioral activation of rats during intraventricular infusion of norepinephrine, *Proc. Natl. Acad. Sci. (U.S.)* **66**:289.

Segal, D. S., Sullivan, J. L., and Mandell, A. J., 1971, Effects of long-term reserpine on brain tyrosine hydroxylase and behavioral activity, *Science* **173**:847.

Segal, D. S., Kuczenski, R. T., and Mandell, A. J., 1972, Strain differences in behavior and brain tyrosine hydroxylase activity, *Behav. Biol.* **7**(1):75.

Segal, D. S., Knapp, S., Kuczenski, R. T., and Mandell, A. J., 1973, Effects of environmental isolation on behavior and regional rat brain tyrosine hydroxylase and tryptophan hydroxylase activity, *Behav. Biol.* **8**:47.

Segal, D. S., Kuczenski, R., and Mandell, A. J., 1974*a*, Theoretical implications of drug-induced adaptive regulation for a biogenic amine hypothesis of affective disorder, *Biol. Psychiat.* **9**:147.

Segal, D. S., McAllister, C., and Geyer, M. A., 1974*b*, Ventricular infusion of norepinephrine and amphetamine: direct versus indirect action, *Physiol. Behav.* **2**:79.

Sjostrom, R., and Roos, B. E., 1972, 5-Hydroxyindoleacetic acid and homovanillic acid in the cerebrospinal fluid in manic-depressive psychosis, *European J. Clin. Pharmacol.* **4**:170.

Wallach, M., Winters, W., Mandell, A. J., and Spooner, C., 1969, A correlation of EEG, reticular multiple unit activity and gross behavior following various antidepressant agents in the cat, *Electroencephalog. Clin. Neurophysiol.* **27**:563.

Chapter 9

Integration and Conclusions

Arnold J. Friedhoff

Millhauser Laboratories
New York University Medical Center
New York, New York

1. INTRODUCTION

The most definite link of a catecholaminergic system to a specific behavioral abnormality is the link between the striatal dopaminergic system
and the motor disturbance involved in Parkinsonism of both idiopathic and
drug etiology. It is not surprising that our first understanding of the role of
catecholamines in the brain came in relation to a disorder of motor function, rather than one involving mentational processes. However, even
Parkinsonism is not solely a motor disturbance. Patients with this disorder
manifest "flat" facies and often disturbances of mood. Further inquiry is
necessary to determine whether the affective and mood changes in this
disease are secondary psychological manifestations related to the incapaci-
tation associated with Parkinsonism, or are specific manifestations of a
disabled extrapyramidal system.

Intriguing correlations have been reported between catecholaminergic
function and emotion, mood, and even drug-craving. Also, aminergic
systems in the brain have been suspect in higher functions, such as those
that are disturbed in psychotic disorders, or involved in learning and
memory. Our ability to further define the relationships between catecholamines and these more complex, or at least more subtle functions
provides a greater challenge to the creativity and technological skill of
neuro- and psychobioligists than any previous efforts.

2. RESEARCH STRATEGIES

It is evident from the preceding pages that our current hypotheses have been derived almost entirely from the observations of drug effects, both those that produce and relieve behavioral malfunction. The discovery of the dopaminergic deficit in Parkinson's disease can be traced directly to early observations that reserpine and chlorpromazine produce Parkinson-like effects. The catecholamine hypothesis of depression was developed after it was found that antidepressant drugs affected noradrenergic function in the central nervous system. The transmethylation hypothesis was evolved because methylated derivatives of catecholamines have a structural similarity to mescaline, and the dopamine hypothesis of psychosis stems from findings that all antipsychotic drugs can produce Parkinsonian side effects, and thus presumably interfere with dopaminergic function.

The heuristic value of these observations of drug effects is self-evident, and the advance in our understanding of the role of catecholamines in behavioral function should not be underestimated. Nonetheless, there are serious limitations in our ability to further refine our understanding without developing new strategies, probably new technology and hypotheses subject to more explicit and definitive tests.

One problem is that drugs produce many effects, not only the one of interest, thus limiting our ability to attribute a specific effect to a specific drug action. This problem can be partly overcome by the utilization of several drugs which affect the same system through different mechanisms, since it is unlikely that drugs which affect catecholaminergic activity through different means will also all have the same effects on other systems. If a given behavioral effect can be accomplished by an agent which increases synthesis of a catecholamine, one which blocks degradation, and one which prolongs the life of the amine at the synapse, then we can have some confidence that this effect is related to enhanced catecholaminergic activity. However, concordance of effects from several approaches only narrows the possibilities. How then can we demonstrate more specifically the way in which the catecholaminergic system is involved in behavioral and mental regulation?

One fact becomes increasingly clear—that the further development of our understanding will not come from any one field, but through the integration of observations from the fields of psychiatry and psychology, pharmacology, biochemistry, neurophysiology, neuroanatomy, cell biology, and probably others. The preceding chapters reflect a great deal of work carried out from each of these vantage points.

3. DETERMINANTS OF BEHAVIOR

Although we know intuitively what we are talking about when we refer to behavior, a formal definition is difficult to construct. In the present context we are referring not only to observable activity of an organism reflected in some type of motor activity, but also to thinking, feeling, learning, remembering, and attentional and attitudinal state. However, the components of these phenomena, which we might agree are the province of those concerned with behavior, are not readily separable from other functions which we commonly regard as physiological or biochemical, rather than behavioral. It is pointless to attempt to draw boundaries between psychological and biological functions, rather than to recognize that these functions are continuous, as is their relationship to the external environment.

An example of this interrelatedness can be drawn from the catecholamine hypothesis of depression. It has been difficult to determine whether catecholamine excretion in depressed patients is affected by decreased motor activity of many depressed individuals, or whether the hypoactivity results from impaired catecholaminergic output. Most likely both are true. Altering catecholaminergic activity may affect motor activity, while modifying motor activity may affect catecholaminergic output.

The answer to this problem will not be found by ignoring behavioral–biological feedback loops, or by failing to recognize that cause and effect may be related in a circular pathway or may interact with each other in a continuous and dynamic manner. The highly adaptive nature of behavioral and mental function requires the most intimate adjustments between immediate effect and immediate effector, and it is the function of investigators in this field to attempt to determine the sequential relationships of these highly interacting systems.

Sequential effects of this type have been difficult to observe in psychiatric illnesses for several reasons. One is the absence of suitable animal models in which various functional parameters can be readily manipulated and higher order behavior observed. For another, it appears that compensatory adaptive changes may occur which delay, in time, the appearance of a behavioral effect following the modification of a biological parameter. Such adaptive effects can be seen during the experimental induction of an amphetamine psychosis by the continuous administration of amphetamine. At a given dose, subjects characteristically begin to develop mental aberrations which quickly disappear. At an even higher dose, the symptoms may again reappear briefly and then disappear again. Ultimately, as the dose is raised, the compensatory capacity of the subject is exceeded, and the symptoms are maintained.

There are a number of possible explanations for this phenomenon. One is that as amphetamine produces its psychotogenic effect (perhaps by increasing dopaminergic activity), a compensatory system is turned on which reverses the mental effects produced by amphetamine. As the dose is increased it reaches the point where such compensations are ineffective.

A similar mechanism may be involved in the disappearance of the effect of morphine on catecholamine turnover during tolerance. Also, it is not uncommon for schizophrenic patients to describe periods during the onset of their illness when they were able to "pull themselves together."

These compensatory mechanisms have been little studied despite their obvious potential in the treatment of psychotic illness. Furthermore, the operation of such mechanisms makes the likelihood of finding a simple cause and effect relationship more remote, even when our ability to manipulate suspected causal factors is unhindered. A temporal lag of substantial nature may intervene between manipulation of the independent variable and the dependent variable. Some of these difficulties can be overcome by carrying out parametric studies and longitudinal studies rather than those involving single observations, and data can then be scrutinized through sequential analytical techniques. This phenomenon of compensation should be of interest to the clinician as well as the investigator since it can operate to obscure effector–effect relationships in all kinds of psychiatric dysfunction.

Workers in the field of neurobiology may have been unduly influenced by the mental deficiency model, in which a malfunction of one enzyme can lead to a severe degree of central nervous system impairment. It seems unlikely that such relationships will be easily found in even severe psychiatric illness of the psychotic type because of the many external and internal factors which are capable of modifying the course of a psychotic illness. In contrast to the mental deficiency syndrome, psychoses come and go, get better and worse, often without specific intervention. A psychosis is a mild disease in many ways, producing no consistent abnormalities in basic physiology and no observable changes in anatomical structure. Only the highest mental functions are disturbed, although the social consequences of this disruption may be severe. In contrast, mental retardation is frequently associated with obvious morphological changes and is not reversible once established. However, even in the case of certain mental deficiencies of clear genetic origin, external events may be critical in determining the expression of symptoms. The best-known example is that of phenylketonuria. In this disorder, the retardation will not occur if the affected subject has a good doctor who advises the parents to withhold phenylalanine, and good parents who follow this advice. Thus, the expression of a genetic trait can always be viewed as a resultant of gene–environment interaction.

Although nearly everyone now agrees that the influences of physiology and environment cannot be separated, laboratory experiments are generally designed without regard for this principle. The behavioral effects resulting from an increase or decrease in activity of a neurotransmitter system are dealt with as though these were independent of the situation, although we know that the same stimulus affecting the same neural system can produce different behavioral effects depending on conditions. A running animal who is startled by a noise may stop to listen, whereas a resting animal who hears the same noise may get up and run. Just as the phenotype is a resultant of gene–environmental interaction, so the behavioral expression of the action of a neural system is a resultant of the interaction of that system with the environment. Future advances in understanding the action of transmitter systems, including the catecholaminergic system, depend on our ability to define not only the biological parameters of a complex neural network, but also the situational parameters with which the organism is interacting.

Another frequently overlooked factor in clinical research is the extent of the differences among individuals. Individual differences are important in functions such as dopamine-β-hydroxylase level in the serum in which there is a wide individual variation. In these cases, it may be impossible to demonstrate abnormalities by considering group means, and it may be necessary to study changes to detect pathology by measuring deviations from an individual's own norm. In most cases, however, subjects come to our attention only after disordered function is established. If the disorder is reversible we can study the subject again in the well state. If it is not, it may be necessary to perturb the system and measure its responsivity.

4. CONCEPTUAL MODELS FOR THE MULTIPLE ROLES OF CATECHOLAMINES IN BRAIN

Reference to the chapter headings in these volumes indicates that cate-cholamines are believed to be implicated in a wide range of functions. There is now extensive evidence regarding the involvement of dopamine in the regulation of extrapyramidal motor function, and accumulating evidence that norepinephrine also plays an important role. There is circumstantial evidence that catecholamines are important in the maintenance of psy-chophysiological function, and evidence is presented that these amines play a role in activation, conditioning, learning, stress, narcotic action, and depression and psychosis. Can catecholamines be involved in so many different functions, or is this a reflection of a fad during which we apply a popular area of research to the study of every conceivable condition? Undoubtedly, the latter factor has stimulated some investigations. However, there is a feature common to most of the states and conditions discussed in these volumes, in that each involves emotions. If catecholamines, as now appears probable, are involved in the regulation of emotions, then they might play an important role in determining all those states and conditions in which emotions are a factor. Although there is widespread acceptance of the idea that catecholamines are important in the regulation of emotional state, definitive evidence for this involvement is lacking. Partly, this stems from the difficulties in assaying states comparable to human emotions in non-human species. In humans we do not have very explicit information about the effects of experimental manipulation of catecholaminergic action on emotions. We know that compounds, such as amphetamine, which increase the action of central catecholaminergic systems, produce activation and arousal, but very little is known about the effects of either increased or decreased catecholaminergic activity on affective responsivity. Inasmuch as the assumption that catecholamines are involved in emotional control appears to be central to most of the clinically oriented catecholamine research, it is essential that we develop more specific information about the role of these compounds in emotional control.

5. NEW CONCEPTUAL MODELS OF PSYCHOPATHOLOGICAL STATES

It is typical of biological science that early research into an area ignores many possible complicated interactions and is dependent on a large number of unwarranted assumptions. In the study of the role of catecholamines in psychopathological states, the earliest studies were unidimensional in character. They were based on the assumption that if catecholamines were elevated, one state would result; if they were lowered, an opposite state would occur. This formulation does not take into consideration a number of possible interactions. We pointed out the need to consider, in any conceptual model, situational factors operating in the environment of the organism. It is also important to consider the plasticity of the central nervous system. Bechtereva *et al.* discuss two kinds of approaches to the treatment of mental disorders. The approach that they use is different from that with which most western investigators are familiar, and the terminology may not be known to non-Soviet readers. However, it is interesting that Arnold Mandell and his co-workers have independently arrived at a somewhat similar concept of central nervous system adaptation using traditional American approaches to research. Bechtereva *et al.* point out that it may be possible to control disease by compensating for deficient mechanisms (the pathogenic approach) or by restoring a CNS balance at a new functional level by suppressing the activity of the unaffected or "healthy" systems (the symptomatic approach). Mandell *et al.* believe that antidepressant drugs may work by stimulating the central nervous system to make a new adaptation to an existing pathological condition. Both teams of investigators point out the necessity for considering that the brain has tremendous plasticity, so that influencing one system through drugs, stimulation, or by disease probably results in complex reciprocal changes in a number of other systems. This may be best demonstrated by the intriguing relationships between the dopaminergic and cholinergic neurons in the striatum, and the possible role of both of these systems in the action of antipsychotic drugs.

6. DEVELOPMENT OF NEW TREATMENTS

For the clinician, the ultimate goal of all research is to facilitate the development of better treatments. The last decade has seen the development of a model of the catecholaminergic neuron. Our increase in understanding of various steps involved in the biosynthesis, storage, release, and inactivation of transmitter has made it possible to design drugs which can specifically affect each step in this process. The better definition of the process opens up possibilities for new therapeutic agents.

7. DIRECTIONS FOR FUTURE RESEARCH

At the present time there are important gaps in our understanding of the central catecholaminergic neuronal systems. We do not know all of the projections of this system in the brain, or its role in other than a few nuclei. We have only limited understanding of the biology of the catecholaminergic neuron and incomplete understanding of the total metabolism of catecholamines. We do not know why mammalian tissues have an enzyme which can catalyze the formation of hallucinogens such as mescaline from transmitter metabolites. Do these hallucinogens have a physiological role in the CNS (in image formation or dreaming?), or is the enzyme only a vestigial reflection of our relationship to the peyote cactus?

The most serious deficit in our knowledge is at the level of behavior. We need a more explicit definition of the relationships of biogenic amine neuronal systems to emotional responsivity, attention, arousal, and mood.

All scientific exploration requires reductionism in order to make a problem manageable. All of the work on catecholamines reflects this necessity. We remind the reader again, that the brain above all organs has enormous adaptive capacity, derived, in part, from its ability to take compensatory action. These compensatory phenomena operate in the behavioral as well as the biological. realm. In the future we will have to deal simultaneously with the relationships of many interacting brain systems. For the present we can try to develop better hypotheses which will consider biological, behavioral, and environmental factors as part of one interacting system.

Index